Evidence into Practice

Integrating Judgment, Values, and Research

LAURITA M. HACK, PT, DPT, MBA, PhD, FAPTA

Professor Emeritus
Department of Physical Therapy
Temple University
Philadelphia, Pennsylvania

•

JAN GWYER, PT, PhD, FAPTA

Professor
Doctor of Physical Therapy Division
Department of Community and Family Medicine
Duke University
Durham, North Carolina

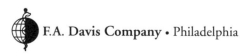
F.A. Davis Company • Philadelphia

F. A. Davis Company
1915 Arch Street
Philadelphia, PA 19103
www.fadavis.com

Printed in the United States of America

Last digit indicates print number: 10 9 8 7 6 5 4 3 2 1

Acquisitions Editor: Melissa Duffield
Manager of Content Development: George W. Lang
Developmental Editor: Peg Waltner
Art and Design Manager: Carolyn O'Brien

As new scientific information becomes available through basic and clinical research, recommended treatments and drug therapies undergo changes. The author(s) and publisher have done everything possible to make this book accurate, up to date, and in accord with accepted standards at the time of publication. The author(s), editors, and publisher are not responsible for errors or omissions or for consequences from application of the book, and make no warranty, expressed or implied, in regard to the contents of the book. Any practice described in this book should be applied by the reader in accordance with professional standards of care used in regard to the unique circumstances that may apply in each situation. The reader is advised always to check product information (package inserts) for changes and new information regarding dose and contraindications before administering any drug. Caution is especially urged when using new or infrequently ordered drugs.

Library of Congress Cataloging-in-Publication Data
Hack, Laurita Mary.
 Evidence into practice : integrating judgment, values, and research / Laurita M. Hack, Jan Gwyer.
 p. ; cm.
 Includes bibliographical references.
 ISBN 978-0-8036-1808-4 (pbk. : alk. paper)
 I. Gwyer, Jan. II. Title.
 [DNLM: 1. Physical Therapy Modalities. 2. Biomedical Research. 3. Decision Making. 4. Evidence-Based Medicine. 5. Professional-Patient Relations. WB 460]
 610.72′4–dc23

2012033718

This book is dedicated to our colleagues in practice who commit themselves to excellence and full engagement with their patients.

And

To Jack and Sarah and to Marty and Lisa—for everything

Foreword

The world's robust health and health care research enterprise produces a burgeoning flow of innovative methods for improving the well-being of people. Unfortunately, this ongoing research bounty poses important challenges for clinicians, including learning about and critically appraising new evidence on the diagnosis, prognosis, prevention, and management of clinical problems; adopting the most validated and efficacious innovations; offering these innovations to clients when appropriate, taking into account their preferences and capabilities; and "exnovation," eliminating practices that research has shown to be ineffective or harmful.

It is only recently in the history of health care that clinicians in any profession have been taught the skills to try to meet these challenges, and it is interesting to reflect on the relatively rapid (and painfully slow) evolution of evidence based clinical practice. Initially, beginning in the 1980s,[1] a decade of publications on "critical appraisal of the medical literature" described the key concepts of science that provide a foundation for valid assessment of screening and diagnostic tests, prognosis and clinical prediction, causal claims, and health care interventions. Although these concepts quickly became popular in health professional education circles, it was obvious that changing the habits of practicing clinicians was much more difficult than just teaching basic principles of critical appraisal.

The term "evidence based medicine" was coined at the beginning of the 1990s to try to galvanize the process of using research evidence in clinical care.[2,3] This was a "call to arms" to abandon traditional ways of clinical practice. It provocatively pitted evidence based medicine against eminence based medicine and denounced the tradition of relying on pathophysiology as the main pillar of practice. This call captured a great deal of attention, but it also raised many antibodies and, at least partially, correctly. Pathophysiology does have much to do with clinical practice. Experience (if not eminence) is essential.

A somewhat more mature model soon emerged, attempting to integrate evidence from research not only with clinical expertise but also with the patients' circumstances and their preferences and capabilities.[4] The authors of *Evidence into Practice: Integrating Judgment, Values, and Research* have embraced this model and advanced it a great deal, delving into what is known of clinical decision making, assessing patient's preferences, working in a team, and many related aspects of current practice.

Recognition of the opportunities for evidence based decision making has now spread worldwide throughout the health professions, but the tools for making this decision making happen effectively and consistently in clinical practice are still under development. One reason is that the resources for evidence based practice must be tailored to the purposes, needs, and mode of practice of each clinical discipline and, ultimately, to the needs and capabilities of each patient. We are still learning how to do this. This volume tackles these challenges for physical therapists, when working individually and in the rapidly evolving teams that are needed to deal with complex disease conditions and the multiple disease afflictions that inevitably arise when life is prolonged, whether it be for premature infants, children or adults with disabilities, or elders with chronic diseases.

Readers will learn a great deal about their profession, ways and means to provide evidence informed care, and how to continue to learn when knowledge for the benefit of patients keeps advancing. Unless someone turns off the faucet of knowledge, this book is a *must* for physical therapists and other health professionals.

R. Brian Haynes, OC, MD, PhD, FRCPC
Professor,
Department of Clinical Epidemiology and Biostatistics
McMaster University

---

[1]Department of Clinical Epidemiology and Biostatistics, McMaster University. How to read clinical journals: I. Why to read them and how to start reading them critically. Can Med Assoc J 1981; 124:555–8.
[2]Guyatt GH. Evidence-Based Medicine. ACP J Club 1991;114:A16.
[3]Evidence-based Medicine Working Group. Evidence-based medicine: a new approach to teaching the practice of medicine. JAMA 1992;268:2420–5.
[4]Haynes RB, Devereaux PJ, Guyatt GH. Physicians' and patients' choices in evidence based practice. Evidence does not make decisions, people do [Editorial]. BMJ 2002;324:1350.

Foreword

"We can't have full knowledge all at once. We must start by believing; then afterwards we may be led on to master the evidence for ourselves."

—THOMAS AQUINAS

•

When I was a physical therapist student in the early 1970s, we were required to conduct a research project. I compared forced passive stretching with "contract-relax," a proprioceptive neuromuscular facilitation technique, for reducing tight hamstrings and used my classmates as experimental participants. In seeking a rationale for the two intervention techniques, I did not go to the literature to determine which technique was more effective—there was none. I went to the library with my 3 × 5 cards and abstracted results from the basic science literature, which discussed theory related to how the Golgi tendon organ and the muscle spindle worked using evidence from experiments in animal models. My purpose in writing the review of the literature was to "guess" how the two receptors worked in the human body when the techniques improved the passive range of motion at the knee. In the classroom, we were introduced to treatment techniques with no thought of evidence to support one technique over another. Instead, we were given a "bag of tricks," and we were told that experience and master clinicians would help us to identify the most effective intervention to achieve our treatment goal. There was no emphasis on consensus as to the best intervention; the emphasis was on our ability to decide what was right. But, today, if physical therapists could agree on the best intervention rather than relying on their own opinion, a consumer would be guaranteed that the best intervention would be offered regardless of which physical therapist provided care.

Now we almost suffer from the opposite problem I faced when I was completing my master's thesis; we have a plethora of evidence! And yet, during his address to congress on behalf of people with disabilities, the actor Michael J. Fox said that if you ask people what their favorite therapy is, they will tell you it is the one that works (http://ptwa.org/Content/Legal/EBP.htm).

Wouldn't it be wonderful if we all selected the same intervention, and it worked? Physical therapists have to reduce unnecessary variation in practice so that they can determine if what the literature indicates is the "best" is in fact the most effective. Imagine a time when our patient records are collected in a common database and that we are all using the same outcome measures. We will then be able to determine if the intervention is effective, if the intervention works only in certain conditions and what they are, if there is residual disability, and if the "best" needs to be better. Clinical decision making is not removed from the therapist who selects the "best practice." The decision making is focused instead on making an accurate diagnosis; classifying the impairments into a set and matching the best intervention with the classification is where we should be honing our expertise. How do we get there in the absence of "best practice" guidelines? We search the literature.

How does a clinician choose within the evidence to select an examination tool or an intervention that will help a patient achieve a goal effectively and efficiently? What sources should be trusted? How do we help patients understand why we have selected one intervention instead of their "favorite"?

I would like to write that all that you have to do is read *Physical Therapy* (www.ptjournal. org). As I am Editor-in-Chief, I know that the editorial board, reviewers, and staff work diligently to provide a venue with immediate clinical relevance. Unfortunately, we do not have all the information that all practitioners need. At this time, there are more than 23,000 biomedical journals. The United States National Library of Medicine at the National Institutes of Health publishes a free database, PubMed (http://ncbi.nlm.nih.gov/pubmed/). Using the Medical Literature Analysis and Retrieval System (MEDLINE), a bibliographic database of life science and biomedical information, PubMed has 21 million citations. Where does one start? You could also use CINAHL (http://ebscohost.com/biomedical-libraries/the-cinahl-database), a cumulative index for nursing and allied health literature that provides indexing for more than 3000 journals. MEDLINE and CINAHL can provide access to original research, but what if you want assistance in reviewing the articles? There is PEDro (Physiotherapy Evidence Database), (http://pedro.org.au/) produced by the Centre for Evidence Based Physiotherapy at The George Institute for Global Health in Australia, a free database of over 22,000 randomized trials, systematic reviews, and clinical practice guidelines in physiotherapy. There is also The Centre for Evidence Based Physiotherapy, based in Maastricht, Netherlands (http://cebp.nl), whose mission is to seek, collect, and disseminate available scientific evidence in the physiotherapy domain for physiotherapists, health care workers, patients, and financiers of health care. This Web site has over 2500 white papers, all free. As well, there is *Hooked on Evidence*, (http://hookedonevidence.org), produced through the American Physical Therapy Association. This database does not restrict itself to randomized controlled trials; it includes clinical trials, cohort studies, case-control studies, case reports, single-subject experimental design, and cross-sectional studies. There are also disease-specific Web sites, such as Stroke Engine (http://strokengine.ca/about.html) developed by the Canadian Stroke Network that provides information on the effectiveness of over 35 interventions used in stroke rehabilitation, including Canadian Best Practice Recommendations for Stroke Care. International best practice guidelines, practical guides, e-learning modules, and pocket guides are also included to assist clinicians. StrokEngineAssess provides information on over 60 assessments related to stroke.

Suppose you want someone else to synthesize the work and provide you with a summary of multiple trials conducted on a particular intervention? The Cochrane Collaboration is an international network of more than 28,000 dedicated people from more than 100 countries. This team helps health care providers, policy makers, and patients and their advocates make well-informed health care decisions by preparing, updating, and promoting the accessibility of the Cochrane Reviews (http://cochrane.org). There are over 5000 so far. In 1997, the Agency for Health Care Policy and Research (AHCPR)—now the Agency for Healthcare Research and Quality (AHRQ)—launched an initiative to promote evidence based practice in everyday care through the Evidence-based Practice Center (EPC) Program (http://ahrq. gov/clinic/epc/). The EPCs develop evidence reports and technology assessments on topics relevant to clinical and other health care organization and delivery issues, specifically those that are common, expensive, and/or significant for the Medicare and Medicaid populations. Within the Effective Health Care (EHC) Program, EPCs conduct comparative effectiveness reviews, effectiveness reviews, technical briefs and future research needs reports, focused on patient-centered outcomes.

The amount of available information is daunting. But we have no choice, in my opinion, other than to search for the optimal method to produce the most effective outcome. It is not only a professional responsibility; it is a mandate. Third-party payers have access to the same information that we do; if we select an intervention because it is "what everyone else is using," we may not get reimbursed if there is evidence that the intervention is not effective. I believe that resources such as *PTNow* (http://apta.org/ptnow/) will provide quick and evidence based answers to clinical questions. This portal will answer a question such as "What is the most effective intervention to treat a grade III ankle sprain?" I believe that you will be able to access an answer to your question from a hand-held device during a treatment sessions.

We do not have access to this type of answer right now. While we await tomorrow's technology, we have to design effective plans of care today. The authors of this textbook have a commitment to helping you find the best evidence to assist you with clinical decision making. They have explored each of these topics in depth to help you make the best possible clinical decisions. They have also placed the evidence in the context of your clinical judgment and your patients. As theologian Thomas Aquinas suggested, you have the belief ... now seek evidence to support or refute that belief.

Rebecca L Craik, PT, PhD, FAPTA
Professor and Chair
Department of Physical Therapy
Arcadia University

Preface

Writing a book successfully needs a spark to begin, a passion to continue, and a determination to finish. The spark for this book came from reflection on the patterns of practice exhibited by the expert physical therapists we studied for the text, *Expertise in Physical Therapy Practice,* written with our colleagues Gail Jensen, and Katherine Shepard.[1] Before the concepts of evidence based practice had become known in the United States, the experts we interviewed were describing a pattern of practice that was deeply imbedded in a unified sense of practice, something we called a philosophy of practice. This philosophy grew from clinical judgment—making good decisions, knowledge—arising from available literature and from patients; virtue—a passion to do the right thing; and movement—using their own bodies and influencing their patients to produce the desired effect. Based on responses from our readers and from colleagues with whom we discussed our results, we knew that this pattern of practice was intriguing and important and that physical therapists wanted to emulate it.

The passion came as each of us began to work in the evidence based practice (EBP) world, teaching both entry-level and experienced clinicians the tenets of EBP. Both of us have been teaching since the days when the accepted way to prepare practitioners to *use* research in guiding their care was to teach them how to *do* research. We remember year after year of doing this and year after year being told by our graduates that they did not use this material because they were not researchers. Clearly there was a disconnect between our goal of producing thoughtful clinicians who use contemporary research and the way we were teaching them to do that. But EBP changed all of that. Graduates were finally reporting that they sought new literature and were asking how they could maintain access to literature databases.

The passion for writing this text really flamed when Dr. Hack had the opportunity to participate in a group of ethics teachers and researchers, known as the Dreamcatchers. One member of this group offered that she thought EBP had the potential to be unethical.[2] This was a surprising comment that caused much reflection. After a time, what became clear was that the application of information from the literature without exercising good clinical judgment and without honoring patient values and circumstances was indeed unethical, as it denied the obligation we have to meet the duties of patient autonomy, beneficence, non-maleficence, and justice. On the other hand, it seems to us, that to practice without using the unified principles of EBP—clinical judgment, patient values and circumstances, and evidence from the literature—was also unethical. So was born the idea for this text, to present the full picture of EBP, not focusing only on evidence from the literature, as other texts have, but providing depth and breadth across all three aspects so that our readers could truly embrace evidence based practice and offer their patients the care they deserve.

The determination to complete the text (and it takes lots of determination!) came from the support we provided each other, first through many visits between Durham and Philadelphia and then through our weekly Skype working sessions. We were able to keep each other going through many life changes and challenges that threatened to eat up our time and energy. It has been said that the only thing harder than doing research with colleagues is doing it alone.

The same can be said for writing a book. We brought different perspectives and experiences to this text, and we think it is richer for our collaboration.

We wish to thank the FA Davis staff who patiently helped us through to completion, including Margaret Biblis, for agreeing with us that this was a good idea; Melissa Duffield, for gently keeping us on the path; and Margaret (Peg) Waltner, for greatly reducing the confusion in our writing.

We hope that you find the book an inspiration in your practice. Providing health care and, for us particularly, physical therapy is a privilege of the highest calling. Providing it by using your best clinical judgment, by understanding and respecting your patients' values and circumstances, and by appropriately applying evidence from the literature means that we all truly honor our calling.

LAURIE HACK
Philadelphia, Pennsylvania

Jan Gwyer
Durham, North Carolina

---

[1]Jensen G, Gwyer J, Hack L, Shepard K; Expertise in Physical Therapy Practice, 2nd Ed, St. Louis, Saunders Elsevier, 2006.
[2]Royeen C, in Purtillo R, Jensen G, Royeen C, Eds, Educating for Moral Action: A Sourcebook for Health and Rehabilitation Needs, F. A. Davis, 2004.

Contributors

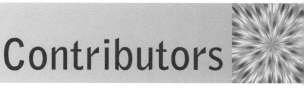

Christopher G. Bise, PT, DPT, MS
Assistant Professor
University of Pittsburgh
School of Health and Rehabilitation Science
Pittsburgh, Pennsylvania

Marian R. Block, MD, ABFP
Consultant, Pittsburgh Regional Health
* Initiative*
Formerly Vice President and Chief Quality
* Officer*
The Western Pennsylvania Hospital
Pittsburgh, Pennsylvania

Jack Coulehan, MD, FACP
Emeritus Professor of Prevention Medicine
Senior Fellow, Center for Medical
  Humanities, Compassionate Care and
  Bioethics
Stony Brook University
Stony Brook, New York

Anthony Delitto, PT, PhD, FAPTA
Professor and Chair
Department of Physical Therapy
Associate Dean for Research
University of Pittsburgh
School of Health and Rehabilitation Science
Pittsburgh, Pennsylvania

Suzanne P. Gordon, PT, EdD
Professor and Director
School of Physical Therapy
Husson University
Bangor, Maine

Alison Bailey Hallam, PT, MS
Lecturer
Arcadia University
Glenside, Pennsylvania
Physical Therapist
Bryn Mawr Rehabilitation Hospital
Malvern, Pennsylvania

John C. Hershey, PhD
Anheuser-Busch Professor of Management
* Science*
The Wharton School
University of Pennsylvania
Philadelphia, Pennsylvania

Michael P. Johnson, PT, PhD, OCS
Division Director
BAYADA Home Health Care
Moorestown, New Jersey
Adjunct Faculty
Arcadia University
Department of Physical Therapy
Glenside, Pennsylvania
Member
National Advisory Council
Agency on Health Care Research and
  Quality (AHRQ)
Rockville, Maryland

Kristin von Nieda, PT, DPT, MEd
Associate Professor
Department of Physical Therapy
Arcadia University
Glenside, Pennsylvania

Kim Nixon-Cave, PT, PhD, PCS
Board Certified Pediatric Specialist
Manager, Physical Therapy
The Children's Hospital of Philadelphia
Physical Therapy Department
Philadelphia, Pennsylvania

Connie Schardt, MLS, AHIP, FMLA
Associate Director
Research and Education Medical Center
  Library
Duke University Medical Center
Durham, North Carolina

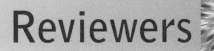

Sarah Blanton, PT, DPT
Assistant Professor
Department of Rehabilitation Medicine
Emory University
Atlanta, Georgia

Phyllis A. Clapis, DHSc, PT, OCS
Associate Professor
American International College
Springfield, Massachusetts

Sherrilene Classen, PhD, MPH, OTR/L
Assistant Professor
College of Public Health and Health
    Professions
Department of Occupational Therapy
Gainesville, Florida

Jeanne Cook, MS, PT, CWS, DCE
*Director, Clinical Education of Physical
    Therapy*
Missouri State University
Springfield, Missouri

Marie Earl, PhD, MSc, BSc (Kin), BSc (PT)
Assistant Professor
Dalhousie University
School of Physiotherapy
Halifax, Nova Scotia, Canada

Coral Gubler, PT, PhD, ATC
Assistant Professor, Physical Therapy
University of Southern Alabama
Mobile, Alabama

Andi Beth Mincer, PT, MS
Assistant Professor, Physical Therapy
Armstrong Atlantic State University
Savannah, Georgia

Diane Pitts, RN, PT, RSN, BS
Instructor in Physical Therapy
University of Southern Alabama
Mobile, Alabama

Frank Underwood, PT, PhD, ECS
Professor, Physical Therapy
University of Evansville
Evansville, Indiana

Contents

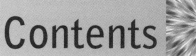

Opening Words

Declare the past, diagnose the present, foretell the future; practice these acts. As to diseases, make a habit of two things—to help, or at least to do no harm. The art consists in three things—the disease, the patient, and the practitioner. The practitioner is the servant of the art, and the patient must combat the disease along with the practitioner.

—ADAPTED FROM HIPPOCRATES, *EPIDEMICS,* BK. I, SECT. II

INTRODUCTION

It is clear that the expectations set by our patients, by society, and ourselves require us to do the best we can with each of our decisions. Imagine a large multispecialty outpatient practice. These four patients are on the schedule, each of whom has caused the patient's physical therapist to question the current plan of care.

Ms. Swenson has been coming in for 3 weeks now, with little progress, and her therapist is beginning to wonder whether her heel pain is actually being caused by plantar fasciitis, as is stated on her referral from a physician colleague, or whether it might have a more central cause. The therapist remembers that he has had a few patients in the past month with severe heel pain related to spinal changes. The therapist has had only a few months' experience with lower-extremity orthopedic problems but has a colleague in the practice for whom it has been a specialty for about 3 years.

The Cho family is coming in with their grandmother, who speaks only Korean. The therapist has not been able to convince the patient that a regular aerobic exercise program is necessary to help her manage her low back pain. The therapist thinks it may be because her family will not let the therapist tell her that her back pain is a chronic, life-long condition that will need continual management. The therapist has become increasingly frustrated with what he perceives as the family's lack of cooperation and thinks today may well be a good time to discharge her if there is no further progress to be seen.

Mr. Washington, who had a stroke about 3 months ago, with some increasing depression, has shown great response to his therapist's use of repetitive tasks in the plan of care. Hand function has improved, the depression seems to be lifting, and the patient is quite pleased with the progress. However, Mr. Washington has not been keeping up with his co-payments for visits, as mandated by his insurance plan, and the therapist knows that Mr. Washington will reach his maximum visit limit in two more visits. Because both the patient and therapist see the progress being made, the therapist wants to arrange for a way to continue care, without taxing Mr. Washington's limited means any further.

When Mr. Davis came in 2 days ago he excitedly showed his therapist a printout from a Web site claiming that ultrasound would be a very successful intervention for his chronic shoulder pain. The Web site, owned by the manufacturer of home ultrasound units, includes some references to research studies that supposedly support this claim. The therapist now wonders whether she should add ultrasound to his plan of care on his return visit today and how she can best determine the truth about ultrasound as an appropriate intervention for chronic musculoskeletal pain.

APPROACHES TO DECISION MAKING

Every day, all day, clinicians in every practice setting face questions such as these. How do clinicians deal with these kinds of questions in the midst of their busy practices? Clinicians often turn to a few "tried-and-true" approaches to help them make decisions, with the following reasoning for their choices:

- Authority—I do it this way because that's the way I'm told to do it by my supervisor, my facility, the physician, or someone else perceived in some position of authority.
- Educational Background—I do it this way because that's the way my teachers taught me to do it when I was in school or at the last continuing education conference I attended.
- Tradition—I do it this way because that's what all the standard textbooks say; it just seems as though that's the way it is. After all, it's what everyone else does.
- Trial and Error—I do it this way because it seems to work for me. It certainly worked the last time I tried it.

Each of these approaches may actually work—some of the time! Their major advantage is that they are all readily accessible and can help us in the moment of actual patient care right when we really need the answer. But upon reflection, we can easily see that none of them can work well on a regular basis and each of these approaches could easily lead us to make less than optimal decisions about our patient care.

Finding the Right Answer at the Right Time

So how do we manage the dilemma of finding the *right* answer at the *right* time? Recently an approach that has been termed evidence based practice (EBP) has been suggested as an answer to this dilemma. The leading proponents of EBP have put forth the following proposition:

When we integrate:

- Our own well-developed *clinical expertise*, with
- An understanding of and a value for each *patient's own values* and and for each *patient's own circumstances*
- The *best research evidence* available about our question
- We create truly evidence based practice[1]

Let's examine each of these terms and see how they might help with the patient questions we've posed.

Clinical Judgment

"Clinical judgment" refers to the ability of the clinician to blend his or her skills and experience to make good clinical judgments in a timely clinical fashion.[1,2] Ms. Swenson's therapist

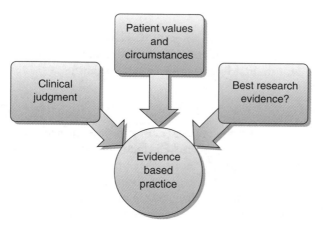

Figure 1 Evidence Based Practice.

was facing a more difficult time because he did not have sufficient experience to be able to categorize Ms. Swenson's signs and symptoms. He did recognize that he could tap into the clinical experience of a colleague who probably also had better psychomotor skills in carrying out specific tests and measures for this patient.

Patient Values

"Patient values" refers to the preferences that each patient, and often the patient's family, brings to the clinical encounter. These preferences can arise from cultural or religious norms, from personal attitudes and beliefs, or from the patient's prior experiences and knowledge.[1,3] Mrs. Cho and her family were displaying a set of values about the patient's understanding of her health care that were different from her therapist's values. For the family, saving a revered member of the family from hearing difficult news was more important, while to the therapist, having the patient really understand her situation was more important. The therapist needed first to recognize this difference and then respect the choice being made while trying to find a way to be successful with the patient's goals.

Patient Circumstances

"Patient circumstances" refers to the situation in which the patient finds him- or herself. This could refer to the location of care; to the resources available to provide the care, including funding for the care; or to the resources for the patient to deal with the short- and long-term sequellae of the illness or trauma.[1,4] Mr. Washington's therapist has identified that his patient does not have the economic means to sustain what the therapist believes is the best course of action based on the research evidence and needs to learn what other resources are available to help mitigate these circumstances.

Best Research Evidence

"Best research evidence" refers to the information available from the basic sciences that underlie our care, but primarily from clinical research, to help us answer specific questions about our patient care.[1,5] For example, the therapist who wants to understand the usefulness of ultrasound for Mr. Davis can identify literature that can answer this question, appraise the validity and relevance of the literature, and apply the information to this specific patient.

Evidence Based Practice

Evidence based practice (EBP) refers to the full integration of each of these elements, which allows the patient and the practitioner, working together, to make joint decisions that result in the ability to achieve the goals needed and desired for reaching optimal health.

Obligations of Care

Good health care has been the goal of the patient and the practitioner from time immemorial. But exceptions to the desired standard of care have also been well documented throughout history. There has always been, as there should be, great concern that practitioner mistakes could result in death or serious morbidity. One of the most recent and thorough examinations, a study conducted by the Institute of Medicine,[6] estimates that 98,000 people die needlessly in the United States each year due to mistakes made by their caregivers. This level of error results in very high costs in lives lost, lives diminished, and dollars spent. There are great efforts being made to help design health care so that the likelihood of making such mistakes is reduced. These efforts include engineering better systems, raising awareness, improving teamwork, and changing reimbursement incentives.[7] All of these efforts hinge on helping clinicians make better decisions.

Although "first do no harm" is a central tenet for all health professions, we have a far higher obligation than to simply avoid costly errors. Health professionals, by virtue of their roles, have implicitly agreed to assume a fiduciary relationship with their patients. In other words, patients and society have the right to believe they can trust the health care professional to act in the patient's best interest, placing that interest above all other interests and concerns. Physicians have expressed these behaviors in many ways. The American Board of Internal Medicine sets the following standard for all those aspiring to board certification in internal medicine: "Professionalism in medicine requires the physician to serve the interests of the patient above his or her self-interest. Professionalism aspires to altruism, accountability, excellence, duty, service, honor, integrity and respect for others."[8]

The profession of physical therapy has articulated a similar set of behaviors that are considered the core values to be displayed by the members of the profession. The values are included in the standards for entry-level education and for specialty certification. These core values are accountability, altruism, compassion/caring, excellence, integrity, professional duty, and social responsibility. Of note here are the definitions of altruism, excellence, professional duty, and social responsibility:

- *Altruism* is the primary regard for or devotion to the interest of patients/clients, thus assuming the fiduciary responsibility of placing the needs of the patient/client ahead of the physical therapist's self interest.
- *Excellence* is physical therapy practice that consistently uses current knowledge and theory while understanding personal limits, integrates judgment and the patient/client perspective, embraces advancement, challenges mediocrity, and works toward development of new knowledge.
- *Professional duty* is the commitment to meeting one's obligations to provide effective physical therapy services to patients/clients, to serve the profession, and to positively influence the health of society.
- *Social responsibility* is the promotion of a mutual trust between the profession and the larger public that necessitates responding to societal needs for health and wellness.[9]

Using This Book

This text will focus on helping clinicians, in all stages of their professional lives, from student to expert, learn to maximize their ability to use each of these elements to truly create an alliance with their patients that results in optimal patient care. The book is divided into four sections, one for each element of EBP and one that discusses applications of EBP. It is difficult to place the three elements into a linear order, when in fact they are completely intertwined. Our clinical expertise helps us identify data that lead us to search the evidence in the literature. The evidence in the literature gives us guidance on understanding our patients' values. But, as some order is necessary, we have chosen to use the following order for each section.

- Section I focuses on the first element of EBP, clinical expertise.
  - Chapter 1 introduces the common language we use in describing physical therapy practice.
  - Chapter 2 includes the ways that clinicians typically think.
  - Chapter 3 shows ways that humans often err in decision making.
  - Chapter 4 explains the reasons for these errors.
  - Chapter 5 will then offer several ways to improve decision making.
- Section II focuses on the second element of EBP, the knowledge of and respect for patient values and circumstances.
  - Chapter 6 emphasizes the importance of cross-cultural communication that fully respects the values of the patient.
  - Chapter 7 shows the value of the interview as a primary means of communication, including communication about values and circumstances.
  - Chapter 8 includes evidence from current literature about patient values, using qualitative research techniques to enlighten our understanding of patient values.
  - Chapter 9 concludes with a discussion of the health care system as it affects patient circumstances and evidence from the current literature about patient circumstances.
- Section III focuses on the third element of EBP: identifying, analyzing, and applying evidence from the literature.
  - Chapter 10 provides a discussion on the process of identifying strong, answerable clinical questions.
  - Chapter 11 highlights the process of searching for answers.
  - Chapter 12 presents the necessary information to appropriately assess the evidence in the literature by understanding research design, methods, and statistics.
  - Chapters 13 to 16 discuss the many ways we find evidence in the literature (studies, synopses of studies, syntheses, synopses of syntheses, summaries, and systems) and show the ways we can assess each of these types of evidence.
- Section IV focuses on implementing the principles of EBP in practice.
  - Chapter 17 explores the many reasons it is difficult to translate evidence into practice.
  - Chapter 18 demonstrates how EBP can enhance patient care documentation and how documentation can enhance our ability to put the principles of EBP into practice.
  - Chapter 19 offers a specific example of integration of EBP into practice.

We will conclude with some final words about where the future may take us as we practice in a fashion that truly integrates all of these elements to achieve the best clinical decision making possible.

Learning Tools Within the Chapters

The text is designed to encourage your learning as much as possible. We introduce each chapter with a question or issue from an actual patient case. The patient, Mr. Sam Ketterman, is a 90-year-old man well known to one of the authors. He presents with the typical complexity of so many of our patients, requiring many decisions to be made to help him achieve the best health possible. (The full case is presented in the Appendix.)

You will find many of these features in each of the chapters:

- Case examples that appear early in the chapter and will often appear in other chapters, some of these will include discussion questions.
- Occasional sidebars throughout the chapter that provide interesting facts about the topic, Web links, or graphic illustrations of certain points.
- Self-assessment questions to help you determine whether you have mastered the material in the chapter.
- Continued learning questions or strategies to help you continue to master the material as you put it into practice.

CONCLUSION

We hope to demonstrate that each of the elements of EBP is necessary but not sufficient by itself to provide the quality of patient care that society has every right to expect of us. If we are to achieve that level of care, we must fully integrate each of these elements into EBP. We look forward to exploring these issues together throughout this text.

REFERENCES

1. Strauss SE, Glasziou P, Richardson WS, et al. *Evidence-Based Medicine*, 4th ed. Elsevier Churchill Livingstone; 2011.
2. Jensen G, Gwyer J, Hack L, et al. *Expertise in Physical Therapy Practice*, 2nd ed. St. Louis: Saunders Elsevier; 2006.
3. Institute of Medicine. *Crossing the Quality Chasm: A New Health System for the 21st Century*. Washington DC: Institute of Medicine; 2001.
4. Kissick WL. *Medicine's Dilemmas*, New Haven: Yale University Press; 1994.
5. Law M. *Evidence-Based Rehabilitation*. Thorofare NJ:, Slack; 2002.
6. Kohn KT, Corrigan JM, Donaldson MS. *To Err Is Human: Building a Safer Health System*, Washington, DC, National Academy Press; 1999.
7. Leape LL, Berwick DM. Five years after *To Err Is Human*: What have we learned? JAMA. 2005;293:2384–2390.
8. American Board of Internal Medicine. Project Professionalism. Philadelphia: American Board of Internal Medicine; 2001. http://www.abim.org/pdf/profess.pdf. Accessed January 11, 2011.
9. American Physical Therapy Association, Professionalism in Physical Therapy: Core Values. http://www.apta.org/AM/Template.cfm?Section=Policies_and_Bylaws&TEMPLATE=/CM/ContentDisplay.cfm&CONTENTID=36073, accessed January 6, 2011.

Clinical Judgment

Clinical judgment has always been a guide for good practitioners. Before physical therapists were able to use theoretically grounded and methodologically tested research hypotheses that provided scientifically sound evidence to guide clinical decision making, they sought guidance from well-developed practice knowledge and clinical reasoning. When good practitioners attempted new interventions, they carefully observed the situation and could recall successes and failures. Studies of expertise in physical therapy have helped us understand this important element in evidence based practice (EBP).[1-5] The deep practice-based knowledge of these experts gives them skill in active reflection.[1] Experts use all three elements of EBP but always modulate what they learn from the literature with their own expert judgment to best meet their patients' needs.

This section begins with Chapter 1, which provides an overview of the language of practice and the important developments over the past decades that allow us to communicate with each other and our health care colleagues. In this chapter we describe two important purposes for a common language in our profession: to describe our patients accurately and to describe our processes and outcomes of care. You will find a useful and context-rich description of models of disability and patient management as well as an introduction to the *Guide for Physical Therapist Practice*.

In Chapter 2 we present an overview of how physical therapists make clinical decisions. The types of decisions required in practice are highlighted along with an array of approaches to clinical reasoning used by physical therapists and some of their colleagues in medicine, nursing, and occupational therapy.

Chapter 3 presents a perspective on errors in clinical reasoning, drawing from reports in medicine, physical therapy, and occupational therapy. An understanding of the types of errors typically found in physical therapy practice and the sources of influences on errors is an important step in improving clinical reasoning.

Chapter 4, written by Jack Hershey, provides an understanding of how biases affect clinical decisions. Detecting bias in one's own thinking is difficult, but if it is done well and consistently, it will result in more accurate sharing of knowledge with patients.

Chapter 5 deals with the tools available to physical therapists to assist with clinical reasoning. You are encouraged to examine the way physical therapists think and their use of practice algorithms that might facilitate the best clinical reasoning. Policies that improve understanding of what good clinical practice is or what evidence to use in clinical decision making are also introduced in this chapter.

References

1. Jensen G, Gwyer J, Hack L, Shepard KF. *Expertise in Physical Therapy Practice.* 2nd ed. St. Louis, MO: Elsevier; 2007.
2. Jones M, Jensen G, Edwards I. Clinical reasoning in physical therapy. In: Higgs J, Jones M, eds. *Clinical Reasoning in the Health Professions.* Boston: Butterworth-Heinemann; 2000.
3. Resnik L, Jensen GM. Using clinical outcomes to explore the theory of expert practice in physical therapy. Phys Ther. Dec 2003;83(12):1090–1106.
4. Smart K, Doody C. The clinical reasoning of pain by experienced musculoskeletal physiotherapists. Man Ther. Feb 2007;12(1):40–49.
5. Zimny NJ. Clinical reasoning in the evaluation and management of undiagnosed chronic hip pain in a young adult. Phys Ther. Jan 1998;78(1):62–73.

chapter 1

The Language of Practice

*Language shapes the way we think, and determines what
we can think about.*

—BENJAMIN WHORF

•

✳ Mr. Ketterman's Case

Mr. Ketterman has just told me 90 years worth of medical and social history. He has
so many problems I just don't know how to organize my thoughts! *(See Appendix for
Mr. Ketterman's health history.)*

INTRODUCTION

As human beings, we use language, all kinds of language, to communicate with each other.
We speak of verbal and nonverbal language; of written, oral, sign, and symbolic languages; of
languages of different peoples, countries, and times. Each occupation has also developed a
language that describes the tools, the processes, and the products of that occupation. Some
of these languages are easily translated or understood by those outside the occupation; others
become more complex, perhaps even obscure and can sometimes serve to exclude others. But
these languages occur for good reason—they serve to provide the framework for a way of
thinking, for clarifying and articulating the lens used by its members to view the world. We
are not speaking here of the many abbreviations, acronyms, or eponyms that have cropped
up in the vocabulary of health care practitioners, but of the basic language that defines the
philosophy of practice. There are at least two central components of a useful language of
practice. We need to be able to *describe our patients* and then to *describe the process and outcomes
of our care* for these patients. This chapter will present systems based on the biopsychosocial
model to describe our patients and a patient management model that describes the process
of our care.

DESCRIBING OUR PATIENTS

Accurate and comprehensive descriptions of patients are essential. The descriptive label given
a patient can help us not only as health care practitioners but as sociologists, health services
researchers, and others, striving to understand the concepts of health and illness and what

they mean in human life. In this instance the label serves as shorthand for explaining the natural progression of the specific patient and the general condition of groups of people. A label also can help us choose proper interventions and predict outcomes for our patients. In this instance the descriptive label serves as a diagnosis.

The Biopsychosocial Model

The World Health Organization (WHO) has defined health as "a state of complete physical, mental and social well-being and not merely the absence of disease or infirmity."[1] Since it was adopted in 1946, this definition, while presenting an ideal, has permeated much of the discussion on health care. It served as the foundation for the overarching model for understanding health and illness known as the biopsychosocial model (Fig. 1-1).[2] This model assumes that the person's response to any state of health or illness is a result of the interaction of the person's psychology and social environment with the biological determinants of disease and trauma.

Despite this long-standing recognition that health and illness exist far beyond the confines of pathology, the primary language used to describe patients has been to label the patient by using the patient's diagnosis of pathology. For example, we speak of the patient with viral rhinitis (the common cold), or the patient with a bladder infection, or the patient with an ankle sprain, or the patient with multiple sclerosis. While these labels do indeed describe the factor that initiates the need for health care, they do not necessarily describe the continuing status of health or illness the patient may experience, so they cannot help us determine the continuing health care needs of the patient. The label of viral rhinitis may well be sufficient to predict the care needs of the patient since it is a self-limiting disease that is "cured" with time. The label of bladder infection may well be sufficient, as long as it is precise enough to prescribe the appropriate antibiotic medication that then "cures" the disease. The label of ankle sprain may not be quite as useful, however, because depending on several factors (patient status, structures involved, nature of the injury, degree of the sprain, etc.) a sprain may never be fully "cured." The patient may well have residual alterations to soft tissue that will always leave him or her susceptible to reinjury. The label of multiple sclerosis becomes yet more problematic both in describing the patient and in contributing to determining the patient's care needs. There is not a known "cure" for this problem, nor is there a known method of

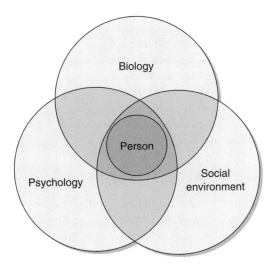

Figure 1-1 The Biopsychosocial Model, demonstrating the interaction of biology, psychology, and the social environment in defining the health status of the individual person.

controlling its progression. The efforts of the health care system related to this pathology are focused on reducing the intensity of the effects of the disease and on helping patients maintain maximum function.

DEVELOPMENT OF MODELS FOR ENABLEMENT/DISABLEMENT

For physical therapy, as for many of the fields in the area of rehabilitation, articulation of the concept of disability has given us the language to more fully describe our patients than the language used previously. Sociologists studying the sociology of health and illness recognized that using pathology to describe patients was simply not sufficient to fully understand and describe the life of a person with a chronic or progressive disease. This led sociologists to begin to develop disablement models. Nagi provided the first organized description of a concept of disablement as distinct from disease.[3,4] He identified that in order to understand disability, it was necessary to make distinctions among four separate but linked concepts: pathology, impairment, functional limitation, and disability.

The first concept is *pathology*, broadly defined to include a wide variety of diseases arising from different etiologies, including infection, trauma, and degenerative processes. Whatever the etiology, the pathology is seen as the start of a cascade of events and only one part of the full picture that explains the health status of the patient. All pathologies have the potential to cause problems in the human organism. The next stage, the consequences of pathology, occurring at the organ or system level, is called *impairment*. For example, the pathology of fracture results in impairments of pain and loss of motion. The next stage of the cascade is *functional limitations*. Impairment often results in the inability to carry out specific functional activities. For example, the pain that results from a fracture can in turn result in reduced ambulation endurance. *Disability* is the next step of the cascade. Disability moves beyond the biological events and begins to look at the person. A disability occurs when the person's functional limitations interfere with the person's role in life, be it work, family, or leisure roles. For example, the limitation of ambulation endurance that results from the fracture becomes a problem when ambulating long distances is part of the person's normal work or leisure activities and cannot be supplemented by the use of personal assistance or assistive devices.

Expansion of the Nagi Model

These concepts were expanded by later authors to add more dimensions to Nagi's work (Fig. 1-2).[5–7] One principal addition is the identification of the factors that can affect the cascade from pathology to impairments to functional limitations. This modified model shows that demographic factors, health history and habits, and personal characteristics can all affect the cascade. In addition, Guccione added the concept of *handicap*. Society places a handicap on a person when it refuses to make adjustments to accommodate the disability. This refusal may be an appropriate response based on available resources, but it still handicaps the person. This model was used to drive the creation of The *Guide to Physical Therapist Practice*[8] and is therefore very familiar to many physical therapists in the United States.

International Classification of Functioning Model

At the same time that the language of the Nagi model and its evolutions were gaining a foothold in the conversation about health care in the United States, the WHO was developing the International Classification of Functioning, Disability and Health (ICF). At the time, the International Classification of Diseases (ICD), which classifies patient care based primarily on the patient's pathology and which was also developed by the WHO, was the most prominent

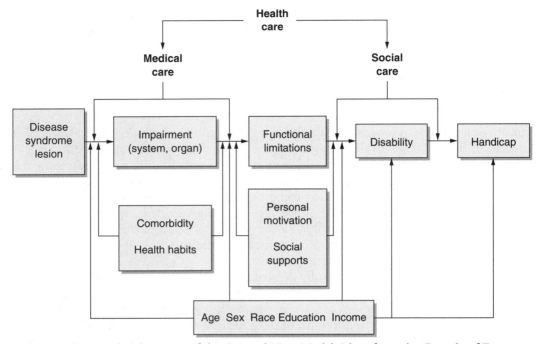

Figure 1-2 Guccione's Adaptation of the Original Nagi Model, Identifying the Cascade of Events That Follow from Pathology, as Modulated by Many Factors. *(Adapted from Guccione AA. Physical Therapy Diagnosis and the Relationship Between Impairments and Function. Phys Ther. 1991;71:499–504 and Guccione AA, Geriatric Physical Therapy, Philadelphia, Mosby, 1993.)*

of the classification systems. In the United States it is widely used to classify patients for many purposes, including reimbursement and categorization for required reporting. It has also been used for research and for prediction of resource allocation, especially for prevention and for management of chronic diseases. Just as with the Nagi-based models, it was recognized that this pathology-based classification scheme was inadequate by itself to meet all the needs of the health care systems around the world. The ICF is the response to this realization and to the recognition that an enablement model is a better way to describe the full continuum of the human health experience. The most recent revision of the ICF (Fig. 1-3) has now been widely accepted across the world as a system for classifying the relationship of health, function, and disability.[9,10]

The ICF is based on the premise that disability is actually a continuum that coexists with health. In other words, everyone is in some state of health and some state of disability. The ICF consists of three parts: the health status (top row of the model); three components of functioning—body structure, activities, and participation (second row of the model); and contextual factors of environment and person (third row of the model). It clarifies that factors related to the person and to the environment can modulate the affect of health status on body structures and functions, on activity, and on participation in one's role. It also provides a model that supports the concept of prevention as a means to maintain the maximum level of health possible. Physical therapists have begun using this system to describe patient care, especially when discussing patients with long-term disabilities.[10–12]

While the Nagi-based models and the ICF use somewhat different language, they have in common a view that pathology is a starting point for a cascade of events and that these events can be modulated by many factors. Table 1.1 provides the definitions of the terms used in

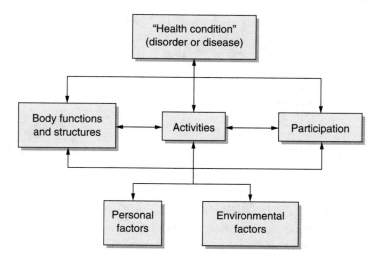

Figure 1-3 The International Classification of Functioning, Disability, and Health (ICF) Model of Functioning and Disability. *(Adapted from International Classification of Functioning, Disability, and Health [ICF]. ICF full version. Geneva, Switzerland: World Health Organization; 2001.)*

Table 1.1	Comparison of Terms in Nagi-Based Models Compared With the ICF Model
Nagi[3,4]	**ICF**[9]
Active Pathology—Interruption or interference with normal processes and effort of the organism to regain normal state	*Health Conditions*—diseases, disorders, and injuries
Impairment—anatomical, physiological, mental, or emotional abnormalities	*Body Function*—physiological functions of body systems *Body Structures*—anatomical parts of the body *Impairments*—problems in body functions or structure
Functional Limitation—limitation in performance at the level of the whole organism or person	*Activity*—the execution of a task or action by an individual *Activity Limitation*—difficulties an individual may have in executing activities
Disability—limitation in performance of socially defined roles and tasks within a sociocultural and physical environment	*Participation*—involvement in a life situation *Participation Restriction*—problems an individual may experience in involvement in life situations

From: Jette, AM. Toward a common language for function, disability, and health. Phys Ther. 2006;86:726–734.

the two models, Nagi (and its derivatives) and ICF, which are most familiar to physical therapists.

These models have given us language which allows us to explore all the sequelae of disease and illness, be they acute or chronic, and which describes prevention activities. Moreover, these models firmly recognize that health is a complex phenomenon that goes well beyond the biological basis of pathology to include the psychological and social aspects of human life.

DESCRIBING THE PROCESS AND OUTCOMES OF OUR CARE

The Guide's Patient Care Management Model

The American Physical Therapy Association's (APTA) *Guide to Physical Therapist Practice* was developed to provide a common language of physical therapy care that could be used by a wide variety of audiences, including physical therapist clinicians, educators, and researchers, and also external groups such as referring sources and payers. One of the most important parts of the *Guide* is the *patient care management model* (Fig. 1-4).[8,13] The process described by this model uses decision making that is very similar to the process used by other health care practitioners, including physicians. It does this through both its organization and its language, as will be pointed out as the model is described.

Examination

This first step in the model uses the term *examination*. This is an important language change from the terms *evaluation* or *assessment* that have been used traditionally in physical therapy. The process of examination is both sequential and iterative and consists of three parts: history, systems review, and specific tests and measures. An examination begins with the *history*. By learning about the patient's past and current status, as reported by the patient and others, the clinician can begin to focus on the specific tests to perform. The history includes not only the typical chief complaint, medical history, and medication history but also demographic data; social history, including employment; growth and development; living environment; general heath status; social and health habits; family history; functional status; and a review of clinical tests performed by other practitioners. (Chapter 7 provides valuable information on conducting the patient interview as the major source of the patient's history.)

Systems Review: All practitioners do a quick *systems review* each time they see a patient. For physical therapists this is a review of the four systems that are in their primary domain: musculoskeletal, neuromuscular, cardiovascular/pulmonary, and integumentary, as well as the patient's communication abilities. A review of a system consists of simple measures that help to decide if further specific testing is needed. For example, if we are seeing a patient who has come to us with an upper-extremity problem and we watch that person walk into the treatment booth with no apparent difficulty, we have just done a systems review for ambulation problems and do not do any specific lower-extremity testing. Most practitioners do this as an almost automatic part of practice. For physical therapists, adopting the patient care management model means documenting the systems review as a formal part of a patient's care.

Specific Tests and Measures: The history and the systems review are used to guide the practitioner in selecting from among the available *specific tests and measures* that seem best indicated for the individual patient. Box 1.1 shows the list of specific tests and measures used by physical therapists. The *Guide* provides a detailed analysis of each area of testing, including clinical

The elements of patient/client management leading to optimal outcomes

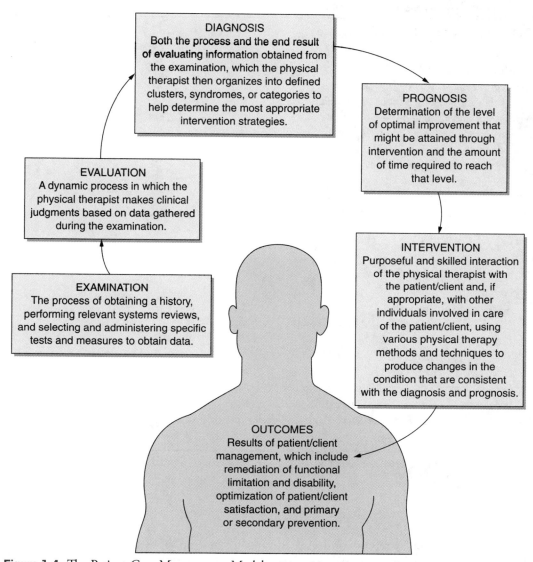

DIAGNOSIS
Both the process and the end result of evaluating information obtained from the examination, which the physical therapist then organizes into defined clusters, syndromes, or categories to help determine the most appropriate intervention strategies.

PROGNOSIS
Determination of the level of optimal improvement that might be attained through intervention and the amount of time required to reach that level.

EVALUATION
A dynamic process in which the physical therapist makes clinical judgments based on data gathered during the examination.

INTERVENTION
Purposeful and skilled interaction of the physical therapist with the patient/client and, if appropriate, with other individuals involved in care of the patient/client, using various physical therapy methods and techniques to produce changes in the condition that are consistent with the diagnosis and prognosis.

EXAMINATION
The process of obtaining a history, performing relevant systems reviews, and selecting and administering specific tests and measures to obtain data.

OUTCOMES
Results of patient/client management, which include remediation of functional limitation and disability, optimization of patient/client satisfaction, and primary or secondary prevention.

Figure 1-4 The Patient Care Management Model. *(Adapted from Chapters 2 and 3, American Physical Therapy Association, A Guide to Physical Therapist Practice, 2nd ed. Alexandria, VA: American Physical Therapy Association; [rev] 2003.)*

indications, the types of tests available, the tools used in gathering data, and the data generated.[8]

The decision about which tests to choose demonstrates one of the interrelationships between the concept of the enablement/disablement model and the patient care management model. We will analyze one of the areas of special tests and measures, flexibility, as an example. A physical therapist would make the decision to use a measure of flexibility when finding clinical indicators from the history and systems review that supported that decision. These indicators could be based in pathology, such as the presence of rheumatoid arthritis. They could be based

Box 1.1	**Categories of Tests and Measures Used by Physical Therapists**

Aerobic Capacity and Endurance

- Anthropometric Characteristics
- Arousal, Attention, and Cognition
- Assistive and Adaptive Devices
- Circulation (Arterial, Venous, Lymphatic)
- Cranial and Peripheral Nerve Integrity
- Environmental, Home, and Work (Job/School/Play) Barriers
- Ergonomics and Body Mechanics
- Gait, Locomotion, and Balance
- Integumentary Integrity
- Joint Integrity and Mobility
- Motor Function (Motor Control and Motor Learning)
- Muscle Performance (Including Strength, Power, and Endurance)
- Neuromotor Development and Sensory Integration
- Orthotic, Protective, and Supportive Devices
- Pain
- Posture
- >Prosthetic Requirements
- Range of Motion (Including Muscle Length)
- Reflex Integrity
- Self-Care and Home Management (Including Activities of Daily Living and Instrumental Activities of Daily Living)
- Sensory Integrity (Including Proprioception and Kinesthesia)
- Ventilation, Respiration (Gas Exchange), and Circulation
- Work (Job/School/Play) Community, and Leisure Integration and Reintegration (Including Instrumental Activities of Daily Living)

Data from Chapters 2 and 3, American Physical Therapy Association, *A Guide to Physical Therapist Practice*, 2nd ed. Alexandria, VA: American Physical Therapy Association, (rev) 2003;24.

in impairments, such as reports of decreased range of motion. They could be based in functional limitations, such as reports of inability to dress. They could be based in disability, such as the report that the patient is no longer able to work. Whatever the indication, and there may be many, the clinician would then need to decide which specific tests of flexibility would be used, choosing from among regional and specific joint measures. Depending on the tests chosen, the therapist would need access to instruments such as goniometers and also skill in correct measurement techniques. Finally, the tests would give the therapist data that specify those joints and regions where range of motion is not normal.

Evaluation

The next step of the patient care management model is *evaluation*. In the patient care management model, evaluation is not the physical act of collecting data, but rather the judgment which the physical therapist uses to transform the data from the examination into clinical decisions about the patient. These decisions include diagnosis and prognosis.

Diagnosis: One decision made through evaluating the examination data is the patient *diagnosis.* The issue of diagnosis is the primary locus of the interrelationship between managing patient care and the concept of disablement. The most common way that patients are classified is by the pathology that begins or has the potential to begin the patient's problems. But a diagnosis is simply assigning a patient to a particular classification. It is this diagnosis, or classification, that helps guide all of the rest of the treatment decisions. So a diagnosis, or classification label, can describe the patient's impairments, limitations, functional limitations, disabilities, or handicaps (using the language of the Nagi model) or describe the impairments, activity limitations, or participation restriction (using the language of the ICF).

There are two parts to this decision that bear analysis. The first part of the equation is the decision to make a classification at all. Why do individual patients need to be assigned to a particular classification? This is the very heart of the diagnostic process. By recognizing that an individual patient is similar to other patients, we can begin to predict with some certainty the likelihood of recovery, the likelihood of various interventions being successful, and the most likely time frame for that level of recovery. If patients are considered only one at a time, we can never develop a sense of these probabilities.

The second part of this equation is the type of diagnosis. As we've discussed, diagnoses of pathology alone are not always useful for physical therapists in designing a plan of care. For example, knowing that a patient has had a cerebral vascular accident (a diagnosis of pathology) tells us very little about this patient's impairments or functional limitations. But it is those very impairments and functional limitations that the therapist wants to address through physical therapy interventions. Classification by impairments and functional limitations allows physical therapists to appropriately choose interventions with the best likelihood of success in ameliorating those impairments or functional limitations.

Prognosis: *Prognosis* is another of the decisions made based on the examination. A prognosis is a prediction of how long it will take to reach certain goals in plans of care. The data from the examination lead not only to a classification but also to a classification that has known probabilities of recovery. The prognosis becomes part of a plan of care that includes achievable goals and outcomes. Goals refer to removing or reducing impairments. Outcomes refer to removing or reducing functional limitations and disability.

Intervention

The final decision made based on the examination is the choice of *interventions.* The *Guide* describes three areas of interventions: documentation and communication, patient/client-related instruction, and procedural interventions. The *Guide* notes that both documentation and communication and patient/client instruction are an integral part of each and every visit, thereby recognizing the importance of these activities for the success of patient care.[8]

Procedural Interventions

Procedural interventions (Box 1-2), the methods used to reach goals and outcomes, vary in each episode of care based on the goals and outcomes established for the patient.[8] The description of each intervention category in the *Guide* includes clinical considerations, again divided by pathology, impairments, functional limitations and disability, specific interventions, and anticipated goals and expected outcomes.

Outcomes

The last step in the model is identifying the *outcomes* anticipated for the individual patient as well as collecting data that help predict outcomes for groups of patients with similar classifications or diagnoses. There are a variety of outcomes of interest to physical therapists, including

> **Box 1.2** **Procedural Interventions Used by Physical Therapists: Therapeutic Exercise (Including Aerobic Conditioning)**
>
> **Functional Training in Self-Care and Home Management (Including Activities of Daily Living and Instrumental Activities of Daily Living)**
>
> - Functional Training in Community and Work (Job/School/Play) Integration or Reintegration (Including Instrumental Activities of Daily Living, Work Hardening, and Work Conditioning)
> - Manual Therapy Techniques (Including Mobilization and Manipulation)
> - Prescription, Application, and, as Appropriate, Fabrication of Devices and Equipment (Assistive, Adaptive, Orthotic, Protective, Supportive, and Prosthetic)
> - Airway Clearance Techniques
> - Wound Management
> - Electrotherapeutic Modalities
> - Physical Agents and Mechanical Modalities
>
> Data from Chapters 2 and 3, American Physical Therapy Association, *A Guide to Physical Therapist Practice*, 2nd ed. Alexandria, VA: American Physical Therapy Association, (rev) 2003;24.

reduction of pathology, impairments, and functional limitations and disability, as well as improving quality of life, patient satisfaction, and cost efficiency.

CONCLUSION

Both the disablement models and the patient care management model provide language to describe care, to communicate with patients and with each other, to facilitate good clinical thinking (see Chapters 4 and 5), and to frame scholarship. Mr. Ketterman's case (see Appendix) is written using the ICF language and the terminology from the patient care management model. This choice of language allows us to organize a complex health history for a patient with multiple problems in a way that allows for a clear understanding of his needs, the therapist's plans for intervention, and the results of those interventions.

SELF-ASSESSMENT

1. Can you describe the cascade of events for one of your patients, or a patient you have observed, using either the Nagi model of disablement or the International Classification of Functioning, Disability and Health?
2. Using this same patient, can you identify diagnoses across the disablement model you are using? Are you using more than a diagnosis of pathology? How do each of the diagnoses across the disablement model affect your clinical decisions and your expectations for the patient's success?

Continued learning

- *The Guide to Physical Therapist Practice*

In addition to the printed version of the *Guide*, which originally appeared as an article in *Physical Therapy*, it is now available in a Web-based format at http://guidetoptpractice.apta.org/. In addition to much more detail about the patient care management model, the *Guide* has several sections with background information on the tests, measures, and interventions used in physical therapy. It also has a section, "Preferred Practice Patterns" which integrates the information on tests, measures, and interventions into an organized set of expectations for over 30 of the most common groups of patients seen in physical therapy. All of this information can be useful to both students and practicing clinicians in reviewing and expanding their own knowledge base and in assessing the care they plan for particular patients.

If you have not used the patient care management model to document your care, try reorganizing one of your current patient cases into the patient care management model. Did you find that some data might be missing? What advantages and disadvantages do you see to using this format for documentation?

• *International Classification of Functioning, Disability, and Health (ICF)*

In addition to the texts that are available from the WHO, a very useful Web site about the ICF is http://www.who.int/classifications/icf/en/. The site includes several useful tools, including a checklist for use in documentation. The World Confederation for Physical Therapy also has a variety of resources about the ICF at its Web site, http://www.wcpt.org/icf. Both the WHO and the APTA offer many opportunities to become better trained in using ICF language to describe and document care. The WHO materials are available for download and use at its Web site. The APTA has developed training modules at its Learning Center, http://learningcenter.apta.org/, to assist in understanding and applying the ICF; one module can be used to earn continuing education credits.

REFERENCES

1. Constitution of the World Health Organization. http://www.searo.who.int/EN/Section898/Section1441.htm, accessed July 31, 2007.
2. Engel GL. The need for a new medical model: a challenge for biomedicine. Science. 1977;196:129–136.
3. Nagi S. Disability concepts revisited: implications for prevention. In Pope AM, Tarlov AR eds. *Disability in America: Toward a National Agenda for Prevention.* Institute of Medicine, National Academy Press, 1991.
4. Nagi S. Some Conceptual Issues in Disability and Rehabilitation. In Sussman M, ed. *Sociology and Rehabilitation.* Washington, DC: American Sociological Association; 1965:100–113.
5. Guccione AA. Physical Therapy Diagnosis and the Relationship Between Impairments and Function. Phys Ther. 1991;71:499–504.
6. Guccione AA, ed. *Geriatric Physical Therapy,* St. Louis, Mosby, 1993.
7. Verbrugge LM, Jette AM. The disablement process. Soc Sci Med. 1994;38:1–14.
8. American Physical Therapy Association, *Guide to Physical Therapist Practice,* 2nd ed. American Physical Therapy Association, Alexandria, VA, 2001.
9. International Classification of Functioning, Disability, and Health (ICF). ICF full version. Geneva, Switzerland: World Health Organization; 2001.
10. Jette AM. Toward a common language for function, disability, and health. Phys Ther. 2006;86:726–734.
11. Steiner WA, Ryser L, Huber E, et al. Use of the ICF model as a clinical problem-solving tool in physical therapy and rehabilitation medicine. Phys Ther. 2002;82:1098–1107.
12. Palisano RJ. A collaborative model of service delivery for children with movement disorders: a framework for evidence-based decision making. Phys Ther. 2006;86:1295–1305.
13. Hack, L. Chapter 1: Principles of Therapeutic Intervention with Modalities, in Michlovitz and Nolan, Modalities for Therapeutic Intervention, 4th ed. FA Davis, 2005.

chapter 2

How Physical Therapists Make Clinical Decisions

If you chase two rabbits, both will escape.
—Author Unknown

By three methods we may learn wisdom: First, by reflection, which is noblest; Second, imitation, which is easiest; and third by experience, which is the bitterest.
—Confucius

•

✳ Mr. Ketterman's Case

Mr. Ketterman appears to have a relatively short life expectancy. What is my role as his physical therapist? Should I provide any care at all? If so, what kind of care? How safe would treating him be? Does he need referral to others? So many questions! *(See Appendix for Mr. Ketterman's Health History)*

INTRODUCTION

Physical therapists are responsible for making many types of decisions with and for their patients. These decisions are elementary components of every aspect of the patient management model discussed in Chapter 1; for example, physical therapists are required to develop a diagnosis and prognosis and to select interventions. The decisions range from thoughtfully considered decisions developed over time, such as an appropriate discharge destination for a patient following an inpatient course of care, to moment-by-moment decisions, such as movements required during a treatment session. Over the century of our profession's history, physical therapists have grown both in the capability and desire to make these clinical decisions. Early in the profession, physicians wrote detailed treatment prescriptions that covered all but the most mundane clinical decisions required of physical therapists. We were viewed as technical assistants who could neither diagnose a patient's impairments or functional limitations nor develop a plan of care. In the 21st century, we view ourselves as autonomous practitioners with significant responsibility for the judicious care and successful outcomes for our patients. Thus, the types of clinical decisions made and the characteristics of the clinical reasoning processes are of great interest to practitioners who wish to improve their approach to practice.

The science that supports theories of clinical reasoning in physical therapy is built upon studies of cognitive processing in nonmedical fields,[1] medical problem solving,[2–6] and expert practitioners in nursing,[7–9] occupational therapy,[10] and physical therapy.[11–22] Expert practitioners provide researchers with the opportunity to study the combination of knowledge and skill acquisition along with the cognitive and metacognitive processes of clinical reasoning.

The most recent attempts to understand the clinical reasoning of experts in contrast to novices have been conducted in the practice environment as the importance of the contextual nature of clinical reasoning has emerged.[23] Grounded theory qualitative case studies have also emerged as the research method of choice for studying the expertise of health care practitioners[8,13,24] as contrasted with earlier research on physician decision making that used standardized stimuli with research subjects in an artificial setting. These innovations in research approaches have provided health care professionals with a richer body of theory for designing strategies with which to increase the clinical reasoning abilities of students and professionals. For example, the majority of studies of decision making by physicians have been conducted to understand diagnostic decisions about the pathology causing the patient's symptoms.[6,25,26] The *Guide to Physical Therapist Practice*,[27] introduced in Chapter 1, has been important in expanding the work on clinical reasoning in physical therapy.[28–30]

This chapter will provide an overview of the types of decisions required of physical therapists and the clinical reasoning strategies that have been identified. In the following two chapters, we will discuss errors or biases that could cause clinical judgment to be flawed. Case vignettes will be presented to encourage you to engage actively in a reasoning exercise and then attempt to identify which of several strategies you find typical of your own thinking.

THE CONTEXT OF CLINICAL REASONING

First Things First: Is This My Patient?

Ken's Experience, Part One: Ken is participating in a weekend neighborhood social event that includes a picnic and games. His neighbors know that Ken is a physical therapist in private practice in the community, and some have sought his services in the past. During a game of volleyball, Michelle, one of Ken's neighbors, falls to the ground and grabs her ankle after jumping to block a ball. She cries out in pain for help, and the neighbors gather around her, several looking at Ken, expecting that he will help.

Ken's experience highlights many decisions that a physical therapist must address before making any further clinical decisions. At this point in the case, Ken has made no decision, but with his first step toward the potential patient, he will have made a plethora of decisions.

*Pause now and list as many decisions as you can that you would make in the first few seconds of your response.

Now review Box 2.1 to see the many questions that have to be answered as Ken prepares to decide about intervening in the situation. Notice that several of the questions that are included are designed to help the therapist refine his decision making: legal, ethical,

---

Box 2.1 **First Things First: Is This My Patient? Potential Decisions to Be Made**

- Legal
  1. Can I legally provide services of a first aid nature to this person?
  2. Can I legally provide services of a physical therapy nature to this person? In this setting?
  3. Is there a Good Samaritan law in this jurisdiction that will protect me if my actions cause harm? Does such a law protect me as a citizen, as well as a health care provider?
- Ethical
  1. Am I obliged by my code of ethics to provide first aid services to this person?
  2. Can I refuse to help this person?
  3. Must I seek the person's permission before giving advice or direct care?
- Practitioner Competence
  1. Am I a qualified first aid provider?
  2. Am I skilled at diagnosing injuries of the ankle?
  3. If I initiate an evaluation of this person, will I know what to do with the information I gather?
- Practitioner Status
  1. Am I impaired in any way at this point in the day based upon what I have done or ingested?
  2. Am I reluctant to become involved to the extent that my judgment might be impaired?

---

competence-based, and status-based. This tool can be helpful in thinking broadly about all the types of decisions required when you are in a similar situation. Ken's experience illustrates the importance of making good judgments before initiating a relationship with a patient; if a poor judgment is made at this point, later decisions will likely become more complex. For example, if Ken's specialized expertise and practice are in cardiac rehabilitation and he decides to help Michelle, he may enter into the diagnostic reasoning process without sufficient knowledge to avoid causing harm. These unexpected, pre-relationship types of decisions have not been studied in the literature, but they share some characteristics with ethical reasoning—the type of reasoning used by physical therapists when ethical and practical dilemmas arise.[31] Experienced clinicians often reflect that the decisions related to whom to treat and when to treat become some of the most challenging clinical decisions in their practice. We all would benefit from more evidence in order to answer questions concerning many of the patients with whom we have the opportunity to interact. In this case, a potential future patient needs emergency care, and the decision to intervene or not becomes one of the most important decisions of the entire case.

DIAGNOSTIC CLINICAL REASONING

Shoe On, Shoe Off: What Has Happened to Your Ankle?

Ken's Experience, Part Two: Ken has decided that he will help Michelle by examining her ankle, with her permission. He wants to help Michelle understand what has happened to her ankle, ease her pain, and determine what level of care she needs immediately and in the next 24 hours. He wants to make helpful recommendations to Michelle; he is not at this moment interested in soliciting her as a patient.

Box 2.2	**Shoe On, Shoe Off: What Has Happened to Your Ankle?** **Potential Decisions to Be Made**

- Legal
    1. Get the patient's verbal consent for your examination.
- Ethical
    1. Determine what will maximize patient comfort first.
    2. Determine what actions would make the injury worse and avoid these.
- Diagnostic
    1. Determine how to perform your examination.
    2. Determine the extent of the injury to the ankle and surrounding tissues.
    3. Assess your confidence in your diagnosis.
- Prognostic
    1. Determine the need for additional medical attention immediately or within the next 24 hours.
- Intervention
    1. Select immediate necessary care and implement.
    2. Identify follow-up care and make recommendations.
    3. Perform the interventions or delegate them to the patient and family.
    4. Seek treatment supplies or delegate this to the patient and family.

Ken has decided to enter into a relationship with his neighbor, and although preliminary, the relationship has the elements of a patient–physical therapist relationship, even though the parties have been cast into these roles suddenly. The next set of decisions calls on Ken to bring his clinical expertise, knowledge, and reasoning together to make correct clinical decisions and recommendations for Michelle.

Pause now and note the clinical decisions that you would make if you were Ken, their purpose, and the order in which you would pursue them.

Now review Box 2.2, and determine if you have made similar choices. Ken has several types of decisions to make as this list indicates, but his primary concern might be to diagnose the patient's pathology. However, doing this prior to discussing with Michelle what he can offer her and gaining her consent would be unnecessarily risky in the context of this case. Some of Ken's options might raise ethical dilemmas. One such dilemma might be captured in his decision to take her shoe off or not for the purposes of examining her ankle. Taking the shoe off might cause more pain or injury, and once off, increased edema is a potential complication unless alternative strategies to control edema are available. But if Ken chooses not to take Michelle's shoe off, he may limit his ability to make an accurate diagnosis of the presence of a fracture.

Once Ken makes a diagnosis, he will be simultaneously assessing his confidence in the diagnosis, given any limitations on his examination or other data-gathering abilities. The greater the limitations, the lower Ken's confidence will be that he has made a correct decision, and this uncertainty will flow into his next set of decisions. Ken must make a prognosis as to whether or not Michelle requires medical care at a hospital emergency room, an urgent medical care center, or in a physical therapist's office on Monday morning.

Sometimes, when we are uncertain of our diagnosis of a patient's pathology and make either overly risky or overly cautious decisions, every other component of care can be affected,

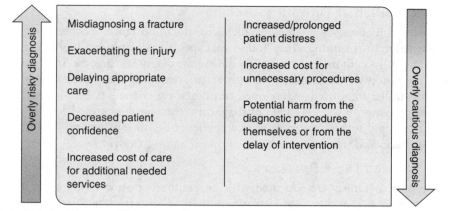

Figure 2-1   Relative Impact of Diagnostic Decisions.

resulting in harm to the patient or unnecessary expense and use of resources (Fig. 2-1). Other times, a less accurate diagnosis of the pathology of an injury may not have negative consequences. For example, if you are incorrect in isolating the specific muscle in the group of wrist extensors that may be experiencing an inflammatory response in a patient with forearm pain, you are still able to proceed with your intervention decisions with some confidence that they will be successful regardless of which muscle is most affected, as your intervention will address the entire group.

We discuss more about possible mistakes in diagnosis and other aspects of care in Chapter 3 and possible reasons for these mistakes in Chapter 4. In Ken's case, if he is uncertain of his diagnosis, this will not deter him from making intervention decisions because the motivation to do something for Michelle is strong, as she has an acute injury. Groopman,[32] in his text entitled *How Doctors Think*, suggests that emergency room physicians, when most uncertain, ask themselves the following types of questions, which might be helpful to Ken right now:

- Is this patient seriously injured?
- What is the worst outcome here?
- How likely is it?

Types of Diagnostic Decision Making

Diagnostic decision making has been studied in physical therapy over the past 20 years, and researchers have found that it shares many similarities to the processes used by physicians, although the nature of the diagnoses made by each professional are different. The research has identified two major processes in decision making: hypothetico-deductive reasoning and pattern reasoning.

Elstein et al[3] identified a model of medical decision making, termed the hypothetico-deductive model of reasoning, as the dominant strategy used by physicians to cluster patient symptoms into diagnostic categories of pathology. Often termed *backward reasoning*, this process consists of gathering cues, generating hypotheses that fit one or more of the cues, and then testing the hypotheses to determine the best fit for the diagnosis. This process is used to turn an unstructured, unfamiliar, or complicated patient problem into one that can be addressed with the use of one or more hypotheses. In physical therapy this process is commonly seen in the practice of reevaluation, where the prevailing hypothesis can be continually confirmed or disconfirmed.[13]

Pattern Recognition or Forward Reasoning

For experienced clinicians, researchers also identified the importance of contextually developed clinical knowledge in reasoning. They found that specialists combined highly organized and accessible knowledge with mental processing during the diagnostic process. In situations where the patient's symptoms were familiar to the physician, reasoning was more rapid or automatic. The specialists utilized knowledge developed from their experiences to build recognizable patterns of patient symptoms.[33] This type of diagnostic reasoning is termed *pattern recognition*, or *forward reasoning*, and is typical of more experienced clinicians whereas the hypothetico-deductive, or backward, reasoning is more common amongst novices.

Choosing Between These Processes

Student physical therapists are educated with an emphasis on mastering basic and applied research knowledge so that they might identify in their patients the likely pathology, functional limitations, and impairments that should be the focus of their physical therapy care. This type of knowledge may, however, fail a novice clinician when faced with a complex clinical scenario that was never discussed while acquiring technical knowledge. With increasing experience, expert practitioners in physical therapy were found to have combined their basic science knowledge with a growing rich resource of practical knowledge. Using techniques called reflection in action,[34] they then transformed their knowledge into a rich pool of information to inform clinical decisions. Reflection in action requires the practitioner to analyze cases that caused doubt and to rethink the choices made to determine what worked and why it worked. Schon[34] suggests that without reflective practice, logical or rational problem solving alone will never be enough to enhance clinical reasoning.

These two primary types of diagnostic reasoning (backward and forward reasoning), as well as reflection, have been identified in studies of novice as well as expert physical therapists.[13,18,35] All agree that physical therapists are not as concerned with a correct diagnosis of pathology as they are with a correct understanding and labeling of the significant impairments and functional limitations the patient is experiencing. Research by Jones et al[36] suggests that physical therapists use a hypothesis-oriented approach while working collaboratively with the patient to understand the functional losses most important to the patient. Edwards et al[31] studied the clinical reasoning strategies of expert physiotherapists in Australia and identified two types of diagnostic reasoning strategies. Diagnostic reasoning using either forward or backward strategies resulted in the identification of physical disabilities and impairments important for guiding the selection of interventions. Narrative reasoning was defined as important in the diagnostic role of the PT as the physical therapist attempted to understand the patient's story, illness experience, context, beliefs, and culture.

If Ken happens to specialize in orthopedic or sports physical therapy, he may move quickly to help Michelle and, with a careful examination of her ankle and well-honed questions about her symptoms, be able to use a pattern recognition clinical reasoning strategy to form his diagnosis. If he specializes in cardiac rehabilitation, he may take a more deliberate route in both his examination and questioning, testing his hypothesis about the likelihood of a lower limb fracture against each finding. In either case, Ken will be able to understand the impact of his diagnosis on Michelle's pain and loss of function over the days to come.

PATIENT MANAGEMENT REASONING

Lisa's Experience: Lisa, a certified clinical specialist in neurological physical therapy, practices in an integrated service delivery facility that provides acute inpatient rehabilitation services, subacute inpatient rehabilitation services, and home health physical therapy services to patients who have significant rehabilitation needs. The philosophy of this health care center is to provide patients with continuity of care from the same practitioners as they progress to lower levels of care requirements and finally to their homes. Lisa is fortunate to be able to follow her caseload of patients who have experienced stroke and traumatic brain injury for a long time and across settings. Lisa believes that this extended contact with her patients helps her clinical reasoning skills as she is able to assess the outcomes of her decisions directly and for a longer-than-average period. She practices with an interdisciplinary team of rehabilitation providers who respect each other's expertise and collaborate on many clinical decisions. For example, Lisa will be presenting Mr. Simon's case to the team today as she has identified a complication of pusher syndrome in his recovery from a right cerebral artery stroke. Lisa has developed a set of intervention techniques but she is reevaluating her decision for discharging Mr. Simon to his home given this complication and the difficulty of teaching the patient and his family safe transfer techniques.

Diagnostic reasoning has received much attention in the medical literature, but more recent research in health professions such as nursing, occupational therapy, and physical therapy has unearthed a wealth of perspectives on the complex decisions required of practitioners who spend a significant amount of time with a patient across episodes of care. A physician may repeat his or her diagnostic reasoning skills every 15 minutes throughout the day with different patients. However, physical therapists and other rehabilitation personnel will practice other types of clinical reasoning during their extended encounters with each patient, often over frequent visits. Table 2.1 contrasts some of the aspects of medical decision making with those found in nursing and occupational therapy.

Lisa's experience with Mr. Simon provides a stimulus for reflecting on the many areas of clinical reasoning in physical therapy patient management.

*Pause now and reflect on Lisa's clinical decisions in Mr. Simon's case. How many different types of decisions for a physical therapist can you identify in this scenario?

Now review Table 2.2, which shows several categories of clinical reasoning related to patient management identified from research on nurses, occupational therapists, and physical therapists. Many of these categories will sound familiar to physical therapists because they describe the types of thinking that is required of them each day. Table 2.2 defines each type of clinical reasoning and gives examples of each type that could be drawn from Mr. Simon's case. The breadth of the categories of patient management reasoning identified speaks to the range of reasoning skills required of a physical therapist.

Continued study of patient management reasoning is crucial to improving understanding of clinical reasoning strategies. As we will discuss in the next two chapters, we are prone to clinical reasoning errors in both diagnostic and patient management. For example, evidence from actual patient experience provides the basis for studying the typical errors physical therapists make in predictive reasoning. Are we overly optimistic in predictive reasoning, perhaps ignoring evidence about typical recovery patterns? The identified categories of patient management reasoning can help us understand which types of reasoning are most easily learned, which types are most valuable to the patient experience, and which types of reasoning are most challenging when practicing outside our area of expertise.

Developing or Improving Clinical Reasoning Skills

How does this research help you develop or improve your clinical reasoning skills? First, these descriptions of clinical reasoning strategies identified in studies of physical therapists can facilitate discussions between novice and experienced clinicians. Questions such as the ones in Table 2.2 can help physical therapists reflect on their clinical reasoning abilities and identify

Table 2.1 Comparison of Clinical Reasoning Approaches in Health Professions

Health Profession	Knowledge Assumptions	Reasoning/Thinking Skills	Practitioner–Patient Interactions
Medicine			
Novices: tend to use hypothetico-deductive model (backward reasoning)	Building knowledge structures	Hypothesis generation and testing deductive thinking	History provides cues for hypothesis generation and testing
Experts: tend to use forward reasoning or a combination of backward and forward reasoning when having difficulty	Highly structured knowledge base informed by experience Specific to clinical specialty area	Pattern recognition Use of illness scripts Intuitive thinking	Listening to patient cues Illness scripts Activities
Nursing			
Cognitive and rational models limit understanding of clinical reasoning	Knowledge socially constructed	Intuitive	Listening and interpreting patients' stories
Practical reasoning part of everyday practice	Knowing the patient and family essential in clinical practice	Engaged (not disengaged) reasoning; emphasis on learning and being with others Deliberative; patient advocacy	
Occupational Therapy			
Clinical reasoning focused on human meaning involving multiple modes of reasoning	"We know more than we can tell" Tacit knowledge essential	Procedural reasoning used for and thinking about the disease and initial treatment (similar to hypothetico-deductive model) Interactive reasoning used to understand the patient; active collaboration Conditional reasoning used to understand experiences of patients (integrative form of reasoning)	Central role of narrative thinking involved in telling patient stories and story making (ways in which the therapist connects therapy to the patients' lives)

Data from: Benner P, Tanner CA, Chesla CA. *Expertise in Nursing Practice.* New York: Springer; 1996; Patel VL, Kaufmann D, Magder S. The acquisition of medical expertise in complex environments. In: Ericsson KA, ed. *The Road to Excellence.* Mahwah, NJ: Lawrence Erlbaum; 1996; 127–165; and Mattingly C, Fleming MH. *Clinical Reasoning.* Philadelphia: FA Davis, 1994.

	Table 2.2	**Patient Management Clinical Reasoning Strategies Applied to Lisa's Experience with Mr. Simon**	

Type of Reasoning	Definition	Examples as Applied to Mr. Simon's Case
Procedural Reasoning[§] Procedural Reasoning[†]	Decision making about selecting and implementing treatment procedures Identifying functional problems and selecting procedures to reduce the effects of the problems	Will Mr. Simon respond to visual cues of vertical to aid his unsupported sitting balance?
Interactive Reasoning[§] Interactive Reasoning[†]	Establishment and monitoring of patient rapport Understanding the patient	Will Mr. Simon trust my feedback on his safety in transfers?
Collaborative Reasoning[§]	A consensual approach to interpreting exam findings, goal setting, and implementing interventions	Joint decisions made with the interdisciplinary team concerning the best practice for Mr. Simon's pusher syndrome.
Teaching Reasoning[§]	Decisions about content and methods to effectively teach patients and families	What method should I use to teach Mrs. Simon how to safely transfer her husband from the wheelchair to the bed?
Predictive Reasoning[§]	Active envisioning of future scenarios with patients and the implications of choices	Should I delay Mr. Simon's discharge to his home?
Ethical Reasoning[§]	Understanding ethical and practical dilemmas in practice and evaluating appropriate actions	If Mr. Simon has reached the end of his reimbursed time in sub-acute rehab, can I discharge him if he is not safe at home?
Narrative Reasoning[†]	Understanding the unique lived experience of patients	How does Mr. Simon think his function will be different when he goes home?
Conditional Reasoning[†]	Placing the person and the physical problem in a contextual big picture; thinking about the whole condition, how it could change and what is necessary for it to change	What was Mr. Simon like before his stroke and how can I help him pursue that status again?
Practical Reasoning[c]	Practical reasoning in an evolving, open-ended situation; reframing the problem	Are Mr. Simon's symptoms indicative of new pathology?

[§]Reasoning categories from Edwards, Jones et al. 2004.[31]
[†]Reasoning categories from Mattingly and Fleming.[10]
[c]Benner from 1999.[8]

areas in which they would like to improve. Ask yourself which types of decisions come easily, and which types of decisions are typically more difficult? Second, describing these types of reasoning allows us to articulate the complexity of prolonged interactions with patients. Most researchers found that physical therapists, as well as nurses and occupational therapists, are adept at thinking or reasoning along multiple lines of thought simultaneously. Mattingly and Fleming identified this behavior in occupational therapists and termed it "the therapist with a three-track mind" (p. 133). Such therapists can monitor their *procedural reasoning* as they select treatment procedures and their *interactive reasoning* as they assess their communication with the patient and, using *conditional reasoning*, they can pull it all together to create an individualized treatment session for the patient.[10] Jensen et al,[13] studying 12 physical therapist experts across four specialty areas, also found this fluidity during treatment sessions with patients. To the observer it is often difficult to determine which type of reasoning is occurring at any particular moment; this makes mentoring students in the clinical setting more challenging. Students can see what the clinician is doing, but they cannot see what the clinician is thinking. The categories can help mentor and student alike make clinical reasoning more explicit and thus allow both to improve their thinking.

CONCLUSION

To understand clinical reasoning in physical therapy requires one to consider the context in which physical therapists practice, the types of decisions that they make, the type of reasoning they use, as well as the development of these skills across a professional career from student to novice to expert practitioner. We have illustrated in this chapter that our limited research suggests that physical therapists share some common thinking processes with other health care practitioners. Jensen et al[13–16] were the first to propose a model of expert practice in physical therapy by contrasting the thinking of novice and expert physical therapists. Clinical reasoning was identified as a key component of the model of expertise. The physical therapist who achieves this level of practice has developed a context-rich, multidimensional base of knowledge through reflective practice, paying close attention to the patient as a source of knowledge. Their clinical reasoning processes are characterized by a strong value for and use of collaborative reasoning with patients for management decisions. They can efficiently recognize patterns in diagnostic reasoning by matching their patient's examination findings to their mental library of patient illness scripts. What is more difficult for expert and novice clinicians alike is describing their thinking processes, or being aware of the nuanced changes that accompany their experience. Research in this area is vital to the profession so that clinicians can develop a lifelong practice of enhancing clinical reasoning abilities.

Physical therapy experts also confirm that patients' values as they relate to their own health care should constitute the primary focus of the clinician's reasoning processes. The second section of this text will delve further into strategies to uncover and value patient preferences in all clinical reasoning.

SELF-ASSESSMENT

1. Identify some experiences that you have had that are similar to the cases presented in this chapter and then use the questions in Tables 2.1 and 2.2 to reflect on your decision making.
2. Think about a patient you have treated recently and identify three decisions you made about that patient's care. If you haven't treated any patients, think about a

patient whose care you have observed. Then use the categories in Table 2.2 to think about what kind of reasoning you used in making these decisions.

3. After these reflections, try to describe your own personal decision making process. Some of us are more graphically oriented than others, so perhaps you would prefer to draw this process rather than write about it.

CONTINUED LEARNING

Choose one of the articles in the reference list, read it carefully, and share what you have learned with your colleagues.

REFERENCES

1. Newell A, Simon H. *Human Problem Solving*. Englewood Cliffs, NJ: Prentice-Hall; 1972.
2. Elstein AS, Schwartz A. Clinical reasoning in medicine. In: Higgs J, Jones M, eds. *Clinical Reasoning in the Health Professions*. Boston: Butterworth-Heinemann; 2000.
3. Elstein AS, Shulman L, Sprafka S. *Medical Problem Solving: An Analysis of Clinical Reasoning*. Cambridge, MA: Harvard University Press; 1978.
4. Elstein AS, Shulman L, Sprafka S. Medical problem solving: A ten year retrospective. Eval Health Professions. 1990;13:5–36.
5. van Gessel E, Nendaz MR, Vermeulen B, Junod A, Vu NV. Development of clinical reasoning from the basic sciences to the clerkships: A longitudinal assessment of medical students' needs and self-perception after a transitional learning unit. Med Educ. Nov 2003;37(11):966–974.
6. Young JS, Smith RL, Guerlain S, Nolley B. How residents think and make medical decisions: Implications for education and patient safety. Am Surg. Jun 2007;73(6):548–553; discussion 553–544.
7. Benner P. *From Novice to Expert: Excellence and Power in Clinical Nursing Practice*. Menlo Park, CA: Addison-Wesley; 1982.
8. Benner P, Tanner C, Chesla C. *Expertise in Nursing Practice: Caring, Clinical Judgment and Ethics*. New York: Springer; 1996.
9. Ritter BJ. An analysis of expert nurse practitioners' diagnostic reasoning. J Am Acad Nurse Pract. Mar 2003;15(3):137–141.
10. Mattingly C, Flemming M. *Clinical Reasoning: Forms of Inquiry in a Therapeutic Practice*. Philadelphia: FA Davis; 1994.
11. Higgs J. A programme for developing clinical reasoning skills in graduate physiotherapists. Med Teach. 1993;15(2–3):195–205.
12. Higgs J, Jones M. *Clinical Reasoning in the Health Professions*. Boston: Butterworth-Heinemann; 2000.
13. Jensen G, Gwyer J, Hack L, Shepard KF. *Expertise in Physical Therapy Practice*. 2nd ed. St. Louis, MO: Elsevier; 2007.
14. Jensen G, Gwyer J, Hack L. Attribute dimensions that distinguish master and novice physical therapy clinicians in orthopedic settings. Phys Ther. 1992;72:711–722.
15. Jensen G, Shepard KF, Hack L. The novice versus the experienced clinician: insights into the work of the physical therapist. *Phys Ther*. 1990;70:314–323.
16. Jensen GM, Gwyer J, Shepard KF. Expert practice in physical therapy. Phys Ther. Jan 2000;80(1):28–43; discussion 44–52.
17. Jones M, Edwards I, Gifford L. Conceptual models for implementing biopsychosocial theory in clinical practice. Man Ther. Feb 2002;7(1):2–9.
18. Jones MA. Clinical reasoning in manual therapy. Phys Ther. Dec 1992;72(12):875–884.
19. Noll E, Key A, Jensen G. Clinical reasoning of an experienced physiotherapist: Insight into clinician decision making regarding low back pain. Physiother Res Int. 2001;6(1):40–51.
20. Payton OD. Clinical reasoning process in physical therapy. Phys Ther. Jun 1985;65(6):924–928.

21. Resnik L, Jensen GM. Using clinical outcomes to explore the theory of expert practice in physical therapy. Phys Ther. Dec 2003;83(12):1090–1106.
22. Zimny NJ. Clinical reasoning in the evaluation and management of undiagnosed chronic hip pain in a young adult. Phys Ther. Jan 1998;78(1):62–73.
23. Schon D. *The Reflective Practitioner: How Professionals Think in Action*. New York: Basic Books; 1983.
24. Embrey DG, Guthrie MR, White OR, Dietz J. Clinical decision making by experienced and inexperienced pediatric physical therapists for children with diplegic cerebral palsy. Phys Ther. Jan 1996;76(1):20–33.
25. Redelmeier DA, Schull MJ, Hux JE, Tu JV, Ferris LE. Problems for clinical judgement: 1. Eliciting an insightful history of present illness. CMAJ. Mar 6 2001;164(5):647–651.
26. Redelmeier DA, Tu JV, Schull MJ, Ferris LE, Hux JE. Problems for clinical judgement: 2. Obtaining a reliable past medical history. CMAJ. Mar 20 2001;164(6):809–813.
27. American Physical Therapy Association. *Guide to Physical Therapist Practice*. 2nd ed. Alexandria, VA: APTA; 2002.
28. Daykin AR, Richardson B. Physiotherapists' pain beliefs and their influence on the management of patients with chronic low back pain. Spine. Apr 1 2004;29(7):783–795.
29. Dieruf K. Ethical decision making by students in physical and occupational therapy. J Allied Health. Spring 2004;33(1):24–30.
30. O'Sullivan PB, Beales DJ. Diagnosis and classification of pelvic girdle pain disorders, Part 2: Illustration of the utility of a classification system via case studies. Man Ther. May 2007;12(2):e1–12.
31. Edwards I, Jones M, Carr J, Braunack-Mayer A, Jensen GM. Clinical reasoning strategies in physical therapy. Phys Ther. Apr 2004;84(4):312–330; discussion 331–315.
32. Groopman J. *How Doctors Think*. Boston: Houghton Mifflin Company; 2007.
33. Patel V, Groen G. Knowledge-based solution strategies in medical reasoning. Cognitive Science. 1986(10):91–116.
34. Schon D. *Educating the Reflective Practitioner*. San Francisco: Jossey-Bass; 1987.
35. Edwards I, Jones M, Hillier S. The interpretation of experience and its relationship to body movement: A clinical reasoning perspective. Man Ther. Feb 2006;11(1):2–10.
36. Jones M, Jensen G, Edwards I. Clinical reasoning in physical therapy. In: Higgs J, Jones M, eds. *Clinical Reasoning in the Health Professions*. Boston: Butterworth-Heinemann; 2000.

chapter 3

Mistakes and Errors: When Clinical Decisions Go Wrong

To make no mistakes is not in the power of man; but from their errors and mistakes the wise and good learn wisdom for the future.

—PLUTARCH

•

✳ Mr. Ketterman's Case

Mr. Ketterman has a fairly unstable cardiac status. If I push him too hard, I could risk a serious cardiac event; if I don't push him hard enough, I will be increasing his morbidity. I don't want to make either mistake. *(See Appendix for Mr. Ketterman's health history)*

INTRODUCTION

We all hope we have chosen health care practitioners who have a good amount of expertise, who can get things right. The issue of a practitioner's clinical expertise has been reinforced as crucial to good decision making by authors throughout the development and implementation of the evidence-based medicine movement. Straus et al[1] define the clinical expertise element of evidence-based medicine as "the ability to use our clinical skills and past experience to rapidly identify each patient's unique health state and diagnosis, their individual risks and benefits of potential interventions, and their personal circumstances and expectations."[1, p1] Similarly, physical therapists must make important choices in practice not only in determining the correct diagnosis and intervention but in performing many hands-on interventions, predicting outcomes of care, setting goals with patients and families, and coordinating resources and personnel to maximize the functional outcomes for the patient. Expertise in all these elements of practice reassures us that our physical therapist will also make good decisions regarding our care and get things right.

However, in clinical practice we all acknowledge that sometimes things don't go right. Sometimes cognitive skills, manual skills, and past experiences are insufficient for the task at hand. In these situations, clinical practice errors of varying magnitudes can occur. Of course, poor outcomes in clinical practice can also occur in a random fashion, as biological events are probabilistic in nature. More often, errors occur when the current level of scientific knowledge used to inform choices is inadequate, or when the clinician lacks knowledge, violates the patient trust in a purposeful manner, or uses faulty logic. Whatever the cause, an examination of clinical practice errors provides a source of knowledge to help us improve our level of practice.

Providing physical therapy care in a manner that reduces errors and increases patient safety should be the goal of every clinician, but it is not an easy goal to attain. Weingart[2] states that the 1999 Institute of Medicine report *To Err is Human*[3] provided evidence that medical errors pose daily risks throughout the health care system in this country but also elucidated the difficulty in estimating the magnitude and attribution of these risks. While injury of various types may occur to patients under our care, determining that these injuries are a result of clinician error is a complicated process. Weingart[2] suggests that harm can result from many complex factors, including: the natural history of the patient's disease, comorbidities, the risks or negative effects of selected interventions, clinical misjudgments, technical performance errors, and bad luck. Given this complexity, it is not surprising that independent reviewers of patient safety events are able to identify when a harmful event has occurred but are not good at analyzing the degree of harm caused in the event nor if the event is a result the presence of a medical error.[4]

In this chapter we will provide an overview of research on errors in medicine, physical therapy, and occupational therapy. An understanding of the type, frequency, causes, and harm associated with errors is a good first step in our attempts to increase patient safety. We will examine errors and the causes of errors, for example, faulty clinical reasoning. In the previous chapter we identified the typical reasoning strategies used by physical therapists in making many types of decisions. Here, we will focus on learning how we might categorize and learn from errors of clinical reasoning. Our increasingly complex health care system can contribute to a clinician's sense of uncertainty when the clinician is making difficult decisions. The ability to recognize those situations in which our uncertainty is heightened should be an important component of reflection in our clinical reasoning process.

DESCRIBING MISSES AND MISTAKES IN HEALTH CARE

Although bad medical outcomes that happen to famous people garner much public attention, researchers find that good epidemiological data on errors is limited. Weingart et al[5] report that the majority of information on medical errors is derived from a few academic medical center studies, and in general the literature suffers from a lack of standardized research methods, definitions, and systems for monitoring and reporting errors. Their review of this literature does reflect increased risk for those patients who are sicker, over 64 years of age, undergo multiple interventions, remain in a hospital longer, and are treated through an emergency department or in an intensive care unit. The estimates of medical errors outside of the hospital setting is low, with prevalence rates for medical errors in physicians' offices found to be 8% to 9% of all errors.

Methods for monitoring and analyzing medical errors in these studies range from medical chart reviews, adverse drug event records, clinician self-reports, and observational studies. Adverse events are defined differently, allowing underestimation of the error rate. For example, when a mistake is made but caught prior to injury to the patient, how should it be labeled? In many settings these events are termed near misses, rather than mistakes or errors, an event that was recognized and recovered in time to prevent an adverse event. Much less is known about near misses than about true adverse events. In 2000, Weingart et al[5] found several additional terms for categorizing medical errors. Some examples are:

- Surgical adverse events versus medication errors
- Preventable versus unpreventable errors
- Diagnostic errors versus therapeutic mishaps
- Fatal versus life-threatening versus serious errors
- Errors of omission or commission

Clearly any efforts to improve the rates of medical errors are dependent upon a common language for describing and reporting them.[4,6]

Creating a Taxonomy

In 2005, researchers with the Joint Commission, previously known as the Joint Commission on Accreditation of Health Organizations (JCAHO), conducted a systematic review of the literature on patient safety terminologies and classifications of errors.[7] Their work resulted in a proposal for a standardized patient safety event taxonomy. The goal was to create a multi-dimensional taxonomy that could be used in various settings and by various practitioners to report incidents of patient safety. The resulting taxonomy includes five primary classification groups, categorizing data that will describe the following aspects of a patient safety event:

- Impact
- Type
- Domain
- Cause
- Prevention and mitigation of the event

Impact

The impact schema describes the degree of harm caused to the patient in medical and non-medical contexts. The levels in this taxonomy, shown in Table 3.1, include psychological and physical medical injury, and progress from no harm, to temporary harm at various levels, to permanent harm, to death or profound psychological harm.

Type

The taxonomy for type of error includes three categories:

1. Communication
2. Patient management
3. Clinical performance

The inclusion of these three categories illustrates the comprehensive nature of the delivery of patient care and the wide scope of activities in which errors can occur. Communication errors could result from inaccurate and incomplete information, questionable advice or interpretation, questionable consent or disclosure processes, or questionable documentation. Patient management errors can be categorized as emanating from questionable delegation, tracking or follow-up, referral or consultation, or use of resources. The clinical performance errors are grouped into three temporal categories, pre-intervention, intervention, and post-intervention (Table 3.2). Table 3.2 also illustrates the various levels of clinical performance errors, including determining incorrect diagnoses and prognoses.

Table 3.1 Standardized Descriptions of Impact of Patient Safety Events[7] Based on the Degree of Resulting Harm

Medical			Nonmedical
Psychological		Physical	Legal/Social/Economic
No Harm and No Undetectable Harm		No Harm and No Undetectable Harm	
No Detectable Harm		No Detectable Harm	
Temporary	*Permanent*	*Temporary*	*Permanent*
Mild	Mild	Mild	Mild
Moderate	Moderate	Moderate	Moderate
Severe	Severe	Severe	Severe
Profound Mental Harm		Death	

Adapted from Chang A, Schyve PM, Croteau RJ, O'Leary DS, Loeb JM. The JCAHO patient safety event taxonomy: A standardized terminology and classification schema for near misses and adverse events. Int J Qual Health Care. Apr 2005;17(2):95–105.

Table 3.2 Standardized Descriptions of Clinical Performance Type of Patient Safety Events

Pre-intervention A mistake that happens during a history interview, or any time prior to intervention with a patient may be in one of these four categories.	Intervention A mistake that happens during a patient intervention may be in one of these seven categories.	Post-intervention A mistake that happens after a patient intervention may be in one of these four categories.
Make a correct diagnosis, but choose a questionable intervention	Correct procedure, with complications	Correct prognosis
Make an inaccurate diagnosis	Correct procedure, incorrectly performed	Inaccurate prognosis
Make an incomplete diagnosis	Correct procedure, but untimely	Incomplete prognosis
Make a questionable diagnosis	Omission of essential procedure	Questionable prognosis
	Procedure contraindicated	
	Procedure not indicated	
	Wrong patient	

Adapted from Chang A, Schyve PM, Croteau RJ, O'Leary DS, Loeb JM. The JCAHO patient safety event taxonomy: A standardized terminology and classification schema for near misses and adverse events. Int J Qual Health Care. Apr 2005;17(2):95–105.

Domain

The domain taxonomy provides a description of the setting of the event, the staff involved, certain patient characteristics, and the targeted type of patient care intervention In this JCAHO taxonomy, descriptions are included that will provide information on patient safety events occurring in several locations in which physical therapists practice, including the rehabilitation component of a hospital, nursing home, rehabilitation facility, and practitioner office. The listing of categories for staff includes physical therapists and occupational therapists. Intervention types include therapeutic, diagnostic, rehabilitation, preventive, or palliative.

Cause

The cause taxonomy has two main categories: systems (organization and technical) and human. *Systems errors* are often not proximate to the patient-clinician relationship but can play a significant role in the context of the safety event. Examples of organizational system causes are the culture—for example, the value for patient safety—or organizational management—for example, the monitoring of unsafe practices. Organizational processes can also affect patient safety, including productivity demands and safety oversight procedures. Technical systems errors typically are found in equipment or materials design, malfunction, or availability. *Human errors* are categorized as those attributable to the patient, the clinician, or to individuals external to the patient-clinician relationship. Patient errors result from behaviors that are not controllable by the clinician. External human failures are behaviors that are beyond the control of the entire organization. Practitioner errors can be skill-based, rule-based, knowledge-based, or unclassifiable. This classification scheme can be used to identify prevention and mitigation actions that can decrease the rate of medical error by selecting from a variety of procedures that will trigger alerts or alarms for practitioners prior to implementation of services. Techniques are suggested, for example, to improve the accuracy of patient identification, reduce acquired infections, and prevent medication errors.

The authors of the JCAHO patient safety event taxonomy recommend its usage in a wide variety of health care systems, including electronic medical records, to enhance the quality of data on medical errors available to researchers on health care quality and to policy makers. However, they recognize the limitations of such a system to fully capture the nuances of accurately describing medical errors in the following statement:

> One source of difficulty we encountered in choosing logical data variables to link disparate terminologies and classifications is that they are all loosely attached in an intricate network of information characterized by events, settings, individuals, and teams of people, protocols, procedures, policies, and communications that function in an uncertain environment.[7, p.101]

Weingart[4] recommends that such a taxonomy will enhance our detection of patterns of medical mistakes; he also acknowledges that "[i]t is not obvious, however, that a classification scheme can reliably capture the 'story' of the event and how it unfolded."[4, p.93]

COGNITIVE ERRORS IN PHYSICIAN DECISION MAKING

Several studies in medicine attempt to focus specifically on the cognitive errors made by physicians as they practice clinical reasoning. Such studies have created categories of cognitive errors by attributing incorrect choices during simulated patient encounters to the patterns of thinking observed in subjects. Young et al[8] studied the cognitive processing abilities of 15 residents as they responded to a recall task and two clinical decision scenarios presented as sample cases by a researcher. A variety of cognitive processing errors could be identified, including:

- Knowledge factors:
  - Inaccurate knowledge or incomplete knowledge about some aspect of a complex system, defined as buggy knowledge
  - Knowledge calibration errors—seen when the residents could not identify gaps in their own knowledge;
- Simplifications—using rules of thumb in complex situations;
- Attentional dynamics such as situational awareness—the inability to track processes and data in time or across more than one topic
- Fixations—inability to reassess a situation in light of new information

Typically, residents with less experience make a greater number of cognitive errors than those with more experience. Studies of cognitive reasoning such as this are often conducted in a laboratory setting, not a clinical setting. (See Chapter 4 for a more detailed discussion of cognitive errors in decision making.)

Studying cognitive processing skills in decision making is one approach to avoiding reasoning errors. Students who struggle with a repeated deficiency in one aspect of knowledge transfer or attentional dynamics may seek help with specifically planned learning experiences to enhance their thinking skills.[9] A student or novice clinician might master these cognitive processes in the classroom but have difficulty demonstrating sufficient performance in a busy clinical environment. The guidance of a more experienced clinician can assist the novice to identify errors such as his or her gap in knowledge or the tendency to ignore new exam findings. However, these analytical experiences are often difficult to incorporate into a busy clinician's schedule.

Kempainen et al[10] suggest that improvements in clinical reasoning will only happen if physicians have knowledge of cognitive processing and use it to internally monitor their thinking. This requires a commitment of time for reflection on the quality of one's thinking in situations where no known errors have been committed as well as when they have. Borrell-Carrio and Epstein[11] have called for physicians to increase self-awareness of their errors in practice through reflection on their abilities to tune or calibrate both their thinking and their emotional responses to the decision confronting them. The habit of self-questioning during clinical work is recommended to increase one's awareness of the personal conditions under which they function during difficult clinical decisions. Mamede et al[12] suggest that reflective physicians are those who can examine a decision from a broader perspective and can tolerate or even enjoy the internal tension created when working with complex cases.[12] Box 3.1 presents some provocative self-reflective questions drawn from the work of these authors.

ERRORS IN PHYSICAL THERAPY AND OCCUPATIONAL THERAPY PRACTICE

The best description of practice errors has been provided by the medicine, nursing, and pharmacy professions, and most of this work describes medication errors.[13] While not as comprehensive, a few authors have reported useful information about the types of errors made by occupational therapists and physical therapists. Scheirton and Mu[14,15] have studied errors in

Box 3.1	**Questions to Enhance Self-awareness of Errors in Clinical Reasoning**

1. How open am I to my patient's view of his/her symptoms?
2. How motivated am I to solve this problem?
3. Do I have sufficient energy or focus at this time to make the best decision?
4. What factors in the patient's response to me are influencing my thinking; for example, is the patient hostile or desperate?
5. Did I close the alternative options for this patient too soon?
6. Is any previous negative outcome with a similar patient affecting my decision making abilities?
7. What am I assuming about this patient that may not be true?
8. Am I being judgmental about this patient in a negative or positive way?
9. What is my frustration level, and how is it influencing my thinking?
10. What surprised me about this patient?

Adapted from Borrell-Carrio F, Epstein RM. Preventing errors in clinical practice: A call for self-awareness. Ann Fam Med. Jul–Aug 2004;2(4):310–316, and Mamede S, Schmidt HG, Rikers R. Diagnostic errors and reflective practice in medicine. J Eval Clin Pract. Feb 2007;13(1):138–145.

occupational therapy practice in physical rehabilitation and geriatric settings, using focus groups and survey research. The majority of practice errors identified by occupational therapists were preventable errors that occurred during patient interventions. Misjudgment and insufficient experience and preparation were identified as potential causes of errors made by the occupational therapists in these studies. These researchers have further investigated the response to errors among these therapists, finding that they reported a significant amount of emotional distress. Coping strategies were used to help the therapist recover from the effects of the error, including: a corrective action plan for the therapist, volunteering to spend extra time with the injured patient, and making constructive practice changes to prevent a similar error in the future. These authors have included physical therapists in some of their focus group research on patient safety and reported an ethical analysis of six cases of error committed by physical and occupational therapists in a recent report.[16] They identified that the cases illustrated what they termed technical and moral errors; analysis of moral errors focused on the ethical responsibilities of the clinicians in each case.

Much less research has been conducted on the types of errors that characterize physical therapist practice. In 1992, Deusinger[17] reported the results of telephone interviews with 119 physical therapists in Missouri who agreed to discuss clinical errors in their practice careers. The author attempted to develop a typology to categorize the reported errors as to:

• Type—defined as an error of omission or commission
• Action—defined as decision making, interpersonal communications, technical or psychomotor skills, or cognitive factors related to knowledge
• Consequences—defined as potential versus actual, and as social or physical

The typology demonstrated reliability only in categorizing the error type and the consequences. Sixty-one different tasks were described by the subjects as associated with errors in practice, 13 of which accounted for 65% of the errors. The majority of errors occurred during intervention tasks (29%) such as gait, modalities, and exercise. Eighteen percent of the errors were attributed to mistakes in planning the patient's program or delegation of care. Only 7% of errors were reported during the action of examination or evaluation, perhaps attributable to the time frame of data collection (1986). Subjects were asked to report the likely cause of the error, and these data appear to reflect findings similar to those in medicine, with the most frequent causes reported including inadequate knowledge or clinical experience and cognitive failures including inaccurate assumptions and failure to consider consequences of the decision. Environmental factors were also identified, including time pressures and inadequate staffing or supervision.

Errors and Error Prevention Across Patient/Client Care Management Model

As seen in the research efforts in medicine, the types of errors and the consequences of these errors should be of specific interest to physical therapists who wish to improve their clinical expertise. One perspective for studying the type of errors physical therapists make is to consider the management model developed by the APTA,[18] discussed in Chapter 1. Using this model to evaluate errors in practice may focus attention on the elements of patient management activities that place patients at the most risk. This perspective may also be helpful for analyzing cognitive errors or problems with thinking, as the patient management model represents actions performed with the patient in a temporal fashion. For example, what are the consequences for clinical decisions about interventions, if diagnosis is incorrect?

Examination

The physical therapist patient management model begins with clinical decisions about how to examine the patient. The therapist must conduct an appropriate history interview, select which systems to screen and examine, and then select the correct tests and measures to perform with the patient. Each test must be performed accurately and interpreted correctly to inform the evaluation of the patient's condition. This is not only the first interaction between patient and therapist but, some would say, the most important element of the model in which to strive for clinical expertise. Groopman[19] suggests many cognitive errors that happen during the medical interview derive from poor physician communication skills. A few of these include failing to actively listen to the patient, ask open-ended questions in a manner that communicates interest in the patient, and follow up on aspects of the patient's story. Roter et al[20,21] found that physician's use of good communication skills can enhance the patient's involvement in problem posing and problem solving collaborations during the interview. In Section Two Coulehan and Block discuss ways to improve the interview process to overcome these types of errors and Gordon, Nixon-Cave, and Johnson all provide information about exploring patients' values as a component of the therapeutic alliance.

Tests and Measures   As clinicians with over 800 physical performance tests and measures at our disposal, physical therapists face a challenge in selecting a test with the best diagnostic properties for each patient problem reported. Evidence regarding the diagnostic accuracy of many of these tests has increased significantly over the past decade.[22-25] Physical therapists who increase their knowledge of these studies, especially for the most frequently used tests in their practice, will enhance their ability to avoid the errors of selecting inappropriate tests, in applying and interpreting the tests, and in over- or underutilization of tests. The consequences of errors in decision making during the examination phase include overtesting that can cause increased pain to the patient, undertesting that can cause the physical therapist to make an incorrect diagnosis, and poor communication that can create an adversarial patient-therapist relationship.

Evaluation

Once the examination data have been collected, the physical therapist evaluates the data to determine the patient's diagnosis. These data will be used in developing a prognosis and a plan of care. Diagnostic errors may result in incorrect or incomplete diagnoses, such as when one aspect of the diagnosis is missed completely. How might these errors occur? Perhaps the physical therapist misinterprets the data from the examination due to not being able to conduct the test accurately; for example, a test appears to produce normal results but the clinician may not have had sufficient strength to administer the test on a particularly large patient. Other sources of cognitive diagnostic errors include incorrectly identifying a pathological structure or movement pattern or miscategorizing the nature of the patient's movement impairments. Diagnostic errors also might be a result of cognitive, communication, or technical errors occurring during the examination phase of patient management. Thus an error occurring earlier in the patient management process will likely influence the next phase of decision making. For novices, diagnostic errors may occur due to the inability to put all the examination data together into a cogent hypothesis that fits.[26]

The ability to see patterns emerging from examination data is developed through reflective practice by expert physical therapists.[27] Experts are skilled evaluators, as they combine their content knowledge, their knowledge of the patient and of self, and their practice knowledge to make diagnostic decisions. The consequences of a misdiagnosis in physical therapy are not precisely known, but may include inappropriate selection of interventions that may cause injury to the patient or extend the time needed to reach a successful conclusion of care, delayed referral of the patient to an appropriate practitioner for further diagnostic evaluation, or labeling and treating patients unnecessarily when misidentifying their movement patterns as abnormal.

Prognosis

Prognostic errors occur in practice when the physical therapist does not accurately predict the natural course or progress of the patient's pathology or impairments, or the recovery of functional performance, or future disability level. Perhaps a client might be advised to return to work or sports activity at too early a point in his or her recovery. Prognostic errors might also result in either over- or underutilization of health care resources of all types, including durable medical equipment or disposition placement for continuing care. Avoiding prognostic errors is difficult for physical therapists because our health care system partitions the continuous care of our patient among more than one physical therapist, passing the patient along to the physical therapist practicing in the acute care setting, the home health setting, or the outpatient setting. These disconnected care patterns make it difficult for the physical therapists to gain information on patient outcomes that can inform their decisions during their interactions with the patient. Physical therapists must work to discover methods to monitor the long-term outcomes of their patients in order to build the experiential knowledge base that will enhance future prognostic decisions.

Intervention

Errors that occur during physical therapist interventions are perhaps the most obvious clinical practice mistakes because they may risk the physical safety of the patient. In addition to the psychomotor skills required of many clinical interventions, the physical therapist must know which intervention to choose, when and where to apply them, and with what force. Any misjudgment of one of these aspects of the intervention can change the right treatment into a dangerous treatment rather quickly. An accessible store of knowledge of past patients' reactions to interventions, coupled with close monitoring of the patient during treatment, may reduce the occurrence of intervention errors in clinical practice.

Outcomes

Errors that may accompany the outcomes of physical therapy care can best be described as a mismatch between the outcome measures selected by the physical therapist and the patient's goals or circumstances. The physical therapist may believe the care delivered was successful based upon an improvement in the patient's pain scores, but the patient may have functional goals that were never identified or addressed. The assumption that a patient's function will automatically return once pain is reduced can represent an error of faulty logic on the therapist's part. If the therapist does not fully consider the patient's circumstances, this may also lead to a mismatch in treatment outcomes. For example, the therapist may underestimate the aerobic or muscular endurance required for mobility by a patient living in a very rural environment.

Implications of Errors in Physical Therapy Practice

We are just beginning to understand the importance of learning about practice errors in the physical therapy profession. It can be a difficult topic to discuss, as physical therapists cannot avoid their natural human tendency to deny fault, blame others including the patient, and refuse to acknowledge that an error has been made, whether or not injury to the patient has occurred. Ethicist Ruth Purtillo[28] reminds us that despite the best training physical therapists are not immune to situations where harm occurs. She then challenges the profession and individual clinicians to confront tendencies to deny the errors we make, to acknowledge them to ourselves and to the affected patient, and further to offer an apology and request forgiveness. Only when these steps in response to an error are taken, suggests Purtilo, can the therapeutic relationship between patient and therapist be restored.

The benefits of studying errors in clinical practice are significant for both clinicians and the profession. Knowing more about the effects of errors or near misses in physical therapy can enhance our understanding of practice in ways we do not often pursue. For example, if a clinician gives a patient a diagnosis of a labral tear at the shoulder, without the assistance of diagnostic imaging, and treats her conservatively for instability, pain, and decreased function, but the patient actually has a bicepital tendonosis, will the error in diagnosis make any difference in the short- and long-term outcomes for this patient? Likely not, as the conservative treatment approach for both of these pathologies is similar. How precise are our diagnostic categories in physical therapy, and how precise do they need to be, given the interventional options? To move our science and practice to a higher level, we can study our diagnostic errors and identify which diagnostic mistakes carry the most risk for our patients. In some diagnostic groups, it is the missed diagnosis that presents the most risk, for example, failing to refer a patient with a suspicious skin lesion for further testing. In some diagnostic groups, it is the misdiagnosis that places the patient at risk, for example, diagnosing an ankle sprain versus a fracture of the talus.

Occasionally a clinician will conclude a course of physical therapy with a patient, fighting a nagging concern that neither the patient's diagnosis nor the intervention was quite right, and that the patient got better anyway. This might be referred to as a good outcome that is robust to both diagnostic and interventional errors. It also might be considered inappropriate treatment of a pathology that has a natural history of improvement without care. Or the good outcome might be the result of the placebo effect that results from the attention and care of the physical therapist and has little to do with the direct effects of the interventions chosen. Our practice would be enhanced if we knew which of the explanations was accurate.

Placebo: really there or just imagination? The term *placebo* often causes much confusion. We often first think of "placebo" as the label used to describe a sham treatment in an experiment that studies the efficacy of an intervention. In this context it often connotes "nothing," as in one group receiving ultrasound and exercise and the other group receiving a "placebo." But the placebo effect is quite different. It has been described as the measurable positive response to an inert intervention; therefore the responses are thought to be due to factors related to the patient's belief in the positive outcomes of the intervention. In contrast, the nocebo effect is described as the measurable negative response to inert interventions that patients believe will have negative effects. More recently, authors of a systematic review of over 200 articles on the placebo effect concluded that there is little evidence of a true placebo effect in observer-reported outcomes but that there may be in patient-reported outcomes, particularly pain.[29] The concept of the placebo effect remains a matter of some interest in physical therapy, since so much of our care is directed toward improving patient-reported outcomes.

DECISION MAKING UNDER UNCERTAINTY

Many of the errors that we have discussed can find their basis in the uncertainty that surrounds the data we use to make decisions. Those who write about decision making under uncertainty advocate improving our knowledge by learning more about a few key variables.

Expected Value of Alternatives

One variable is the expected value of alternatives. For example, knowing whether a patient prefers more normality by learning ambulation after a serious stroke or faster functionality by using an electric wheelchair can help us decide more accurately what our course of intervention should be. Also, knowing the level of risk aversion or risk seeking our patients and we are comfortable with can also reduce errors. It is especially important to know if there is a disparity between our patient's preferences and our own.[30] As stated by an expert pediatric physical therapist, "I think one of the things I have learned over the past couple of years ... is that the parents' goals are *the* goals, and the child's goals are *the* goals. It's not that the therapist's goals are *the* goals."[27]

Concept of Probability

But perhaps the most important variable we must understand to reduce error is the concept of probability, along with the actual probabilities associated with the options in each clinical decision. The concept of probability helps us recognize that our decisions are not based on certainty. This by itself improves decision making. And identifying specific probabilities improves it even more.

Base Rate

There are a few pieces of data that help us understand probability. For example, we first need to know the base rate of the event with which we are concerned: just how many people have this problem? Base rate is measured by both the prevalence (how many people have this problem now) and incidence of the problem (how many people get this problem in any given time period).

> Without knowing the base rate, a comment such as "people in a particular group who received a particular drug are twice as likely (100% increase) to commit suicide" means almost nothing. We need to know just how many people in the group commit suicide without the drug. If the suicide rate is 10,000 per 1,000,000 (1%), then a 100% increase means 20,000 per 1,000,000. This might be a very acceptable increase if the drug provides relief from serious symptoms in the remaining 980,000 people. But if the suicide rate is 250,000 per 1,000,000 (25%), then a 100% increase means 500,000 per 1,000,000. That much mortality may be unacceptable!

In addition to base rate, we also need to know the likelihood that an intervention will lead to either an improvement or decrement in the patient's status. These measures include things such as absolute and relative risk. These types of data and the statistics that analyze them are discussed in the epidemiology literature.[31,32] We discuss more detailed ways to understand the research on specific probabilities in Chapter 12. Chapter 4 contains many examples of the faults in decision making that we can all experience. Understanding the concept of probability and knowing actual probabilities can assist us in avoiding these faults.

CONCLUSION

We all make mistakes! As we have discussed in this chapter, there are many sources for the mistakes that we make.

- First, we know that biologically based events are inherently probabilistic; almost nothing about illness and disease can be known with absolute certainty. The best way to deal with this source of error is to understand what is known about probabilities and take that into account in decision making.
- Second, the level of knowledge about the topic may not be currently sufficient; science may not yet have discovered the information necessary to understand what is happening. The only way to deal with this source of error is to remain vigilant about new knowledge as it appears.
- Third, knowledge might exist about the topic but we, personally, have not yet learned it. Again, vigilance about identifying knowledge new to us is essential.
- Fourth, we know what the best option for the patient's problem is but choose not to take that option because it is not in our best interest; we violate the patient's trust in us. The remedy for this source of error is to always make the ethical choice.
- Fifth, we do not think in a logical way about the information we have available to us. A remedy for this is to understand the errors we humans typically make in our logic.

The first two causes are beyond our control, as we cannot change the nature of biological events, nor can we know something not yet known. But we can work to reduce the impact of the latter three causes of errors. Section Three of this book provides many tools to overcome deficiencies in our own knowledge. Section Two provides ways to reflect on actions to overcome the temptation to violate the patient's trust. The remaining chapters in Section I identify ways to improve our logic in our patient care–related decision making.

SELF-ASSESSMENT

1. Think about a mistake that you have made in patient care. Apply the categories from the JCAHO taxonomy and then determine if this can lead you to identify ways to prevent similar mistakes in the future.
2. Use the questions listed in Box 3.1 to reflect on the characteristics of your own thought processes as you approach patient care.
3. Identify a specific patient whom you have treated lately and follow the patient across the patient/client management model. At each phase identify a potential error and then determine what the results of that error would have been.

CONTINUED LEARNING

Choose one of the many nonfiction books written about medical errors. After reading it, and after reading this section of the book, reflect on what can reasonably be learned from these books. Do they simply tell scary or interesting stories, or do they teach lessons that can be applied to your patients? The list below is just a small sample of these books.

- Banja J, *Medical Errors and Medical Narcissism*
- Geller ES, Johnson D, *The Anatomy of Medical Error: Preventing Harm with People-Based Patient Safety*
- Groopman J, *How Doctors Think*
- Nuland S, *The Soul of Medicine*

REFERENCES

1. Straus S, Richardson W, Glasziou P, Haynes R. *Evidence-based Medicine: How to Practice It and Teach It*, 4th ed. Edinburgh: Churchill Livingstone; 2011.
2. Weingart SN, Iezzoni LI. Looking for medical injuries where the light is bright. JAMA. Oct 8 2003;290(14):1917–1919.
3. Kohn L, Corrigan J, Donaldson M, eds. *To Err is Human: Building a Safer Health System*. Washington, DC: National Academy Press; 1999.
4. Weingart SN. Beyond Babel: prospects for a universal patient safety taxonomy. Int J Qual Health Care. Apr 2005;17(2):93–94.
5. Weingart SN, Wilson RM, Gibberd RW, Harrison B. Epidemiology of medical error. BMJ. Mar 18 2000;320(7237):774–777.
6. Leape LL, Berwick DM. Five years after *To Err Is Human*: What have we learned? JAMA. May 18 2005;293(19):2384–2390.
7. Chang A, Schyve PM, Croteau RJ, O'Leary DS, Loeb JM. The JCAHO patient safety event taxonomy: A standardized terminology and classification schema for near misses and adverse events. Int J Qual Health Care. Apr 2005;17(2):95–105.
8. Young JS, Smith RL, Guerlain S, Nolley B. How residents think and make medical decisions: Implications for education and patient safety. Am Surg. Jun 2007;73(6):548–553; discussion 553–544.
9. Elstein AS, Schwartz A. Clinical problem solving and diagnostic decision making: Selective review of the cognitive literature. BMJ. Mar 23 2002;324(7339):729–732.
10. Kempainen RR, Migeon MB, Wolf FM. Understanding our mistakes: A primer on errors in clinical reasoning. Med Teach. Mar 2003;25(2):177–181.

11. Borrell-Carrio F, Epstein RM. Preventing errors in clinical practice: A call for self-awareness. Ann Fam Med. Jul–Aug 2004;2(4):310–316.
12. Mamede S, Schmidt HG, Rikers R. Diagnostic errors and reflective practice in medicine. J Eval Clin Pract. Feb 2007;13(1):138–145.
13. Nicholson D, Hersh W, Gandhi TK, Weingart SN, Bates DW. Medication errors: Not just a few "bad apples". J Clin Outcomes Manag. Feb 2006;13(2):114–115.
14. Mu K, Lohman H, Scheirton L. Occupational therapy practice errors in physical rehabilitation and geriatrics settings: A national survey study. Am J Occup Ther. May–Jun 2006;60(3):288–297.
15. Scheirton L, Mu K, Lohman H. Occupational therapists' responses to practice errors in physical rehabilitation settings. Am J Occup Ther. May–Jun 2003;57(3):307–314.
16. Scheirton LS, Mu K, Lohman H, Cochran TM. Error and patient safety: Ethical analysis of cases in occupational and physical therapy practice. Med Health Care Philos. Sep 2007;10(3):301–311.
17. Deusinger S. Analyzing errors in practice: A vehicle for assessing and enhancing the quality of care. Int J Technol Assess Health Care. 1992;8(1):65–78.
18. American Physical Therapy Association. *Guide to Physical Therapist Practice*, 2nd ed. Alexandria, VA: APTA; 2002.
19. Groopman J. *How Doctors Think*. Boston: Houghton Mifflin Company; 2007.
20. Roter D. The medical visit context of treatment decision-making and the therapeutic relationship. Health Expect. Mar 2000;3(1):17–25.
21. Roter DL, Hall JA. Physician gender and patient-centered communication: A critical review of empirical research. Annu Rev Public Health. 2004;25:497–519.
22. Arab AM, Salavati M, Ebrahimi I, Ebrahim Mousavi M. Sensitivity, specificity and predictive value of the clinical trunk muscle endurance tests in low back pain. Clin Rehabil. Jul 2007;21(7):640–647.
23. Cook C, Hegedus E. *Orthopedic Physical Examination Tests: An Evidence Based Approach*. Upper Saddle River, NJ: Prentice Hall; 2007.
24. Cook C, Massa L, Harm-Ernandes I, et al. Interrater reliability and diagnostic accuracy of pelvic girdle pain classification. J Manipulative Physiol Ther. May 2007;30(4):252–258.
25. Walsworth MK, Doukas WC, Murphy KP, Mielcarek BJ, Michener LA. Reliability and diagnostic accuracy of history and physical examination for diagnosing glenoid labral tears. Am J Sports Med. Jan 2008;36(1):162–168.
26. Jensen G, Shepard KF, Hack L. The novice versus the experienced clinician: Insights into the work of the physical therapist. Phys Ther. 1990;70:314–323.
27. Jensen G, Gwyer J, Hack L, Shepard KF. *Expertise in Physical Therapy Practice*, 2nd ed. St. Louis, MO: Elsevier; 2007.
28. Purtilo RB. Beyond disclosure: Seeking forgiveness. Phys Ther. Nov 2005;85(11):1124–1126.
29. Hróbjartsson A, Gøtzsche PC (20 January 2010). Placebo interventions for all clinical conditions. *Cochrane Database Syst Rev*106 (1): CD003974.
30. Bazerman MH. *Judgment in Managerial Decision Making*, 5th ed. John Wiley &Sons; 2002.
31. Norman GR, Striener DL. *Biostatistics: The Bare Essentials*, 3rd ed. Shelton, CT: People's Medical Publishing House; 2008.
32. Haynes RB, Sackett DL, Guyatt G, Tugwell P. *Clinical Epidemiology: How to Do Clinical Practice Research*, 3rd ed. Philadelphia: Lippincott Williams and Wilkins; 2005.

Biases in Clinical Reasoning: "Most of My Patients Are Helped by This Treatment."

John C. Hershey, PhD

*It has been said that man is a rational animal.
All my life I have been searching for evidence which could
support this.*

—BERTRAND RUSSELL

•

✳ Mr. Ketterman's Care

Mrs. Ketterman wants to know what I think of the recommendation from Mr. Ketterman's physician to initiate a glutamate pathway modifier as a treatment for his Alzheimer's disease. She knows that I see many patients with Alzheimer's disease in my practice. *(See Appendix for Mr. Ketterman's health history.)*

INTRODUCTION

In this chapter, we will examine some important questions that health care practitioners should consider before stating a diagnosis or prognosis. Embedded in each diagnosis or prognosis are a number of assumptions, possibly shared, between the clinician and patient. In addition, there may well be biases that serve to undermine the accuracy of the prognosis, biases that may work entirely subconsciously on the clinician. In Chapter 2 we described two ways in which clinicians typically make decisions:

- the classic differential diagnosis known as hypothetico-deductive reasoning, or
- the expert's ability to use pattern recognition as a shortcut to a diagnostic or intervention decision.

Neither one of these decision making styles or other types of clinical reasoning is wrong in and of themselves, but each can lead to faulty reasoning and errors in judgment. Biases, defined as inaccurate beliefs that affect decision making,[1] coupled with any clinical reasoning strategy can result in errors. Can we ever free our clinical reasoning of biases? While the answer to that question is unavailable, we do know that if we do not recognize our biases, we cannot work to avoid their negative impact on our decision making. Let's examine the case example of Jack Watson.

✳ **Case Example**—Jack Watson

Jack Watson, a 64-year-old patient with a history of left knee pain, has returned to his orthopedic surgeon in December for the fourth time in 6 months. His pain had appeared without warning the previous March, following a day when he put much greater strain on his knee than usual. A long-time weekend warrior, Jack played his usual strenuous Saturday morning game of tennis, proceeded to spend 3 hours weeding in his garden that afternoon, and then decided to try out some new hamstring-stretching exercises he had heard about from his tennis partner. With his first step the following morning, he had acute left knee pain, and it has continued to a greater or lesser degree ever since.

Jack had a mild case of polio at the age of 9, with modest muscle loss in his back and legs. While his musculoskeletal system no doubt compensated for this muscle loss in a variety of ways throughout his life, Jack nevertheless has been able to remain quite active physically. He played varsity tennis in college, continued to play tennis throughout his adult life, jogged regularly starting at the age of 48, and has led a generally active life for someone with a middle-management job in a Fortune 500 company. Aside from his musculoskeletal problems, his health is excellent.

Jack waited 3 months before finally seeing an orthopedic surgeon in June. The surgeon ordered an MRI, which showed a chronic torn meniscus and Grade 4 chondramalacia in Jack's left knee. As the first line of attack, the physician recommended physical therapy, NSAIDs, and acetaminophen, with instructions to return in 6 weeks. After some improvement, physical therapy was continued for another 6 weeks, but with little further improvement.

In December, following several intervening visits, the physician suggested that it might be time for arthroscopic surgery, although there was not much hope given the problem. It would be mostly for diagnostic purposes. A second possibility was to try injections of sodium hyaluronate (Hyalgan). The physician leaned toward trying the injections and said, if they failed, Jack could decide later whether or not to have the surgery.

Hyalgan is a sterile mixture that is made up mostly of a natural, highly purified sodium hyaluronate that comes from rooster combs. The body's own hyaluronate acts like a lubricant and a shock absorber in the joint, and it is needed for the joint to work properly. In osteoarthritis, there may not be enough hyaluronate, and there may be a change in the quality of the hyaluronate in joint fluid and tissues. Hyalgan is given as a shot directly into the knee.

The most common side effects of Hyalgan therapy are injection-site pain, swelling, heat and/or redness, rash, itching, or bruising around the joint. Any such effects are generally mild and usually do not last long. Patients are advised to consult their physician if they are allergic to products from birds such as feathers, eggs, and poultry.[2] Jack has no such allergy, and the physician thought that a series of five injections, spaced one week apart, would be the logical next step in Jack's care. The out-of-pocket cost for Jack would be $400.

Before making his decision, Jack asked his physical therapist for his prognosis. "Do you think these injections will decrease my pain?" The physical therapist quickly responded, "This treatment seems to help many of my patients." When pressed, he estimated that, in his experience, maybe 60% to 70% got better. This encouraged Jack, since he also knew that the physician had said her experience was that 75% show at least some improvement.

In essence, each of Jack Watson's health care practitioners is saying, *"Most of my patients are helped by this treatment."* This is surely offered as an honest assessment of treatment efficacy, based on the practitioners' recall of personal experience. In turn, patients are no doubt encouraged by such a positive endorsement. They will have every reason to think that they are more likely than not to benefit from the treatment.

BIASES IN DECISION MAKING

In this chapter, we will discuss five types of biases. Any one of these biases can influence the clinician's assessment of the efficacy of treatment. In each case, we start by showing how it applies to the Hyalgan therapy decision. We will also cite other specific clinical examples, mostly from the practice of physical therapy.

Confirmation Bias

"It is the peculiar and perpetual error of the human understanding to be more moved and excited by affirmatives than by negatives." —Francis Bacon

Suppose you believe Hyalgan works really well, and you want to learn more about your beliefs by talking to patients and former patients with joint problems. If some of these patients are doing better, you may be inclined to ask them if they took Hyalgan (since it fits with your model of what works). This is confirmation-seeking behavior, and we are all naturally inclined to engage in it. If, on the other hand, other patients are not doing better, you may not be so inclined, again because it doesn't fit with your model. You therefore assume they didn't try Hyalgan, and therefore never ask if they did. If you did ask, it would be an example of disconfirmation seeking. Disconfirmation seeking is not as natural as confirmation seeking.[3–6]

But notice that you can learn just as much about the effectiveness of Hyalgan by asking for disconfirmation as by asking for confirmation. Suppose those with injections and those without had the same high success rate? If you only seek to confirm, you will conclude that Hyalgan was the cause. Table 4.1 summarizes this tendency. Patients in the first row, who are feeling better, are more likely to be asked if they have tried injections than are patients in the second row. The selective questioning serves to undermine the possibility for true learning, because the results from patients who are not doing better, or are doing even worse, are not taken into account. But if you seek to disconfirm as well, you might soon discover that there

❋ Table 4.1	**How Confirmation Bias Occurs**	
	Patient Has Injection	**Patient Does Not Have Injection**
Patient Is Feeling Better	"Did you try injections?"	"Did you try injections?"
Patient Is Not Feeling Better	Patient is not asked about injections	Patient is not asked about injections

is no *relative* contribution being made to patients' well-being from the treatment you so earnestly believe in.

Consider again the statement, "Most of my patients are helped by this treatment." The next time you find yourself about to say this, ask how much you really know about patient outcomes when the treatment is not given. Is it possible that you are attributing to the treatment something that can just as easily be attributed to something else, such as nature's natural healing process?

Confirmation Bias in the Selection of Interventions

Confirmation bias can also affect a physical therapist's selection of interventions. Physical therapists who are strong proponents of a certain type of physical therapist intervention, for example, joint mobilization for musculoskeletal pain relief, may be susceptible to taking note of the times this treatment decreases a patient's pain, while paying less attention to the frequency with which pain is reduced when another treatment is used. When we have invested our time and resources in developing certain aspects of our practice, we are less likely to ask ourselves, "Should I take another approach to the care of this type of patient?" Perhaps our most difficult problem with confirmation bias is our belief that doing something is better than doing nothing. After all, our patient has often come to us because doing nothing has not worked. We are well advised to be aware of our own decisions that are most vulnerable to our avoidance of disconfirming evidence.

Follow-up Bias for Patients You Treat

There is usually incomplete information from patients who received our treatment. As a clinician, you should ask if you observe all the outcomes from all your patients and, if not, from whom you are more likely to learn the outcome. Consider for now just those patients who get the intervention. If you had a chance to learn the impressions of all of these patients, you would have an unbiased sample, but you may not hear from many of your patients. This lack of complete information could work either way. In saying "Most of my patients are helped by this treatment," you must consider the patients who have been treated who don't return for further evaluation or therapy. If you assume that all of these patients have not returned because they were helped by the Hyalgan and are now with reduced pain, then this will lead you to think the intervention is more beneficial than it really is. If, on the other hand, the patients who are not helped by the intervention are more likely to return, your impressions of the intervention could be the opposite.

Consider Table 4.2. This table classifies the n patients for whom the Hyalgan injections have been given. Your estimate of effectiveness may well be based on the ratio of (a/n_{learn}), which is the percentage of all patients from whom you have feedback, who have improved. The problem is that patients you have observed may have very different results, on average,

Table 4.2 | **Learning and Not Learning the Success Rate of Injections**

	You Learn the Outcome	You Do Not Learn the Outcome	
Patient Improves	a	c?	$n_{improve}$
Patient Does Not Improve	b	d?	$n_{not\ improve}$
	n_{learn}	$n_{not\ learn}$	n

Table 4.3a | **Hypothetical Practice 1: Low Learning, Low Improvement for Patients Absent Feedback**

	You Learn the Outcome	You Do Not Learn the Outcome	
Patient Improves	65	60	**125**
Patient Does Not Improve	35	140	175
	100	200	300

Note the overall improvement rate is 125/300 = 42%.

Table 4.3b | **Hypothetical Practice 2: Low Learning, High Improvement for Patients Absent Feedback**

	You Learn the Outcome	You Do Not Learn the Outcome	
Patient Improves	65	160	**225**
Patient Does Not Improve	35	40	75
	100	200	300

Note that the overall improvement rate is 225/300 = 75%.

from the patients you don't observe. You are estimating the ratio ($n_{improve}/n$), the overall improvement rate, with a biased sample of patients you have learned about, n_{learn}. In giving advice to a new patient, you must recognize this follow-up bias that derives from your own experience.[8]

In Table 4.3, we show how this might work out for four hypothetical physical therapists. Each one has seen 300 patients over the past 3 years who have had injections. Each one has also learned that 65% of those patients from whom they have learned the outcome report improvement.

The first two hypothetical practices shown in Tables 4.3a and 4.3b, have low learning (100 patients out of 300), while the second two hypothetical practices shown in Tables 4.3c and 4.3d, have high learning (200 patients out of 300). Furthermore, the improvement rate for those patients not seen varies across these four hypothetical practices. It is low in the first and third practice (30%), and high in the second and fourth (80%). Note that these variations lead to wide variations in the true overall improvement rate. The lowest overall improvement

Table 4.3c	Hypothetical Practice 3: High Learning, Low Improvement for Patients Absent Feedback		
	You Learn the Outcome	You Do Not Learn the Outcome	
Patient Improves	130	30	**160**
Patient Does Not Improve	70	70	140
	200	100	300

Note that the overall improvement rate is 160/300 = 53%.

Table 4.3d	Hypothetical Practice 4: High Learning, High Improvement for Patients Absent Feedback		
	You Learn the Outcome	You Do Not Learn the Outcome	
Patient Improves	130	80	**210**
Patient Does Not Improve	70	20	90
	200	100	300

Note that the overall improvement rate is 210/300 = 70%.

rate is 42%, in Table 4.3a, while the highest is 75%, in Table 4.3b. The point is that distortions in estimates of success rate can come from both incomplete samples and differences in improvement between those patients who give feedback and those who do not.

Finally, recall the physician who told Jack Watson that 75% of the patients improved with injections. The physician could be more susceptible to a bias caused by incomplete information than is the physical therapist. The physical therapist will typically have more ongoing contact with the patient and can learn over time whether an intervention seems to be helping. However, the physician's plan is to reconsider arthroscopic surgery in the event of treatment failure and no surgery if the treatment succeeds. If a patient does not return, the physician (possibly unconsciously) may count this treatment as a success. Yet many factors besides treatment success could lead patients not to return. Patients might reconsider the idea of having surgery and simply live with the pain. They might be upset that the physician recommended this treatment and go elsewhere for follow-up. They might move. The point is to think about follow-up bias whenever relying on your own experiences with patients. Those whose outcomes you don't actually learn about could have either better or worse outcomes than do those you do learn about. Multiyear clinical studies are often confronted with follow-up bias. One can imagine a successful intervention for which the patients in the control group, seeing no improvement, are less motivated to continue in the study.

Because physical therapy care is segmented in our health care system, patients are often passed from an inpatient physical therapist to an outpatient or home health physical therapist as the course of their injury or illness progresses. All physical therapists that transfer care of their patients to another practitioner are likely to be exposed to follow-up bias for many of the decisions they make for their patients. Imagine a physical therapist practicing in a hospital that makes an error in predicting a safe discharge location for a patient. Unless the patient is readmitted to the same hospital and the care system allows the PT to learn of this, the therapist has no ability to learn how to avoid that error of judgment in the future. In outpatient physical therapy care, we could benefit from structured follow-up of patients who cancel appointments and all patients who conclude a course of treatment so that we may learn the long-term outcomes of our care decisions. In the absence of real outcome information, our natural tendencies to fill the void, combined with our tendencies toward optimism or pessimism, may take over. At the least, we should be honest with ourselves and our patients in recalling what we know and what remains unknown about a specific clinical decision.

Spectrum Bias

Is this patient typical of previous patients who have tried the treatment? Are they more or less likely to be helped? If they are different in any important way, this is known as "spectrum bias," because it refers to how a given patient presents relative to the entire spectrum of patients who have tried the treatment.[9,10]

Again consider the statement, "Most of my patients are helped by this treatment." Think about all the patients who have received the treatment. How does your patient compare with this entire spectrum? If some kinds of conditions, or clinical presentations, are more amenable to treatment success than others, where does your patient fit in? There may be good reason to think the response of your patient is unlike the response of the average patient. For example:

- You may think your patient is more or less likely to be compliant with all the other parts of the treatment plan.
- You may think your patient's condition is more or less likely to be helped. After all, Jack has both a chronically deficient meniscus and severe chondromalacia, and the injections may work best for those with only chondromalacia.
- You may even be less sure of the underlying problem for your patient than for the average patient who receives the treatment.
- You might have a practice that sees lots of difficult cases, so difficult cases are more likely to be referred to you.

Perhaps you are fortunate enough to have good evidence from a controlled clinical trial. Even here, you must be careful to see how your patient compares with those in the trial. Consider the evidence from an investigation of Hyalgan described in the Hyalgan labeling.[2] This study was a double-masked, placebo- and naproxen-controlled, multicenter prospective clinical trial of Hyalgan as a treatment for pain in osteoarthritis of the knee. One issue is whether your patient would meet the entry requirements. But another is where your patient fits into the baseline level of pain spectrum. Hyalgan showed some improvement relative to the controls, but the relative improvement might have been greater for some baseline pain levels than for others. The published results of the study make it impossible to see where these relative differences are, so, as a clinician, you are left only with a sense of caution about how your patient will fare.

Trying to avoid spectrum bias can paralyze a clinician's thinking. While each patient is unique, we are serving that individual patient well when we consider how similar her or his case is to the evidence available to us for our choices. If we limit ourselves to consider the *most likely* predictive factors that recommend one treatment over another for a group of patients similar to the patient we are currently treating, we will avoid the errors that accompany spectrum bias.

Spectrum bias should also be considered as we sort among the various diagnostic tests available to us. The dichotomization of outcomes and groups that is typically used in sensitivity and specificity analysis for diagnostic test accuracy promotes a problem of spectrum bias in that the intermediate-range subjects are often not included in the analysis. Section Three provides more information about many of these issues.

Wishful Thinking or Value-induced Bias

"People say they love truth, but in reality they want to believe that which they love is true." —Robert Ringer

We all, at one time or another, engage in wishful thinking. And our hopes can sometimes influence our beliefs. We want to believe that our diagnoses are accurate and that our treatment recommendations will work, and this may color our interpretation of what we see and what our patients tell us.

It is useful to distinguish between two kinds of wishful thinking: self-centered events and events in which the world at large is seen optimistically.[11] In the former case, one may think, "If I try this intervention, it will work well, even though the evidence shows it doesn't work so well when others try it." There is an illusion of control, not unlike the lottery ticket owners who place higher value on tickets they have personally selected than on tickets they have not selected. In the latter case, many people are simply too inclined to be optimistic generally, rather like Dr. Pangloss, the self-proclaimed optimist in *Candide*.

In applying the idea of wishful thinking to medical decision making, some researchers have labeled this phenomenon as "value-induced bias."[12–15] With value-induced bias, the value or importance of a medical outcome can influence judgments of its likelihood of occurring. For example, smokers may convince themselves they are especially immune to the harmful effects of smoking (self-centered wishful thinking) or that the overall data on smoking is inconclusive (general optimism).

This can apply to our patient contemplating taking Hyalgan. Because we want it to work, we may unconsciously exaggerate our view of its success rate in the overall population (general optimism). Alternatively, we may unconsciously feel that we somehow have a better success rate when we support it than when it is recommended by others (self-centered wishful thinking). Value-induced bias could even lead us to overestimate the likelihood of success for treatments with high transaction costs. For example, a treatment that is expensive, and has significant side effects, or that involves a cross-country trip, might be judged to have a higher probability of success. In the present case, if you know you have a patient for whom the $400 monetary cost plus the time taken from work to get the treatment represents a high burden, you might place greater faith in the treatment than you would for a patient for whom this is not a heavy burden.[14,15]

The next time you think, "Most of my patients are helped by this treatment," ask yourself if you might be influenced, at least in part, by wishful thinking. Yes, we really want our patients to be helped by the intervention. Yes, we don't want patients to pay for unnecessary treatment. But we should not let overall optimism or self-centered wishful thinking color our beliefs. Expert clinicians know that the value or importance of finding the right intervention for a given patient cannot, by itself, influence its likelihood of success.

Physical therapists may find themselves vulnerable to this bias when successive treatment attempts have consistently failed. Each subsequent treatment decision, prefaced by "let's try this," carries an increased hope for a successful outcome. Value-induced bias may be introduced in the clinical decision process when someone other than the PT or the patient recommends the course of action. If you find yourself thinking, "I'm doing this against my better judgment," ask yourself whose judgment has influenced your decision and what real evidence is being presented to support the decision.

Ease of Recall

Our estimates of the likelihood of a given event are often based, at least in part, on how easily we can recall instances of that event or similar events. Events that are easy to recall are judged to be more common than those that are hard to recall. Often, this is not a bad rule of thumb. After all, commonly occurring events are the ones that are more likely to be recalled and hence more likely to be judged common.

The problem occurs when ease of recall doesn't line up with how common the event is. Some highly unusual events might get undue media coverage, leading one to believe they are more common than they are. A recent experience may be more likely to be remembered and thus weighed more heavily. Vivid, or highly salient, events are harder to forget. The availability bias[16-18] is the human tendency to overestimate probabilities of events associated with these overexposed, recent, vivid, or salient events. Perhaps the most famous example is mortality from shark attacks. The United States averages only about one such death per year,[19] yet many of us might guess a much larger number based on coverage in the media and the image presented by a shark attack.

The same goes for cause-and-effect relationships. For example, our recommendation about Hyalgan to a patient might be unduly influenced by a particularly dramatic or recent success (or failure) that actually represents a low-probability association. If our 400-pound patient with 20 years of osteoarthritis of the knees found complete pain relief after these injections, this unlikely outcome could make an impression on us. Because it is at the forefront of our memory, we place undue weight on it in estimating treatment success for our next patient.

Ease of recall does not necessarily mean that a probability estimate is biased. In many cases, common events *are* experienced more frequently and make a greater impression, and this can be helpful in judging the likelihood of future such events. But it is when the availability of information is *not* related to actual frequency that we must be most cautious. Detmer et al[20] asked surgeons to estimate the in-hospital mortality rate for their entire service. Surgeons from high-mortality specialties gave estimates that were more than double those given by low-mortality specialties. The point is that we must be careful not to rely on our own memory or experiences in making judgments about treatment efficacy, side effects, or risks.

CONCLUSION

The five biases described in this chapter are summarized in Table 4.4. In any given clinical situation, we might see more than one of these operating. In fact, in our clinical example in which the patient and his health care providers are trying to decide whether to try Hyalgan for an arthritic knee, all five could potentially be at work. As a result, it is virtually impossible to make definitive statements about the exact probability of success of this intervention.

The important point is to recognize that at least one of these biases can be at work in every clinical diagnosis or treatment decision and to be wary of their perverse effect on judgment and decision making. Simply knowing these biases, thinking of how they can influence your thinking whenever there is uncertainty, considering their implications at least qualitatively, and sharing their consequences with your patients can go a long way to improving your practice of physical therapy.

Table 4.4 Summary of Five Biases Presented in Chapter 4

Bias	Description	Physical Therapy Example
1. Confirmation bias	A tendency to search for or interpret new information in a way that confirms one's prior beliefs and to avoid or discount information that contradicts one's preconceptions	When we personally prefer a controversial treatment, we may take greater note of times when the treatment was successful than when it was not
2. Follow-up bias for patients you treat	A tendency to assume that people who do not return for follow-up have the same distribution of outcomes as those who do return	In the absence of real outcome measures for all patients, we may believe that those patients we follow over time have success rates similar to those we do not follow
3. Spectrum bias	A tendency to forget that a given patient may not be representative of the entire spectrum of patients who present for diagnosis or treatment	When we know the sensitivity and specificity of a given diagnostic test, we must remember that these values typically come from biased groups of patients; intermediate-range groups are often not used in calculating these test characteristics
4. Wishful thinking/ Value-induced bias	A tendency to form beliefs or make decisions based on what is most desired instead of by appealing to the best evidence	We should not let what we want most for our patients color our objective evaluation of the pros and cons of various interventions
5. Ease of recall	A tendency for the ease of recalling similar instances of an event to unduly influence our estimate of its likelihood	We should not place unjustified confidence in a particularly dramatic or recent success (or failure) when designing a treatment plan for our patient

SELF-ASSESSMENT

1. Consider some advice you have given or seen given to patients over the past few weeks. Can you identify any examples of these biases in your decisions about the advice? If you have not recently been involved in patient care, reflect instead on advice you or a family member may have received from a health care practitioner.
2. Identify three changes you might recommend in a physical therapist's practice to help you and your colleagues reduce the likelihood of these biases.

CONTINUED LEARNING

Select and read one of the books described below. These texts also describe other biases at work in human decision making. Using this information, continue the process of assessing your practice to see how you can change it to reduce the likelihood of allowing these biases to negatively influence your decision making.

- Baron, J. *Thinking and Deciding*, 4th ed. Cambridge, UK: Cambridge University Press; 2007.

This is a very impressive textbook covering the full range of psychological research into the nature of thinking and decision making. The presentation is remarkably thorough and clear.

- Hoch, SJ, Kunreuther, HK. *Wharton on Making Decisions*. Hoboken, NJ: John Wiley & Sons; 2004.

This collection of articles written by professors at The University of Pennsylvania's Wharton School addresses both intuitive and analytical approaches to decision making. The major topic headings are Personal Decision Making (Chapters 2–4), Managerial Decision Making (Chapters 5–8), Multiparty Decision Making (Chapters 9–12), and Impact of Decision Making on Society (Chapters 13–17).

- Kahneman, D, Tversky, A. *Choices, Values, and Frames*. Cambridge, UK: Cambridge University Press; 2000.

This is another collection of readings, representing both experimental and empirical studies of human judgment and choice. Many of these readings have become classics.

REFERENCES

1. Elstein AS, Shulman LS, Sprafka SA. *Medical Problem Solving: An Analysis of Clinical Reasoning*. Cambridge, MA: Harvard University Press; 1978.
2. Hyalgan Prescribing Information. products.sanofi-aventis.us/hyalgan/hyalgan.html. Accessed March 27, 2011.
3. Einhorn HJ, Hogarth RM. Confidence in judgment: Persistence in the illusion of validity. Psych Rev. 1978;85:395–416.
4. Wason PC. On the failure to eliminate hypotheses in a conceptual task. Quar J Exper Psych. 1960;12:129–140.
5. Wason PC. Reason about a rule. Quar J Exper Psych. 1968a;20:273–283.
6. Wason PC. On the failure to eliminate hypotheses … a second look. In: Wason PC, Johnson-Laird PN, eds. *Thinking and Reasoning*. Harmondsworth: Penguin; 1968b.
7. Frost R. The road not taken. In: Untermeyer L, ed. *Modern American Poetry, An Introduction*. New York: Harcourt, Brace and Howe; 1919.
8. Brookmeyer R. Accounting for follow-up bias in estimation of HIV incidence rates. J Royal Stat Soc A. 1997;160(1):127–140.
9. Ransohoff DF, Feinstein AR. Problems of spectrum and bias in evaluating the efficacy of diagnostic tests. N E J Med. 1978;299(17):926–930.
10. Goehring C, Perrier A, Morabia A. Spectrum bias: A quantitative and graphical analysis of the variability of medical diagnostic test performance. Stat Med. 2004;23(1):125–135.
11. Bar-Hillel M, Budescu D. The elusive wishful thinking effect. Thinking and Reasoning. 1995;1(1):71–103.

12. Poses R, Cebul RD, Collins M, Fager SS. The accuracy of experienced physicians' probability estimates for patients with sore throats. JAMA. 1985;254(7):925–929.

13. Wallsten T. Physician and medical student bias in evaluating diagnostic information. Med Decision Making. 1981;1(2):145–164.

14. Gurmankin-Levy A, Hershey, JC. Value-induced bias in medical decision making. Med Decision Making. 2008;28:269–276.

15. Gurmankin-Levy A, Hershey JC. Distorting the probability of treatment success to justify treatment decisions. Org Behav and Human Decision Processes. 2006;101:52–58.

16. Tversky A, Kahneman D. Availability: A heuristic for judging frequency and probability. Cog Psych. 1973;5:207–232.

17. Dawson NV, Arkes HR. Systematic errors in medical decision making. J Gen Int Med. 1987;2:183–187.

18. Hershey JC, Baron J. Clinical reasoning and cognitive processes. Med Decision Making. 1987;7:203–211.

19. International Shark Attack File. The relative risk of shark attacks to humans. Florida Museum of Natural History, University of Florida. 2010.

20. Detmer DE, Fryback DG, Gassner K. Heuristics and biases in medical decision making. J Med Educ. 1978;53:682–683.

chapter 5

Clinical Decision Making Tools

If we always do what we've always done, we will get what we've always got.

—ADAM URBANSKI

•

✳ Mr. Ketterman's Case

It seems as though other people must have had patients with all of Mr. Ketterman's problems, even though I don't very often see anyone like this. Maybe I can find some recommendations in the literature about how to treat him. *(See Appendix for Mr. Ketterman's health history.)*

INTRODUCTION

Early physicians learned the art of medicine by tutorial, observing their mentors and discussing the decisions they made.[1] In this manner the rich wisdom of practice was passed from one generation to the next. Of course, errors in thinking were also passed on. Our current health care system has formalized this process of passing on knowledge through organized education that includes both formal academic preparation and well-defined clinical education requirements. During this formal education students are often asked to explain their clinical decision making, but experienced teachers and mentors seldom explicate their own. In addition, explicit processes to explain or improve clinical decision making are considerably diminished once the practitioner has met entry-level requirements. Licensed practitioners, be they physicians or physical therapists, usually make their clinical decisions in isolation, often with only the patient as a fellow participant in the process. This means that there are few opportunities to articulate, examine, and validate the clinical decision making process. We continue to support behaviors that often are just as likely to lead to the continuation of poor decision making as to better decision making. Some would even say that our current health care system forces us to work against the process of making clinical decisions explicit for practitioners, thus forcing isolated and isolating practice environments on young practitioners.

Many systems have been developed in response to this problem. They are primarily divided into two approaches. The first is a process approach that provides templates that encourage good decision making—helping us with *the way we think*. The second is a content approach that provides guidelines about what the decisions should be—suggesting to us *what to think*. When used together these two approaches can be very successful in helping us reflect on and improve our decisions.

PROCESS APPROACHES TO THE WAY WE THINK

The linguist B. L. Whorf has said, "Language shapes the way we think, and determines what we can think about."[2] In Chapter 1 we discussed the language of physical therapy practice, focusing on enablement/disablement models and on the patient care management model as sources of the language we use to communicate. We can also view these models as guides to our thinking processes, leading us to organize our clinical decisions in certain ways, to adopt *new ways to think*.

Enablement/Disablement Models

The use of a disablement model as a basis for our thinking leads us first to recognize that we should be thinking about our patients on multiple levels of pathology and all of its sequellae. If we consider only the pathology or etiology-related diagnosis, we will not consider the need to assess the patient's impairments or functional limitations. The promulgation of the Nagi model and its related forms made possible the development of the *Guide to Physical Therapist Practice* (which we will return to below) by allowing its authors the ability to think about the physical therapist's care in that organized framework.[3]

The International Classification of Functioning, Disability, and Health (ICF; see Chapter1) extends the somewhat linear thinking of the Nagi-related models to the more complex inter-relationships among function, disability, and health, recognizing the impact of environmental and personal factors.[4–6] In particular, the World Health Organization (WHO) states that the ICF was designed to help reformulate the concepts of health and disability by making it clear that all people have some elements of disability, no matter how healthy, and that all people have some elements of health, no matter how disabled. This shift is accomplished by giving us a common metric for measuring both health and disability. This certainly provides a new way of thinking about describing, improving, and measuring health status.[7]

Patient/Client Management Model

We also have the patient/client management model to help us think about patient care.[3] In Chapter 1 we discussed the common language the patient/client management model provides us to document what we do with patients. But the model also provides us a framework for the process of our patient care. The very presentation of the model (see Fig. 1-4) shows that this is a model of a sequence of events and thought processes. There is an order to each part of the model that represents the process that is used in interacting with our patients. For example, examination is generally the first step in the process. The logic of examination means we start with a history; we augment the history with the systems review to identify possible problem areas; we then use both the history and the systems review to focus the selection of specific tests and measures. All these data lead us to the diagnosis and prognosis, which in turn lead us to choose the appropriate interventions designed to achieve certain outcomes. The model includes a step labeled evaluation that is clearly not a behavior but a cognitive process where integration of data to derive conclusions takes place. Therefore, the patient/

client management model is clearly a process of thinking that we can use in our patient interactions.

The Hypothesis-Oriented Algorithm for Clinicians

Rothstein and Echternach proposed the Hypothesis-Oriented Algorithm for Clinicians (HOAC) in 1986 to explicate the hypothetico-deductive process in physical therapy.[8] As we have discussed (see Chapter 2), the hypothetico-deductive process consists of gathering cues, generating hypotheses that fit one or more of the cues, and then testing the hypotheses to determine the best fit or the diagnosis. This process is used to turn an unstructured, unfamiliar, or complicated patient problem into one that can be addressed with the use of one or more hypotheses. The HOAC was a branching process that led clinicians from initial data gathering to problem statements to hypotheses that could be tested by further data collection or treatment. This model became widely adopted in teaching the clinical reasoning in physical therapy education.

The HOAC has been recently modified as the HOAC II,[9] which adds the language of the patient care management model and also recognizes the role of physical therapy in prevention of impairments and disabilities, thereby updating to the current language of our care. As with the original HOAC, the HOAC II offers a series of steps or an algorithm that starts with history and examination, moves through identification of problems, to generation of hypotheses, and to development of a plan of care. It culminates in implementation and then reassessment. Figure 5-1 demonstrates the detail inherent in the HOAC II. By using this algorithm, therapists, especially when dealing with patient problems with which they are unfamiliar, can be more efficient in their clinical care.

The utility of all of these models (the ICF, the patient/client management model, and the HOAC) for guiding our clinical thinking can be seen in the integration of them into a framework for decision making with neurological patients (Fig. 5-2).[10] The authors intend the framework to apply to both the hypothetico-deductive process and the forward reasoning or pattern recognition seen in more experienced clinicians. Shenkman et al state that "by building from simple principles to the entire framework, experienced clinicians and educators can use this framework to assist students and novice clinicians to better understand and incorporate all aspects of decision making necessary for effective care of patients. This framework also provides the experienced clinician with a structure for articulating intuitive decisions."[10]

As can be seen by reviewing each of these models, they do not prescribe what to think, but offer us ways to go about the clinical decision making process. The patient/client management model and the HOAC II come from physical therapy. The first was designed by a large group of physical therapists working under the auspices of the American Physical Therapy Association to articulate the process of good clinical care.[3] The second is an important contribution from its authors to very explicitly describe the use of the hypothetico-deductive process in physical therapy.[8,9] The ICF also has its roots in the field of rehabilitation, with widespread input from member countries of the World Health Organization over a number of years.[7] The most recent framework, the integration of the other three into one model,[10] was done as part of the III Step Conference that was conducted by the Neurology Section and the Section on Pediatrics of the American Physical Therapy Association in 2005 to integrate the science of motor control into the selection and application of interventions in physical therapy.[11]

Although each process is unique in its origins, they have much in common. All are based on review of the literature in decision making, especially by health care practitioners. All speak directly to the decisions that physical therapists need to make each and every day with each

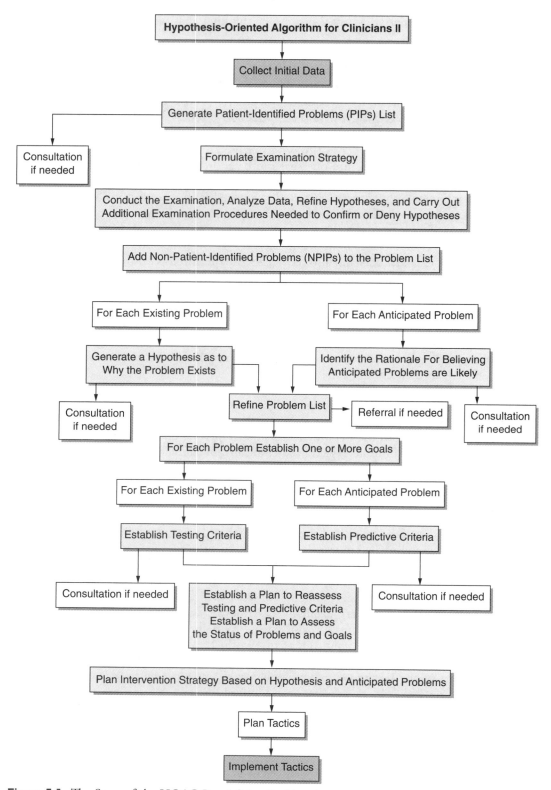

Figure 5-1 The Steps of the HOAC Part I (New Problems). *[As presented in Rothstein JM, Echternach JL, Riddle DL. The hypothesis-oriented algorithm for clinicians II (HOAC II): A guide for patient management. Phys Ther. 2003;83:455–470. Please see reference for Part II (Existing Problems.)]*

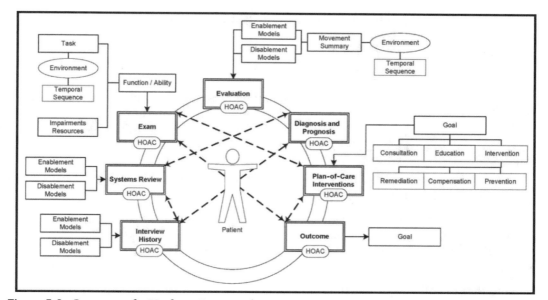

Figure 5-2 Overview of a Unifying Framework Demonstrating Steps in the Clinical Decision making Process. This framework is designed to be patient centered, integrating the enablement and disablement perspectives of the ICF and incorporating a variety of models and analyses at various points in the patient care management process. *(From Schenkman M, Deutsch JE, Gill-Body KM. An integrated framework for decision making in neurologic physical therapist practice. Phys Ther. 2006;86:1681–1702.)*

and every patient. As we have discussed in Chapters 2 through 4, clinical decision making is a complex topic. Good clinical decision making is also very difficult. These tools assist all clinicians, be they novice or experienced, by providing useful and valid frameworks. As we go about our clinical care, we can incorporate these processes into our thought processes. This can be done informally and personally by choices made by each clinician in his or her own thinking. They can also be included in more formal ways into our practices through documentation systems (see Chapter 18), which also serve as a means of communicating with other practitioners, and in the organization of in-service presentations and other forms of professional development.

As we said earlier, the language we use and *the way we think* are inexorably linked. By adopting the language of these models we will change our thinking patterns. By these useful paradigms, we will change our language. Of course, the desired outcome of both is better patient care.

CONTENT APPROACHES TO WHAT WE THINK

If our goal is to improve patient care, then finding recommendations for our behavior that assure we are doing the right thing would be very welcome. After all, if we know that one option is clearly superior to another, we would certainly take that option. The literature is full of recommendations to health care practitioners about what decisions they should make about every aspect of care from the smallest of care issues to decisions that can have immediate effects on mortality. Recommendations exist across the range of decisions we need to make, from screening to diagnosis to intervention. But not all of these recommendations are created equal! Some may come from the makers of various medications or devices, some may come from professional groups with particular political perspectives, some may come from consumer groups with a strong advocacy agenda. And some may come after years of rigorous examination that supports the conclusions drawn as having a positive effect on our patients' health.

It is important that clinicians choose from among these many recommendations wisely or the very goal of improved care will be lost. Therefore we should use an explicit framework to guide our selection of recommendations. Such a framework can help us to be sure that when we are accepting a recommendation about our choices in patient care we have made the right decision.

Eddy has developed just such a framework.[12] In it he describes these types of patterns to guide practice. They include:

- *standards*—when there is clear agreement across the profession that everyone should, even must, make particular clinical decisions;
- *guidelines*—behaviors that are recommended as the best choice; and
- *options*—a range of acceptable behaviors, all equally acceptable, from which to choose.[12]

Note that this discussion refers to standards of specific clinical care, not to standards of general professional practice, such as codes of ethics.

Guidelines

There are no known published standards of care in physical therapy. As is true in most health professions there is little if any agreement about clinical choices that can meet the level of scrutiny that defines a standard of care. However, many types of guidelines have been developed that are available and sometimes used by physical therapists. The agencies that have developed these guidelines range from large national organizations to individual practices. The guidelines also vary greatly in their reliance on evidence from the research as opposed to practitioner opinion. There are many examples of guidelines that have been developed by both governmental and professional advisory groups.[13–15] Many of these guidelines are written with the patient diagnosis as the focus, so they apply broadly to many practitioners, regardless of discipline. Guidelines have also been developed by many facilities and other clinical entities, often in the form of critical or clinical paths.[16,17] Some of these types of guidelines are intended to apply across a wide spectrum of practices, but some, such as guidelines for postsurgical care, are idiosyncratic to the preferences of specific practitioners.

Options

There is a growing body of literature about certain guidelines that are termed clinical decision rules or clinical prediction rules.[18,19] A clinical decision rule is a tool the clinician can use to increase the accuracy of diagnoses and prognoses and therefore improve the selection of specific interventions. These rules are developed and published in the literature as *options* for clinical practice. The rules are developed by testing the results from previously published evidence with specific patient populations. We discuss the development of clinical decision rules, as well as the development of other types of guidelines, in Chapter 15.

In addition, we have a major source for acceptable *options* in physical therapy, the *Guide to Physical Therapist Practice*.[3] The *Guide* contains over 30 descriptions of preferred practice patterns for patients with dysfunction or the potential for dysfunction in the musculoskeletal, the neuromuscular, the cardiovascular and pulmonary, and the integumentary systems (Table 5.1). These patterns represent the profession's first attempt to identify broad

Table 5.1 APTA Guide to Physical Therapy Practice Preferred Practice Patterns

Category of Condition	Practice Pattern Name
Musculoskeletal	A. Primary Prevention/Risk Reduction for Skeletal Demineralization
	B. Impaired Posture
	C. Impaired Muscle Performance
	D. Impaired Joint Mobility, Motor Function, Muscle Performance and Range of Motion Associated with Connective Tissue Dysfunction
	E. Impaired Joint Mobility, Motor Function, Muscle Performance and Range of Motion Associated with Localized Inflammation
	F. Impaired Joint Mobility, Motor Function, Muscle Performance and Range of Motion Associated with Spinal Disorders
	G. Impaired Joint Mobility, Muscle Performance and Range of Motion Associated with Fracture
	H. Impaired Joint Mobility, Motor Function, Muscle Performance and Range of Motion Associated with Joint Arthroplasty
	I. Impaired Joint Mobility, Motor Function, Muscle Performance and Range of Motion Associated with Bony or Soft Tissue Surgery
	J. Impaired Motor Function, Muscle Performance, Range of Motion, Gait, Locomotion, and Balance Associated with Amputation
Neuromuscular	A. Primary Prevention/Risk Reduction for Loss of Balance and Falling
	B. Impaired Neuromotor Development
	C. Impaired Motor Function and Sensory Integrity Associated with Nonprogressive Disorders of the Central Nervous System—Congenital Origin or Acquired in Infancy or Childhood
	D. Impaired Motor Function and Sensory Integrity Associated with Nonprogressive disorders of the Central Nervous System—Acquired in Adolescence or Adulthood
	E. Impaired Motor Function and Sensory Integrity Associated with Progressive Disorders of the Central Nervous System
	F. Impaired Peripheral Nerve Integrity and Muscle Performance Associated with Peripheral Nerve Injury
	G. Impaired Motor Function and Sensory Integrity Associated with Acute or Chronic Polyneuropathies
	H. Impaired Motor Function, Peripheral Nerve Integrity, and Sensory Integrity Associated with Nonprogressive Disorders of the Spinal Cord
	I. Impaired Arousal, Range of Motion, and Motor Control Associated with Coma, Near Coma, or Vegetative State

Table 5.1	APTA Guide to Physical Therapy Practice Preferred Practice Patterns—con'd
Category of Condition	**Practice Pattern Name**
Cardiovascular/Pulmonary	A. Primary Prevention/Risk Reduction for Cardiovascular/Pulmonary Disorders B. Impaired Aerobic Capacity/Endurance Associated with Deconditioning C. Impaired Ventilation, Respiration/Gas Exchange, and Aerobic Capacity/Endurance Associated with Airway Clearance Dysfunction D. Impaired Aerobic Capacity/Endurance Associated with Cardiovascular Pump Dysfunction or Failure E. Impaired Ventilation and Respiration/Gas Exchange Associated with Ventilatory Pump Dysfunction or Failure F. Impaired Ventilation and Respiration/Gas Exchange Associated with Respiratory Failure G. Impaired Ventilation, Respiration/Gas Exchange, and Aerobic Capacity/Endurance Associated with Respiratory Failure in the Neonate H. Impaired Circulation and Antrhopometric Dimensions Associated with Lymphatic System Disorder
Integumentary	A. Primary Prevention/Risk Reduction for Integumentary Disorders B. Impaired Integumentary Integrity Associated with Superficial Skin Involvement C. Impaired Integumentary Integrity Associated with Partial-Thickness Skin Involvement and Scar Formation D. Impaired Integumentary Integrity Associated with Full-Thickness Skin Involvement and Scar Formation E. Impaired Integumentary Integrity Associated with Skin Involvement Extending into Fascia, Muscle, or Bone and Scar Formation

Data from: APTA, *Guide to Physical Therapist Practice*, 2nd ed. Alexandria, VA: American Physical Therapy Association; 2001.

diagnostic categories that group together patients with similar impairments, in order to describe options for care for these groups of patients. Each practice pattern is comprised of specific content in seven general areas, which are derived from the patient/client management model (Table 5.2).

1. The Patient/Client Diagnostic Classification area provides inclusion and exclusion criteria for that particular pattern and some related diagnoses of pathology.
2. The Examination area lists the range of items a clinician should consider in conducting the history, systems review, and specific tests and measures; this is not meant to be a list of what should be done, but rather a fairly complete list of what could be done to provide the information to arrive at diagnoses and prognoses for a given patient who fits this pattern.

Table 5.2 Elements of the APTA Preferred Practice Patterns

Category	Elements
Patient/Client Diagnostic Classification	Inclusion and Exclusion Criteria for the Pattern ICD-9 International Classification of Diseases, 9th Revision Codes for Patient Diagnosis
Examination	Patient/Client History General Demographics Social History Employment/Work (Job/School/Play) Growth and Development Living Environment General Health Status Social/Health Habits Family History Medical/Surgical History Current Conditions (chief complaint) Functional Status/Activity Level Medications Other Clinical Tests Systems Review Musculoskeletal Neuromuscular Cardiovascular/Pulmonary Integumentary Communication/Cognition/Affect/Language/Learning Style Tests and Measures (1 or more from 24 categories)
Evaluation/Diagnosis/ Prognosis	Predicted optimum level of improvement and the time required to reach that level Expected range of visits per episode of care Factors that may influence frequency of visits or duration of episode
Intervention	Coordination, communication, and documentation of care Patient/client instruction Procedural interventions (1 or more from 9 categories) Anticipated goals and expected outcomes for each intervention
Reexamination Global Outcomes Criteria for Termination of PT Services	Reasons for and timing of reexamination Pathology, impairments, functional limitations, disabilities, risk reduction/prevention, health, wellness and fitness, societal resources, patient/client satisfaction Discharge/Discontinuation

Data from: APTA, *Guide to Physical Therapist Practice*, 2nd ed. Alexandria, VA: American Physical Therapy Association; 2001.

3. The Evaluation/Diagnosis/Prognosis area provides expected outcomes for patients in this pattern, length of care, and reasons why a particular patient may depart from these expected norms.
4. The Intervention area lists a range of interventions that are appropriate for a patient who fits this pattern; again, it is not intended that any patient receive all of these interventions, but rather they represent a fairly complete list of what could be done to help achieve the patient's intended outcomes.
5. The Reexamination area provides the reasons for and timing of reexamination.
6. The Global Outcomes area lists outcomes that are applicable to all patients.
7. The Criteria for Termination of PT Services area describes the reasons why patients should be discharged or care should be discontinued.

The elements of these practice patterns can help clinicians evaluate the comprehensiveness of their clinical thinking.

Clinical Guidance

Eddy points out the necessity to move cautiously from options to guidelines to standards. Since standards can be used to hold practitioners accountable for various specific behaviors by forming the basis for malpractice claims or loss of licensure, they require very strong evidence and widespread professional and patient acceptance. However, another important reason to move slowly is to preserve what is termed "warranted variation." When we are not certain of the best course of events, some variety across practitioners and across regions gives us a natural laboratory to explore the outcomes of these various options for our patients. Moving too rapidly to reach a conclusion can result in adoption of a test or intervention that has a less than optimal outcome.[12]

Another benefit of providing options is that they allow the possibility of mistakes. Although we do not want to make mistakes that have lasting harm to patients, mistakes are a powerful way of learning. It has been shown that recognizing a mistake, analyzing it, and adapting behavior accordingly are all hallmarks of the clinical expert.[20]

CONCLUSION

By understanding the typical processes of decision making, recognizing the result of our decisions, and using some tools to improve our decision making process, we are in a better position to understand and use the disablement model, the patient care management model, and evidence based practice to improve patient care.

These descriptions of best clinical practice go by a variety of names, serve a variety of purposes, and have a variety of formats. Some are descriptions, at varying levels of urgency, of what to do with certain patients, and others are descriptions of processes of thinking, without obvious plans of care. When selected wisely, these tools can help clinicians make better clinical decisions. In later chapters we will explore more deeply what a clinician needs to know to make wise choices.

SELF-ASSESSMENT

1. Identify a patient whom you have seen lately. Determine which practice pattern the patient represents, and then compare the care you provided with the care described in the pattern. Why was your care different from that in the pattern? After reviewing the pattern, would you change your care?

---

2. Identify a patient whom you have seen lately. Outline the decision making process for this patient using the format of the HOAC. How was your process different from the HOAC process? Would you change your process with similar patients in the future? Why or why not?

CONTINUED LEARNING

Identify some practice recommendations that influence your care. Determine if they are standards, guidelines, or options. Identify the background information that was used to develop them.

1. Can you find expert opinion and evidence from the literature, or are they based on one person's preferences?

2. As you move through this text, come back to these recommendations to evaluate their quality.

REFERENCES

1. Groopman J. *How Doctors Think.* Boston: Houghton Mifflin; 2007.
2. http://thinkexist.com/quotations/thinking/. Accessed May 18, 2008.
3. APTA, *Guide to Physical Therapist Practice,* 2nd ed. Alexandria, VA: American Physical Therapy Association; 2001.
4. *International Classification of Functioning, Disability, and Health (ICF),* ICF full version. Geneva, Switzerland: World Health Organization; 2001.
5. Jette AM. Toward a common language for function, disability, and health. Phys Ther. 2006;86:726–734.
6. Field MJ, Jette AM. *The Future of Disability in America.* Washington, DC.
7. http://www.who.int/classifications/icf/en/ Accessed October 30, 2011.
8. Rothstein JM, Echternach JL. Hypothesis-oriented algorithm for clinicians. Phys Ther. 1986;66:1388–1394.
9. Rothstein JM, Echternach JL, Riddle DL. The hypothesis-oriented algorithm for clinicians II (HOAC II): A guide for patient management. Phys Ther. 2003;83:455–470.
10. Schenkman M, Deutsch JE, Gill-Body KM. An integrated framework for decision making in neurologic physical therapist practice. Phys Ther. 2006;86:1681–1702.
11. http://www.pediatricapta.org/iiistep/index.cfm Accessed May 19, 2009.
12. Eddy, DA. *Manual for Assessing Health Practices and Designing Practice Policies: The Explicit Approach.* Philadelphia: American College of Physicians; 1992.
13. National Guideline Clearinghouse, Low Back Disorders. http://www.guideline.gov/summary/summary.aspx?view_id = 1&doc_id = 12540 Accessed September 25, 2008.
14. Stiell I, Wells G, Laupacis A, et al. Multicentre trial to introduce the Ottawa ankle rules for use of radiography in acute ankle injuries. Brit Med J. 1995;311:594–597.
15. Philadelphia Panel evidence-based clinical practice guidelines on selected rehabilitation interventions for low back pain. Phys Ther. 2001;81:1641–1667.
16. Kim S, Losina E, Solomon D, Wright J, Katz J, Effectiveness of clinical pathways for total knee and total hip arthroplasty. J Arthroplasty. 1999;18(1):69–74.
17. Schunk C, Reid K. *Care Connections' Clinical Practice Guidelines,* 3rd ed. Therapeutic Associates, year unknown.
18. Childs JD, Cleland JA. Development and application of clinical prediction rules to improve decision making in physical therapist practice. Phys Ther. 2006;86:122–131.
19. McGinn TG, Guyatt GH, Wyer PC, Naylor CD, Stiell IG, Richardson WS. Users' guides to the medical literature XXII: How to use articles about clinical decision rules. JAMA. 2000;284:79–84.
20. Jensen G, Gwyer J, Hack L, Shepard K. *Expertise in Physical Therapy Practice,* 2nd ed. St. Louis, MO: Saunders Elsevier; 2006.

Understanding and Respecting Patient Values and Circumstances

The second element of evidence based practice is fully respecting and integrating our patients' values and circumstances into our collaborative decision making. We bring our expertise as clinicians (Section I) and our knowledge and appraisal of the available evidence (Section III) to working with our patients to make these clinical decisions. Patients and their families bring their own preferences and choices. These preferences and choices are based on cultural norms, personal attitudes and beliefs, and prior knowledge (patient values); and on their own situations related to the location of care and the resources available and needed to provide care (patient circumstances). This element of evidence based practice is often underrepresented in the literature. We regard it as critically important in making evidence based practice all that it can and should be.

The conceptualization of the three elements of evidence based practice applies to all health professions, but it is perhaps even more meaningful to physical therapists. As previous studies have demonstrated, experts in physical therapy make the patient the center of their clinical reasoning.[1] Perhaps this is necessary because so much of what we do requires that patients voluntarily agree to changes in their own behavior in order to achieve success. Cohen speaks of certain professions as being practices of human improvement. He defines them as professions that seek to improve human minds, enrich human capacities, and change behavior. He goes on to say that unless the intended recipients of these improvements—be they student, patient, or client—embrace the changes being sought, then the changes are unachievable.[2]

In this section we strive to provide the reader with the necessary background to fully engage in this element of evidence based practice. The section begins with

Chapter 6, "Bridging the Differences of Diversity: Communicating in the Border-lands," by Suzanne Gordon. This chapter describes how to communicate with our patients across the many cultural and social differences that might tend to separate us. Gordon reviews available knowledge about the therapeutic relationship and describes the communication skills necessary to create that relationship. She does this by focusing on the conditions needed to create a cross-cultural relationship, on the impact of differences in power and prestige, and on the complex interaction of our social identity with our personal identity.

John Coulehan and Marian Block follow that with Chapter 7, "The Patient Interview." They discuss the interview not only as the primary source of information that can help us understand patient values and circumstances and develop the therapeutic relationship but also as the primary source of information in the diagnostic process. They identify the attributes of the interview process that improve its effectiveness as the most powerful and important tool available to the clinician in his or her practice.

These background chapters are then followed by two chapters that lay out very clearly the specific issues related to patient values and circumstances. Kim Nixon-Cave, in Chapter 8, "Learning About Patients' Perspectives: Qualitative Research," reminds us that we make choices about the type of relationship we wish to have with our patients, ranging from paternalistic approaches to fully patient-centered care, and that each of these approaches takes a different view of patient values. She also provides clear examples of the work being done by qualitative research-ers to help document actual patient values, thus showing that we can learn about our patients' values one case at a time through our care, and collectively through sound research.

Finally, Michael Johnson in Chapter 9, "The Health Care System and Patient Circumstances," uses a model from Kissick to help bring some organization to what might be seen as the chaotic state of the health care system in the United States.[3] He also uses the well-established model from Anderson to organize the aspects of patient circumstances that can affect a person's ability to actually access and use health care services.[4]

By linking what we learn of personal values from Nixon-Cave with what we learn of patient circumstances from Johnson, we can begin to fully understand the interplay of all of these factors in our ability to help our patients actually access and receive the best care possible.

References

1. Jensen G, Gwyer J, Hack L, et al. Expertise in Physical Therapy Practice, 2nd Ed, St. Louis, Saunders Elsevier, 2006.
2. Cohen DK. Professions of human improvement: Predicaments of teaching. In M. Nisan & O Schremer (Eds.), Educational Deliberations. Jerusalem: Keter Publishers, 2005.
3. Kissick W. Medicine's Dilemmas: Infinite Need Versus Finite Resources. New Haven: Yale University Press, 1994:185.
4. Andersen RE. Behavioral Model of Families' Use of Health Services. Center for Health AdministrationStudies. Chicago, IL: University of Chicago, 1968.

chapter 6

Bridging the Differences of Diversity: Communicating in the Borderlands

Suzanne P. Gordon, PT, EdD

Diversity: the art of thinking independently together

—Malcolm Forbes

•

✳ Mr. Ketterman's Case

Mr. Ketterman has indicated to me that he no longer wants to be treated by the therapist who covers for me when I am away. She is a 25-year-old woman who speaks with an accent and who has recently decided to share with everyone that she is gay. She also enjoys a rather casual approach to her wardrobe and her interaction with patients. I noticed she has been calling Mr. Ketterman Sam. I want to figure out why Mr. Ketterman has made this request and what if anything I might need to do about the therapist's behavior. *(See Appendix for Mr. Ketterman's health history.)*

✳ Case Example—Sarah

Sarah is excited by her new job in a women's health clinic, particularly since this opportunity allows her to apply her manual therapy skills specifically to women's health issues. She is particularly pleased that the owner of the women's health clinic, Marsha, has a well-articulated philosophy about the importance of health education for everyone who receives services through her clinic. In fact, Marsha is a strong advocate for improving the health of lesbians, bisexual women, transgender people, and their families. Yet, Sarah is anxious. She has always lived in small, rural communities of people just like her and her family—white, middle-class, blue-collar, or professional people who are independent thinkers and either Jewish or Christian. She wonders how she will be able to connect with the patients and clients she will see weekly at an outreach clinic in a community health center in the most run-down neighborhood of her new town. How effective will she be in instructing people who have poor education and few resources? Earlier today, Marsha told her that the community health clinic also serves the Somali immigrant population that has swelled in numbers over the past 10 years. Despite being reassured that the Somali community has emphasized learning English, she worries about how she will be able to establish a therapeutic relationship with women who are so unlike herself.

Sarah knows that she has excellent reasons for being concerned. She, like virtually every other physical therapist, knows that a positive patient-practitioner relationship is pivotal to effective therapeutic outcomes. The physical therapy profession posits that positive therapeutic outcomes emerge from the interaction between the practitioner's technical therapeutic skills and the therapeutic relationship with the patient or client. While the degree to which the therapeutic relationship contributes is legitimately questioned,[1,2] its importance to patient and client improvement is strongly promoted in physical therapy literature[3-5] and education.[6] The question Sarah asks herself is not *should* she develop therapeutic relationships with her patients and clients; instead, she asks *how* to develop the therapeutic relationship across the cultural differences of gender, age, class, race, ethnicity, religion, sexual orientation, and ablement (ability/disability). More important, she wonders how to advocate for the health care and educational resources that are limited for the people relying on the community health clinic's services.

Sarah is well aware that her professional responsibility to develop a therapeutic relationship is informed by evidence based practice. Evidence based practice is a process that begins with the patient and involves asking answerable questions, finding "the current best evidence in making decisions about the care of individual patients."[7,p71] The decisions about the use of best evidence involves assessing available knowledge; integrating into an intervention plan the results of that knowledge assessment with clinical expertise, the patient's unique biology and expectations, and patient values; and, finally, evaluating one's performance through reassessment and reflection.[8,9] Inherent in the multiple definitions of evidence based practice offered by Sackett and his colleagues is the concept of individualized patient care that meets the "patient's unique expectations" and "patient values." Establishing a therapeutic relationship that takes into consideration a patient's unique expectations and values becomes more complex when it requires communicating across the differences of cultural beliefs, values, life experiences, worldview, and assumptions about health and illness. Sarah is determined to develop the skills she needs not only to communicate with her diverse patient and client population but also to advocate for the health care that would best serve them. More importantly, she realizes that to overcome her anxiety about working with people of difference, she needs to explore her own values and attitudes about diversity.

INTRODUCTION

This chapter presents one view of how to communicate across cultural, power, and privilege differences through the creation of a therapeutic alliance. Since cross-cultural communication is based upon solid interpersonal interactions, we review the communication skills necessary for establishing a therapeutic relationship and the therapeutic alliance. A summary of the current research defining therapeutic alliance outlines its characteristics and illustrates how the therapeutic alliance supports the expectations of evidence based practice for meeting patient's unique needs. As Sarah notes, meeting a patient's unique needs when those needs are culturally different complicates the therapeutic alliance.

The first section of the chapter provides evidence of the need for cross-cultural therapeutic alliances in health care. The second section reviews the communication skills and relational conditions that both support and hinder the development of the therapeutic alliance; the third section offers research identifying those specific conditions essential to an effective therapeutic alliance. The fourth and final section provides guidelines for bridging the challenges of cultural difference and for overcoming the disruptive forces created by dissimilarity in power and privilege, by implicit biases and prejudices, and by discrepancies in social identity development. Evidence based practice demands that physical therapists organize their practice around the unique, individualized needs of all patients and clients. Our goal is to explain how to build the therapeutic alliance that supports evidence based practice and bridges the differences of diversity.

CONTEXT FOR CROSS-CULTURAL COMMUNICATION AND THE THERAPEUTIC ALLIANCE

It is important to note that the therapeutic alliance occurs within the context of the U.S. health care system, described in Chapter 9, which also describes how the system creates health disparities. Two decades of research have led the Office of Minority Health (www.omhrc.gov), Institutes of Medicine (www.iom.edu), the Office of Minority Health & Health Disparities (www.cdc.gov/omhd), and the National Center on Minority Health and Health Disparities (ncmhd.nih.gov) to uniformly agree that there are significant differences between populations with regard to health quality, interventions, access, and outcomes. In addition, there are health disparities that emerge from differences in treatment provided to members of racial, ethnic, or other minority groups which are not justified by the underlying health conditions or treatment preferences of the patient. All of these governmental offices and institutes have based their conclusions on a huge body of archival research substantiating health disparities among racial and ethnic minorities and people of lower socioeconomic status and exacerbated by geography (either rural or inner city), gender, age, religion, disability status, and sexual orientation.

This research, as well as other reviews of health disparities,[10–13] consistently documents inequities in the quality of health care experienced by various minority groups even when taking into account variations in insurance status, patient income, and other access-related factors. Many of these studies also controlled for other potential confounding factors that could be considered the cause of disparities, such as racial differences in the severity or stage of disease progression, the presence of comorbid illnesses, and other patient demographic variables, such as age and gender. The majority of even the most controlled studies indicated that minorities are less likely than whites to receive needed services, including clinically necessary procedures. After careful review and analysis, a 2002 Institute of Medicine (IOM) report concluded that "[al]though myriad sources contribute to these disparities, some evidence suggests that bias, prejudice, and stereotyping on the part of healthcare providers may contribute to difference in care."[13]

A 2002 IOM report titled *Unequal Treatment: What Healthcare Providers Need to Know about Racial and Ethnic Disparities in Healthcare* asked, "how could bias, prejudice, and stereotyping contribute to unequal treatment, particularly given that healthcare providers are sworn to beneficence and cannot, by law, discriminate against any patient on the basis of race, ethnicity, color, or national origin?"[12,p1] The IOM answered its own question using information gleaned from a three-year review of hundreds of studies: the three sources of health disparities are society, the patient, and the provider.[13] Society contributes by supporting segregation through the fragmentation of health care, limiting where minorities access and receive care, and through language barriers and systems (regulations and policy) of disparity across socioeconomic status (which includes level of education). The patient, or the patient's family, contributes to health disparities through lifestyle (e.g., tobacco use, alcohol consumption, diet, level of physical activity, and stress) and less utilization of services due to mistrust—a mistrust acquired through direct experiences of discrimination within the health care system. Providers contribute to health disparities through their own, frequently unconscious, bias, stereotyping, racism, prejudice, and discrimination.[13]

We assume that caring and respectful physical therapists hold dear the egalitarian attitude that every patient and client deserves the best care. This professional value is so strong that given evidence that unconscious biases are typically held by those health care providers who espouse few explicit prejudices,[10–14] most physical therapists would be self-motivated to explore their own implicit attitudes, attitudes that may unintentionally interfere in the care provided to people of difference. We begin in the spirit of openness and discovery necessary for exploring how to build the therapeutic alliance across cultural differences. Our aim is not to offend, but to introduce information and concepts that lead to a path of self-exploration and to increase awareness of strategies that will better serve all of our patients and clients.

COMMUNICATION SKILLS AS A SCAFFOLD FOR THE THERAPEUTIC ALLIANCE

Verbal and Nonverbal Communication

Sarah's resolve to learn how to communicate across differences begins with a review of the therapeutic relationship. Communication skills make up the scaffold upon which the therapeutic relationship is built.[3–5] Both verbal and nonverbal skills are used by the patient and the health care practitioner as each reciprocally and mutually interact to send and receive messages. Patients depend primarily upon words, gestures, and body language to send the message that they are seeking help and information. Their expectation is that health care practitioners will receive the information through active listening and consider both the facts presented by the patient and the affective, nonverbal information accompanying the words. In return, the health care practitioner uses verbal language, employing clear and concise lay terminology, along with nonverbal language to convey helpfulness and a willingness to engage with the patient in the pursuit of healing, health, and wellness.

When congruent, the interaction between verbal and nonverbal communication conveys the seriousness of the patient's health needs and concerns and his or her willingness to enter into the caring relationship that will facilitate the attainment of health and wellness. Concomitantly, the practitioner's congruent verbal and nonverbal messages relay attention and caring. Congruency is achieved when the words match the emotions expressed by paralinguistics (those cues conveyed by tone of voice, pitch, speed, and volume that relay the feelings behind the words), facial expressions, gestures, posture, touch, physical appearance, and proxemics.[4,5]

Proxemics refers to the use of spatial relationships in human interactions to communicate social meanings. Authority is implied when one person stands over or above another; respect and willingness to interact are implied when communication occurs at eye level and body postures move in synchrony; caring is implied by gentle touch. For example, the patient who is feeling disenfranchised and insecure may unconsciously position himself lower than the therapist and speak indistinctly and softly with only fleeting eye contact. Or the patient who is intent on clarifying a point and gaining validation will align his eyes with and move closer to the practitioner. Body proximity communicates a relationship intent. The norm in U.S. society is to engage in, or limit, communication within four distance zones[15]: intimate, personal, social, and public. Intimate distance or direct contact is used in such activities as lovemaking, comforting, protecting, or athletics. Personal distance (at 1 to 4 feet) conveys personal interest and the willingness to risk either a caring touch or a harming touch. Social distance (of 4 to 12 feet) is employed in formal business and social discourse; public distance (of 12 to 25 feet) signals an unwillingness to engage in communication, direct eye contact, or physical contact.

Miscommunication

Miscommunication will likely occur when the level of communication is inappropriate in the interaction between patient and practitioner.[3–5] The therapeutic relationship is stymied when communication by either the sender or the receiver remains at a superficial level where no genuine sharing occurs, exemplified by clichéd language and the tendency arising from each individual's self-absorption to tell stories in a spirit of one-upmanship. When communication stagnates at this level or at the level of reporting facts, nothing personal is revealed. The patient's uniqueness remains invisible, and the individualized caring so essential to the therapeutic relationship is blocked. Relying upon interview questions to stimulate conversation may create just this type of limitation. The therapeutic relationship depends on a middle level of communication where some mutual personal information is shared in conversation around a common idea (such as an understanding of the health problem, agreement on the plan of care, or a decision on the intervention goals). The therapeutic relationship ethically dictates a balance between caring engagement and professional distance.[4,5,16] Professional distance requires that the practitioner manage emotions and attitudes, thereby circumventing or preventing the deeper levels of mutual sharing and personal revelation that more typically define a friendship or intimacy.

Another major cause of miscommunication is the distortion of the message itself by the environment or context. The unfamiliar clinic may overwhelm, frighten, and disorient a patient unused to the health care system; the patient then communicates a confused and incomplete accounting of the health problem. Imagine how these emotions are exacerbated when immigrants who have no concept of what the U.S. health care system can provide first seek access. Fear and disorientation, pain, and inattentiveness can also prevent the patient from receiving the therapist's messages of caring, encouragement, intervention, and instruction. The therapist's ability to carefully attend and actively listen to the patient may also be diminished by workplace distractions and productivity pressures. Multitasking, fatigue, and burnout all take their toll on the therapist's ability to manage emotions and interact therapeutically.

Barriers to Communication

Miscommunication between practitioner and patient may occur due to ineffective interpersonal and communication skills, but individuals who pride themselves on their excellent communication abilities may also miscommunicate. Multiple individual psychosocial characteristics—such as personality type, teaching and learning style, cognitive ability and educational level, physical energy and emotional drive—enter into the therapeutic relationship and contribute to the understandings, and misunderstandings, that develop between the therapist and patient. While the health care practitioner's education and knowledge are necessary for effective practice, they can also act as barriers to the patient who feels diminished by his or her lack of understanding. Other potential sources for miscommunication are values, beliefs, attitudes, rituals, and traditions that are culturally acquired through membership in socially determined groups defined by age or generation, gender, class, religion, ethnicity, race, occupation, sexual orientation, and ablement (ability/disability). Effective communication across differing cultural values, beliefs, and rituals takes thoughtfulness and care to find those that are held in common by the practitioner and the patient. Commonly held values and beliefs may become the agreed-upon center around which the patient and practitioner can come together in a therapeutic relationship.

When she heard that she would be working closely with Somali women in her new town, Sarah immediately panicked over cultural and language barriers that would interfere with her ability to communicate effectively. Despite assurances that the Somali community is working to learn English and that the community health clinic is staffed with interpreters, Sarah was aware that differing cultural understandings of eye contact, body proximity, touch, gestures, body language, and openness to revealing personal information and emotions also risk misinterpretation.

Fortunately, multiple community resources are available for learning about the cultural beliefs, values, behaviors, and rituals unique to specific ethnic, racial, and religious cultures. City and state immigration offices and agencies frequently provide resources for exploring the cultural facts about specific ethnic groups. Hospitals and community health centers employ social workers, chaplains, and counselors who serve as cultural brokers. Universities and colleges frequently support institutes that focus on cross-cultural exchange. And there are many books, several of which are listed at the end of this chapter, that help to explain specific cultural characteristics and their implications for health and wellness. As Sarah explored these multiple resources, she began to appreciate the value of creating her own support group and network for understanding the lives and health needs of the Somali population in her town.

As each person enters the health care system, whether as patient, administrator, or practitioner, he or she is granted relative positional status that also confers relative positional power. The hierarchy of positional power, by definition, creates power inequities between the practitioner and the patient. This power may act as a barrier to communication as each stakeholder within the health care system performs within his or her expected normative roles.[4,5] Physical therapists and other health care practitioners are granted the position of authority based on their professional knowledge and their professional status within the health care system. Due to their institutional status, it is easy for physical therapists to unconsciously consider themselves superior to the patient. In this dynamic, the person seeking help becomes dependent on the health care practitioner, thereby positioning the patient as inferior to the practitioner. The dynamic becomes more entrenched as the responsibility for communication and the relationship falls primarily upon the therapist for, after all, the patient's self-centered focus is on resolving his or her health problem.[17] The concepts of therapeutic relationship and therapeutic alliance are predicated on mutuality; the hegemony of the therapist's position risks disrupting that alliance.

BUILDING THE THERAPEUTIC ALLIANCE

As early as 1912, Freud described the dynamic relationship between therapist and patient, noting that the patient's "friendly and affectionate" attachment to the therapist was a "vehicle for success."[18] Subsequently, the concept of the therapeutic alliance became part of psychoanalytic therapy and was described as a theory by Roger in 1957.[19] The theory posited that the conditions necessary and sufficient for change to occur, regardless of the therapeutic theory or techniques employed, included counselor congruence or genuineness in the therapeutic relationship, unconditional positive regard for and to the client (warmth), the ability of the counselor to empathize with the client in the relationship, and communication of empathy.[19] In the past several decades, the psychological, counseling, and psychotherapy literature has reflected efforts to provide empirical evidence in support of this theory and has engaged in a debate over the relative contribution to patient outcomes of therapeutic approaches versus the contribution of the therapeutic alliance.[18–22]

"Attunement to client needs is essential, but not sufficient (for positive patient outcomes)."[23,p122] Major reviews of therapeutic alliance research found consistently small but consistently significant evidence that the quality of the therapeutic alliance predicts treatment outcomes regardless of the therapeutic approach used in the counseling sessions.[18,21,24,25] The literature also confirms that the therapeutic alliance is defined by the integration of its three essential components: bond (the extent to which the patient feels understood and respected in the therapist-patient relationship), goals (mutually agreed upon goals that meet the patient or client's expectations), and therapeutic or technical tasks (collaborative or negotiated agreement on intervention tasks).[20,21] Other reviews that examined the use and utility of the therapeutic alliance in producing behavioral change and positive patient/client outcomes across multiple counseling contexts and diagnoses contended that the therapeutic alliance plays a similar role in other therapeutic settings, including medical and hospital environments.[20,22] The characteristics of the therapeutic alliance emerging from this body of research have relevance to the discussion of how to develop the individualized patient care that meets the "patient's unique expectations" and "patient values" in the evidence based practice of physical therapy.

To create the bond necessary for the therapeutic alliance, the needs of the patient or client are primary. Thus, the needs of the therapist remain secondary to those of the patient or client. Through communication, the health care provider signals to the patient that his or her role is to be there for the patient, to be helpful, and to promote healing. To do this, the physical therapist attends to the congruency of the verbal and nonverbal message sent to the patient by:

- Inhibiting his or her own emotional reactions
- Respecting the patient
- Honoring the patient's feelings and perceptions
- Engaging with the patient to solve the health problem

Engaging the patient can challenge communication skills. To do this, the physical therapist:

1. Utilizes the skills of active listening through restatement, clarification, and reflection;
2. Encourages the patient to elucidate further; and
3. Hears what the patient has to say.[5]

The practitioner works together with the patient to identify the problem, gather objective and subjective facts, and guide or facilitate the solution. This process is a collaborative event in which the patient and the practitioner are equal participants in determining the plan of care, the interventions to be used, and the goals to achieve. Practitioners contribute knowledge, skills, and expertise about physical therapy; patients contribute knowledge, skills, and expertise about living their lives. In such a collaborative alliance, the practitioner and the patient empower each other to explore, discuss, and come to an agreement about the course and outcomes of an intervention.

But in some situations, the patient is not quite willing, or able, to enter into a collaborative agreement. Because the therapeutic alliance functions as a two-way relationship dependent on contributions from both the patient and the practitioner, the practitioner is responsible for nurturing the responsive capacity of the one who is being cared for.[17] "The therapist must not only be aware of the client's relational needs but also must meet them with his or her own appropriate affective response. This appropriate affective response—genuine, spontaneous, caring—is the essence of (the therapeutic alliance). It is what brings the relationship to life and puts flesh on the bare bones of technique."[23,p122] By nurturing the patient or client's ability to engage in the caring two-way relationship, the practitioner empowers the one cared for to embrace and direct behavioral and lifestyle change.[17] Patient participation in the change process then produces the patient's feeling of self-efficacy and motivation.[17] The empowering mutuality of the therapeutic alliance is integral to the change process described as the Transtheoretical Model of Change in physical therapy literature.[26]

The bond within the therapeutic alliance is effective because it is a reciprocal give-and-take between the practitioner and the patient and because its rewards are reciprocal. The patient's major reward is the freedom to be more fully him- or herself in the therapeutic alliance.[17] As the relationship becomes reciprocal and as the patient becomes more willing to risk self-revelation, the emergent mutuality becomes the reward for the therapist.[17] The continued reciprocal nature of the therapeutic alliance then allows the patient to give back by recognizing the practitioner's efforts and the care being provided.

The debates over the relative contribution to quality patient outcomes of the therapeutic alliance versus therapeutic skill pit the two against each other: are outcomes a result of therapeutic intervention, or are they a result of interaction? This question has been answered in the psychology and counseling literature but has only recently been raised in the physical therapy literature.[1,2] The psychology literature notes many studies demonstrating that the therapeutic alliance does correlate positively with therapeutic change.[22] Studies have attempted to quantify the relative contribution of alliance and skill, but it is the interaction of the two, and not a case of either/or, that produces effectiveness and positive outcomes.[21] Researchers in one study commented, "we need to recognize that a variety of elements play an important role (in determining patient or client change), and that these factors are in constant interaction with each other."[22,p277]

The contribution of the therapeutic alliance to quality therapeutic outcomes is supported by research that describes the expert physical therapist.[27-30] In one recent study, using a database that quantified quality therapy outcomes, Resnik and Jensen[30] were able to describe, the common attributes of a sample of physical therapists who performed exceptionally well.[30] This group of expert physical therapists shared a belief in patient-centered, collaborative relationships where "patients are viewed as active participants in therapy and as partners in the therapeutic process who are responsible for making their own informed choices"[30,p103]—a description that sounds very similar to the therapeutic alliance. Resnik and Jensen go on to report that common attributes of the experts' therapeutic relationship with their patients included a commitment to the patient, an ethic of caring, and a respect for individuality.

The three essential components of the therapeutic alliance—bond, goals, and agreement on therapeutic interventions and tasks—are familiar components of two other patient-practitioner communication models promoted in physical therapy and medical literature. These other models are the patient-practitioner collaborative model[29,31] and the shared clinical decision making model.[32,33] The three models share these components: patient-centered care, consideration of the patient's social context, active partnership, and shared decision making based on the mutual exchange of knowledge, values, and expectations surrounding the patient's health care. All of these models of patient-practitioner communication acknowledge that collaborative decision making produces patient autonomy by nurturing the patient's self-confidence and self-management skills to direct his or her own health care. Because these models reflect an ideal patient-practitioner relationship that does not often happen in the clinic, the Institute of Medicine continues to promote patient-centered and equitable care, regardless of the name of the model employed, because of the growing body of research evidence that patient involvement improves outcomes.[32–34] As Weston[33,p438] says, "The most important association with good outcomes is the patient's perception that the [health care provider] and the patient have found common.

BRIDGING DIFFERENCES: COMMUNICATING IN THE BORDERLANDS

"By its very nature 'difference' is discomforting; to engage in dialogue and action with individuals who may have conflicting ideas and construction about the world is hard work. But such work creates the conditions for change and for cultural democracy."[35,p11]

When similarity leads to connection
When in my early thirties, I worked with a woman, also in her early thirties who, like me, had very young children. We made an immediate connection as we worked together for the rehabilitation of her right hemiplegia due to a CVA. She was a teacher to my being a physical therapist. We were both white, women, married, mothers, had college degrees, and lived in the same community. Working together was easy as we planned her treatment and goals and made adjustments in accordance with her progress or new priorities. When communication barriers presented themselves, they could be explained within the framework of her disability, or of her change process, or of her emotional frustrations, anxieties, and fatigue. She, like all patients, and I, like all clinicians, carried our images of self, our social identities, and cultural values into our therapeutic relationship. Because of the similarities in our worldview, beliefs, and understandings about what makes life meaningful, we easily formed a therapeutic alliance without giving the relationship any deep thought.

What happens when you, the clinician, do not form a therapeutic alliance? What happens when you are unable to recognize or understand the worldview, social identity, cultural values, or belief systems of the person you are treating? Then what? How do you form the mutual relationship so necessary for a therapeutic alliance when cultural differences prevent an easy understanding of the patient?

The remainder of this chapter encapsulates the conditions critical to building the cross-cultural therapeutic alliance by offering guidelines for bridging cultural differences. Because these guidelines may not be sufficient for attaining the goal of a mutually reciprocal therapeutic alliance, the chapter offers three other frameworks to aid in understanding and relating to the patient's social context.

The first framework is the sociological theory of privilege, power, and difference that reveals how the persistence of privilege and power within the U.S. social and health care systems creates inequality, thereby explaining contemporary social justice issues.[36] This theory also promotes the development of mutual relationships because it encourages self-awareness of one's own position with regard to social power versus that of one's patients.[36,37] A second framework, describing the impact of microaggressions—implicit biases—as detractors from the therapeutic alliance, further enhances cultural sensitivity. Empirical evidence describes how implicit biases create unintentional discrimination in the medical setting; the literature also provides strategies, such as identifying a common identity with a patient, for developing the collaboration necessary for the therapeutic alliance.[10,11] The third framework is the concept of social identity. Social identity theories explain how issues of power and privilege are enacted personally, as every person acquires, through socialization processes, a social identity that represents a relative position within the social hierarchy.[37-39] Understanding the guidelines and theories that describe interactions across cultural differences offers an opportunity for health care practitioners to develop the strategies and skills necessary for counteracting society's negative influences when providing care.

Conditions Supporting Cross-Cultural Communication

In the story at the beginning of this chapter, Sarah was looking forward to working with women in a women's clinic. As a female athlete, she found it rewarding to work with other women athletes who held beliefs and lifestyle values similar to her own. By sharing the same cultural values concerning activity and exercise, Sarah found that she could easily build effective therapeutic alliances with athletes. Now, she was at a loss in knowing how to connect with women who held differing values and led different lifestyles. Aware of her discomfort in communicating across cultural differences, Sarah sought resources to better understand the cultural characteristics of the Somali (and Muslim) community, the Latino (and Catholic) community, the African American community, and the urban poor. She was interested in how illness, health, wellness, and disability were perceived and practiced in each of these cultural groups.

Despite what she learned, and despite her excitement about exploring different cultures and worldviews, Sarah was surprised to find that she remained uncomfortable with the idea of providing cross-cultural care. What does she do with her awareness of the differences that exist between her and her patients? Is it polite to remain silent about the differences and hope that her silences convey acceptance (even when she may not quite feel that way)? Does she acknowledge and address the differences by questioning the patient? That approach will certainly expose her lack of cultural knowledge! Will exposing her ignorance reduce her professional credibility? Or, will questioning make the patient uncomfortable? Worse yet, what if the patient rejects her because of her cultural ignorance?

When cultural differences are involved in a therapeutic relationship, the history and customs of the patient become an integral part of the interaction—a focus for communication. The exploration and integration of factual knowledge about each other's backgrounds and cultures, however, is not enough. It takes a solid commitment on the part of the therapist, and of the clinic, to willingly take risks and live with the possibility of making embarrassing mistakes. When providing health care services across difference, the goals are to create (1) a clinical space strong enough to hold everyone's differences as well as (2) an effective one-to-one therapeutic alliance. Attention to the following conditions[1] supports cross-cultural communication and promotes the therapeutic alliance across difference.[36,40,41] These conditions are:

- Ensuring an atmosphere of safety
- Developing a mutual relationship
- Understanding the patient's/client's world
- Integrating cross-cultural knowledge
- Respect through nonjudgmental acceptance
- Crossing social barriers
- Confronting microaggressions
- Partnering within a common identity group
- Developing social identity

Ensuring an Atmosphere of Safety

Safety for the patient emerges from the therapist's empathic rapport that includes kindliness, a warmth or positive regard for the patient or client, and acceptance of the patient's feelings and frame of reference.[19,22] Consistent with the communication skills necessary for a therapeutic relationship, the therapist approaches the patient with a genuineness that is verified by congruence between verbal and nonverbal communication. Empirical evidence illustrates that empathy, as a component of therapeutic alliance, contributes to therapeutic change in counseling, regardless of theoretical orientation.[19] The safety that emerges from the empathic relationship encourages the patient to engage in the risk-taking necessary to the mutual sharing inherent in the therapeutic alliance.

One of the goals of providing health care services across difference is to create a clinical space that is safe enough to hold everyone's difference. In identifying difference, engaging with it, and creating safety, we are affecting other people through our modeling of alternative behaviors for relating to people of difference.[36] By modeling behaviors that support patient and client safety, others within our work environments will also do so, thus changing the clinical environment.[36,p134]

Developing a Mutual Relationship

As previously described, mutuality is encouraged when the therapist is available to perceive and react caringly to the patient's interpersonal behaviors. The therapeutic alliance asks the therapist to focus on the patient or client and not on him- or herself. The product of mutuality is partnership in setting goals collaboratively and attaining effective therapeutic outcomes. Yet, developing a mutual relationship across difference poses some unique challenges, particularly if the patient and the practitioner identify with differing social groups.

Differences in social positioning may interfere with developing an equal partnership. As an example, the hierarchical nature of the traditional health care system works against the mutual partnering necessary to the therapeutic alliance. The traditional model of practitioner-patient interaction positions the practitioner in a paternalistic role as she or he identifies problems and prescribes solutions with a focus upon the disease or condition and attributes little weight to the patient's concerns or beliefs.[31] Purtilo and Haddad[5] acknowledge that the traditional model of health care positions the practitioner in a position of authority. They warn that "by strictly following the interview model of communication, the health professional effectively controls the introduction and progression of topics. This pattern of communication involves *the use of power and authority but remains largely hidden from awareness"* (italics added).[5,p159] The power-over practice of positional authority creates a dichotomous "us" (practitioner) versus "them" (patient) mindset that prevents the collaboration and negotiation necessary for mutual decision making about plans of care and treatment goals. This duality interferes with granting autonomous decision making to the patient and, instead, supports the concept of compliance to the detriment of adherence. Consequently, the establishment of an us-versus-them duality acts to undermine the health care practitioner's effectiveness in promoting patient self-responsibility for health and wellness.[5]

Recognizing how the dominant positioning of the physical therapist may prevent patients from mutually participating in the creation of their own treatment goals, physical therapist Sandra Kaplan notes that "the power of the traditional clinician-patient relationship may also leave the patient feeling intimidated."[42,p32] Intimidation risks limiting questions or expressions of disagreement. Studies of therapeutic alliances in counseling environments found that in the presence of therapists who unknowingly, or knowingly, asserted their power dominance, patient adherence that looked like the mutual collaboration indicative of a therapeutic alliance may instead have been a passive submission to the therapist's position of authority.[21,p287] When passive submission replaces mutual agreement, adherence to a plan of care, and hence patient outcomes, are further placed in jeopardy. A conceptual exploration of "power" may help to better understand the conditions necessary for equal participation in a collaborative effort. Power can be viewed in two ways.[43] The traditional configuration of power assumes that power is centralized, so it flows in a top-down direction. Centralized power is primarily prohibitive or repressive, thereby producing resistance.[44] For example, traditional power understands women activists as resisting the oppressive forces of a patriarchal hierarchy.

In contrast to this traditional view, Foucault[45] regards power as something produced in and by social relationships. This productive power can oppress; but, more importantly, it can also produce a power that is transmitted through knowledge and discourse. Productive power regards women activists as active participants in sharing power through collaborative efforts.

In considering the use of power to promote equality, it is useful to think about three distinctions proposed by philosopher Amy Allen[46]: (1) the power-over, (2) the power-to, and (3) power-with. Power-over, or domination, is defined as "... the ability of an actor or set of actors to constrain the choices of another actor ... in a nontrivial way and in a way that works to the others' disadvantage.[46,p125] Power-over is frequently exercised without intention. For instance, power over women is exercised by men "who deliberately intend *not* to do so." Power-over is often unrecognized by the person who holds it. In contrast, the power-to, or empowerment, is described as "... the ability of an individual actor or actors to attain an end or series of ends."[46,p126] Power-to is used by an individual for his or her own benefit, such as empowering the self to challenge a slight; or it can be possessed, delegated, or handed over to someone else, such as when empowering a patient to question his physician. This form of power-to is evident when negotiating. In negotiations, one person is empowered to enter into an agreement with another. The third sense of power, power-with, is the "ability of a collectivity to act together for the attainment of an agreed-upon end or series of ends."[46,p127] Power-with works in concert with others, so it is exercised in interaction and not possessed by an individual.[44] Thus, power-with occurs as a product of dialogue, is characterized by reciprocity, and is a product of partnership, and in that way it becomes an expandable resource.

When the power-with processes of collaboration and equal participation do not work within a therapeutic alliance, empowering and negotiation may. The end product of negotiation is an alternative plan or alternative goals that emerge through compromise. Negotiated compromise may be achieved by using the influence (power-to) gained from within the patient's network of family or friends. Power-to processes are less desirable than the use of power-with, but the resultant mutuality—the working together to determine goals and intervention tasks—can be just as effective whether the togetherness occurs through collaborative efforts or through negotiation.[23] What may be lost is the patient's self-responsibility for determining his own informed choices. The patient's compromised autonomy risks perpetuating the practitioner-patient duality that creates the us-versus-them dynamic in which the "them" is viewed as "less than" in terms of knowledge, skills, experience, and power. This duality defines patients as the problem rather than as partners in a solution, hence preventing the mutuality necessary for bridging difference.

A deeper discussion of how power and authority create privilege and marginalization is presented in Allan Johnson's book *Privilege, Power, and Difference*[36] (listed under recommended readings at the end of this chapter). Privilege exists when one group has something of value that is denied to another group (such as knowledge, professional status, access to health care, a well-paying job, health insurance); hence privilege is understood to occur at "someone else's expense and always exacts a cost."[36,p8] In theories of privilege and power, membership in either the privileged group or the marginalized group is ascribed simply on the basis of social identity or social categories. As a result, privilege is typically unearned and often unconsciously assumed, so its competitive advantage is not acknowledged.[47]

Privilege is also recognized as conferring dominance, meaning that it gives one group power over another, such as men controlling conversations with women based on the cultural belief that men have the right to dominate women.[36,47] Or as noted above, the authoritative power of health care practitioners may confer dominance over patients. Such dominant control then creates a dynamic of oppression by limiting the voice, engagement, and participation of the patient. In our current society, dominance is too often ascribed to those who have membership in the privileged categories of white, male, Christian, educated, middle through upper class, heterosexual, and able-bodied. In situations where the patient and therapist's social positioning is discordant, the potential and unconscious power differential between the two may interfere with establishing the mutual relationship that is so very vital to the therapeutic alliance.

Understanding the Patient's/Client's World

Earlier, Sarah was wondering whether to directly question immigrant patients about their history and customs; she was relieved to learn that exploring those cultural differences should be a focus for communication. Only through the identification of relevant patient attributes can she begin to understand how the patient's health problem interferes with life and role functions. The patient's values, beliefs, identity (including social roles), cultural mores, and rituals and their cultural meanings are best explored in dialogue with the patient through gentle, caring inquiry to better understand the individual's health care customs and assumed roles. An interview is less effective for such a cultural exploration; the interview as a fact-finding mechanism may risk alienating the patient.[5] Instead, anthropologist Arthur Kleinman[48] suggests a series of questions that can sensitively probe how an individual's cultural beliefs and customs influence his or her perception of the health problem. (See Self-Assessment at the end of the chapter for the list of Kleinman's questions.) Since these questions are designed to elicit the patient's explanatory model, they may be more effective once the patient exhibits willingness to share openly.

In facilitating the patient's sharing, Sarah learned to share her own stories that contributed to a relevant therapeutic point. Story-telling, or narrative, is a way to use the personal for understanding and for giving meaning to a situation. Narrative reveals experience, context, motives, emotions, actions, and consequences.[49,50] In using a personal disclosure strategy, the therapist models openness while at the same time using the story to emphasize a therapeutic point, verify the patient's perspective, manage the patient's vulnerabilities and emotions, reiterate a therapeutic instruction, or provide encouragement. Sarah found that her use of narrative prompted the patient's story-telling, which required a different type of active listening since narrative does not explicitly or linearly identify key facts. Instead, stories reveal the patient's perceptions that may only symbolically relate to the health problem and intervention.

Integrating Cross-Cultural Knowledge

Armed with the facts about Somali customs and beliefs, immigration history, and life in the United States, Sarah found that she could use this information with individual patients and their families to question, identify, and build upon commonly held values. She used her cross-cultural knowledge to find common points of agreement, whether addressing a plan of care or goals or a common value or sentiment.

Respecting Through Nonjudgmental Acceptance

Respecting the patient is an ethical responsibility of all physical therapists and other health care practitioners. Health care practitioners also readily assume the professional responsibility of providing the best care possible for each patient. When establishing a therapeutic alliance across cultural differences, respecting the patient and providing best care take on an added dimension. To maximize outcome effectiveness, the health care practitioner must nonjudgmentally accept what the patient is *willing to do* within the therapeutic relationship even if that compromises professional knowledge concerning best care practices. Nonjudgmental acceptance means that we build upon what the patient is willing to do in order to provide the best care that is possible given the unique parameters of that particular situation.

Crossing Social Barriers

Sarah assumed, in working with Somali immigrant women, that she could consciously and intentionally develop the skills needed to form effective cross-cultural relationships with her patients and clients by following the recommendations above. Yet, in reading about health disparities, she realized the power of unconscious attitudes to disrupt the finest intentions to provide the best health care. Sarah wondered how easy it was to be nonjudgmental.

The IOM reports referenced at the beginning of this chapter implicate the psychological factors of provider prejudice and stereotyping as contributors to health disparities,[12,13] despite clear evidence that obvious and blatant racism and other bigotries had decreased substantially in North America over the past 50 years while conscious beliefs in democratic equality and integration had achieved widespread social endorsement.[10,11,51,52] Many social science and psychological research studies have explored the discrepancy between reported reductions in the expression of prejudices, increases in expressions of egalitarian values, and health care disparity. One explanation accepted by many researchers is that egalitarian values operate on a conscious level, thereby mediating overt practices of explicit racism, stereotyping, and discrimination.[10,11,14,51–54] Whites, and members of other dominant groups, have become more aware of the social norms against explicit biases and so have become more guarded about the public expression of prejudice. This explains the consistently high numbers of health care practitioners who self-report no or low racial or minority prejudices.[10,11,51] Consequently, contemporary racism has become a less conscious and more indirect form of prejudice, hence more implicit. Implicit racism and prejudices take the form of anxiety and discomfort, which lead to avoidance rather than open hatred and contempt.[10,11] All of us, regardless of background, are products of our society and as such inadvertently assume and exhibit the implicit biases that potentially interfere in our interactions with people, patients, and clients of difference.

In an attempt to better understand how implicit biases work, psychological research has identified the differing ways that explicit and implicit biases influence behavior.[10,11,14,51–54] Explicit prejudices are those deliberately expressed in social situations with little threat against their expression; implicit biases are generally unconscious and expressed subtly or nonverbally through, for example, gestures, tone of voice, and lack of eye contact. The power of implicit biases to influence interactions lies in their invisibility to the perpetrator, and sometimes to the recipient.[10] Because implicit biases are so hidden, recipients find that they are difficult to confront, leading to greater frustration, stronger perceptions of discrimination, and more anger than when exposed to explicit racism.[10,11,14,51] The invisible and often unintentional nature of implicit prejudices is difficult to describe and quantify, yet recent cognitive studies substantiate IOM's supposition that implicit biases held by health care providers do indeed contribute to minority patients' perception of discrimination in the health care environment.[10,11,14,51–54] (For a demonstration of how implicit attitudes are measured, go to www.implicit.harvard.edu.) Consequently, the implicit biases of health care providers, plus the patients' mistrust of the health care system borne of perceived discrimination, both singly and together contribute to the emergence of health disparities.[10,51]

Confronting Microaggressions

Two well-known diversity research groups describe the everyday behaviors that emerge from implicit biases and contribute to minorities' perception of discrimination. The psychologist Derald Wing Sue and his research team explain that implicit biases tend to produce power inequalities in interactions between two people holding membership in discordant social groups.[52] In the business world, such power differences are called "microinequities," which describe the pattern of being underrepresented, overlooked, and devalued because of one's participation in a minority group. Power inequities may also be perpetuated through subtle forms of racism called racial microaggressions, denigrating and nonverbal messages to people of difference who simply belong to a differing minority group.[52] While these exchanges are frequently viewed by the dominant person as innocuous or inconsequential, the subtle snub, dismissive look, gestures, and tone of voice are perceived by the person of difference as hostile, derogatory, or as a negative slight. Research reveals that such microaggressions happen daily to many people of difference, sapping the psychic and spiritual energy of the recipient and thereby impairing performance.[52] Microaggressions create a dynamic that perpetuates inequities between the perpetrator and the recipient; in the clinic, the inadvertent racial, gender, religious, ethnic, or other discriminatory slight will clearly prevent the mutual and reciprocal bond so essential to the therapeutic alliance and thereby prevent the attainment of therapeutic goals. Table 6.1 provides some examples of racial and other microaggressions that may occur in the clinic.

Partnering Within a Common Identity Group

The research group of John Dovidio, Louis Penner, and Samual Gaertner, plus others, provides substantial evidence that implicit biases emerge from the simple classification of people into ingroups and outgroups, thereby creating an "us"/"they" dynamic.[10,11,14,51,55–57] People acquire a group, or collective, identity based on the perception that they share a common heritage with a particular social group "from which the person acquires a sense of self; by which society

Table 6.1	Examples of Racial (and Other Prejudicial) Microaggressions	
Theme	**Microaggression**	**Message**
Alien in own land The assumption that a person of a different race, ethnicity or religion is foreign-born	A white client does not want to work with an Asian American therapist because "she will not understand my problem." A white therapist tells an American-born Latino client that he/she should seek a Spanish-speaking therapist. A Christian therapist asks a Muslim patient what life is like in the Mid East countries.	You are not an American.
Ascription of intelligence Assigning a degree of intelligence to a person of difference on the basis of race	A clinical instructor reacts with surprise when an Asian American student has trouble with the math in a kinesiology problem. A rehabilitation counselor expresses surprise that a black college student makes straight A's.	All Asians are smart and good at math. It is unusual for people of color to succeed.
Color-blindness Statements indicating that a white person does not want to acknowledge race	A therapist insists that she treats everyone the same, recognizing only similarities and ignoring differences. A client of color expresses concern in discussing racial issues with her therapist. Her therapist replies with, "When I see you, I don't see color."	Race and culture are not important variables that affect people's lives. Your racial experiences are not valid.
Denial of individual racism A statement made when whites renounce their racial biases	A client of color expresses hesitancy in discussing racial issues with his white female therapist. She replies, "I understand. As a woman, I face discrimination also."	Your racial oppression is no different than my gender oppression.
Second-class citizen Occurs when a privileged (white) person is given preferential treatment over a person of difference	A white therapist spends more time treating white patients, and tends to choose white patients over patients of difference. Patients of difference are not welcomed or warmly acknowledged by the clinic's receptionist.	Those belonging to the privileged groups (whites, middle-class, insured, educated) are more valued than people of difference.
Assumption of criminality A person of color is presumed to be dangerous, criminal, or deviant on the basis of race.	The therapist assumes that the Native American patient has a history of alcoholism. The therapist asks another therapist to be present when treating a black patient because she is afraid to be alone in the clinic with him.	You are deviant. You are a criminal.

Data from: Sue DW, Capodilupo CM, Torino GC, et al. Radical microaggressions in everyday life: Implications for clinical practice. Amer Psychol. 2007;62(4):271–286.

socializes, appraises, or makes sense of the person; and by which the person makes sense of herself or himself."[58,p283] A strong, and salient, social identification with an ingroup predicts for prejudicial attitudes toward an outgroup. The bias against the outgroup becomes stronger the more positive the attitude toward the ingroup, but this bias tends, instead, to be expressed as a pro-ingroup bias rather than an anti-outgroup bias.

To mitigate the implicit biases emerging from ingroup allegiances, Dovidio et al suggest a recategorization of the relationship between the health care practitioner and the patient in order to transform their representation of themselves to a more inclusive "we." Their research reveals that the creation of a common ingroup identity reduces implicit biases that threaten interactions between peoples of difference.[10,11,14,51,55,57] These researchers propose that a Common Ingroup Identity Model which unites the practitioner and the patient in collaborative decision making about the nature of the medical problem, the goals of intervention, and the roles of the practitioner and the patient—in other words, a therapeutic alliance—would combat the biases and prejudices that contribute to health care disparities.[10,51] Understanding the normal psychological processes for developing ingroup identities, a process described by social identity theory, will aid in understanding the importance of the Common Ingroup Identity Model to the development of the therapeutic alliance.[37–39,49,50,56,58–68]

Developing Social Identity

Many theories and models[56,58,61–64,68] describe the development of social identities for specific, or for bicultural or multicultural, social groups, but two models, described by Janet Helms,[56,63] illustrate the development of nonminority and minority group identity. Both of these models reveal that race, including whiteness, is a valuable means for understanding and personalizing issues of power and privilege. The developmental process illustrated in Helms's racial identity model is similar to that of other minority and cultural identities.

Given the predominance of white physical therapy clinicians, faculty, and students in U.S. physical therapy clinics and classrooms (Table 6.2), it is instructive to look at the development

Table 6.2	**Percentages of APTA Members, Faculty, Students and Graduates Who Report Being Caucasian**	
	Physical Therapist	**Physical Therapist Assistants**
APTA membership (in October 2005)*	88.8%	88.2%
Core plus Adjunct Faculty (in 2004–2005)**,***	91.4%	92.3%
Graduating Student (in 2005)**,***	81.1%	78.6%
Enrolled Students (in 2006–2007)**,**	81.2%	78.3%

*American Physical Therapy Association. (2006). *Membership demographics: Ethnicity.* Alexandria, VA: American Physical Therapy Association. Retrieved July 8, 2007 at www.apta.org
**American Physical Therapy Association. (2007). *2005–2006 fact sheet: Physical therapist education programs.* Alexandria, VA: American Physical Therapy Association. Retrieved July 8, 2007 at www.apta.org
***American Physical Therapy Association. (2007). *2005–2006 fact sheet: Physical therapist assistant education programs.* Alexandria, VA: American Physical Therapy Association. Retrieved July 8, 2007 at www.apta.org

of white identity as an example of how privilege becomes socially ascribed to individuals. Helms's[56,38,63,67,69] model describes six statuses through which white individuals move as they abandon racist attitudes and develop a nonracist white identity: contact, disintegration, reintegration, pseudo-independence, immersion/emersion, and autonomy.

Status 1: Contact: Individuals in Status 1: Contact make contact with people of color while being unaware of cultural and institutional racism. Consequently, Status 1 individuals view race as unimportant and instead believe that people of color should be treated simply as human beings. These individuals are comfortable with the way things are racially and with their own white privilege until they come in contact with people of difference. Practitioners and patients in the Contact status who are caring and well meaning may consciously adopt a color-blind orientation out of a fear of being termed racist or bigoted; if they deny race, they cannot be accused of racism.[10,11,14] Unfortunately, whites who espouse being color-blind may alienate minority group members by denying the other's social and cultural identity.[10,11,14] People who have limited contact with people of difference may remain in this stage.

Status 2: Disintegration: Once an individual experiences racial dilemmas and acknowledges inequality among races, then that individual moves into Status 2: Disintegration. At the stage of disintegration, an individual is conflicted about being white and so experiences a sense of discomfort, shame, guilt, and anxiety about racial inequalities. To alleviate the incongruity between what society teaches about race (all people are equal) and what is observed (such as racism, sexism, homophobia), this person may adopt the perspective that white privilege is justified (thereby strengthening outgroup biases) or deny that discrimination exists. The practitioner or patient holding the beliefs indicative of the disintegration status may not be able to enter or build the cross-cultural therapeutic alliance.

Status 3: Reintegration: With the conscious acknowledgement of a white identity, the individual moves into Status 3: Reintegration. At this point, the individual succumbs to societal pressure for maintaining the status quo, accepting the belief in white superiority and racial inferiority. The individual in reintegration may hold onto racist values until another event forces the questioning of racial inequality.

Status 4: Pseudo-Independence: Movement into Status 4: Pseudo-Independence is signaled by the intellectual questioning of racist beliefs and unequal treatment. The individual repudiates white superiority but may unwittingly perpetuate institutional and cultural racism by blaming outgroup members for discrimination, thereby holding the victim (instead of the privileged dominant group) responsible for changing society. From this position, advocacy for social change relies upon change in the outgroup member's behavior, such as expecting the person of color to conform to white society, a position that inadvertently risks undermining the outgroup member's own sense of social identity.

Status 5: Immersion/Emersion: With the awareness that whites must engage in changing dominant practices, individuals move into Status 5: Immersion/Emersion to search for a more comfortable way to change not only their own but others' racist beliefs. Sarah, our new therapist, concerned about working with disenfranchised populations, is in the immersion/emersion stage. By acknowledging her lack of experience with interracial and multicultural environments, she also acknowledges her discomfort while firmly committing to best care practices. Her search for more knowledge concerning the language, beliefs, values, and practices of these groups of difference will help her to adapt her behavior to the cultural needs of her patients.

Status 6: Autonomy: The last step in unlearning racism, Status 6: Autonomy, is the acceptance of a newly defined sense of one's own whiteness. With race no longer a threat, privilege can be extended to all others, and oppression can be confronted. The individual in the autonomy status more easily creates alliances with people of color and with other groups of difference in working to eliminate all forms of oppression. Marsha in Sarah's story, who is the owner of the women's clinic and a strong advocate for improving health care for women of differing ethnicities, sexual orientation, and class, is in the autonomy status. Marsha's stage of development of racial identity allows her to support multicultural competency and health equity.[39,56,65,66] She understands that forming alliances across cultural differences is an ongoing process of questioning her own beliefs and of remaining open to the values and practices of groups of difference.

Helms[56,67] expanded her white racial-identity model to include all people of color and ethnic backgrounds. Because all minority groups tend to adopt society's dominant prejudices, Helms maintained that minority identity development involves "overcoming internalized societal racial stereotypes and negative self- and own-group conceptions."[56,p189] The minority identity model describes the resocialization process through five levels of sequential development.

- **Status 1:** Conformity relates to Helms's white-identity contact status, where one's own racial identity is relatively invisible. Because everyone in U.S. society is susceptible to adopting the values of the dominant privileged, individuals in conformity may behave as if allegiance to white standards of merit is more important than allegiance to their own socioracial or other minority group. In the conformity status racial identity may range from a race-neutral position (race is not important) to a blatant anti-black position (the preferred white values are perpetuated).
- **Status 2:** Dissonance when a social encounter challenges his or her current identity and values. Dissonance represents the initial recognition of difference and marginalization but is marked by confusion as the individual attempts to reconcile the wish to be like the white dominant group with the desire to commit to one's socioracial, ethnic or other minority group. The individual in dissonance may exhibit anger toward whites and other dominant cultural groups and so may resist entering the therapeutic alliance with someone who represents a dominant group. This anger may persist, and grow, as the person of difference moves through the third status.
- **Status 3:** Immersion/Emersion represents the development of a strong self-identity with one's social group, which may be reflected by immersion in learning about, and trying on, the images, practices, and values of one's racial, ethnic, religious, gender, age, ability, or sexual orientation group. The consequent strong idealization and own-group commitment creates a strong ingroup bias that creates a concomitant denigration of dominant outgroup standards and values. At this point, immersion in one's culture may be high, but full identity development, representing comfort with oneself within a multicultural society, remains elusive. The person of difference may remain in immersion status, during which racial, ethnic, or other cultural difference create a duality between "us" and the dominant "them."
- **Status 4:** Internalization occurs as the individual of difference achieves comfort with his or her racial or ethnic identity. The person of difference adopts a positive racial image, enabling objective interactions with members of the dominant group. As race and culture become more important to the individual, the person of difference begins to figure out how to interact within the multicultural society without hostility. As the individual's racial or ethnic identity becomes internalized, that person can more easily engage in the mutual and reciprocal interactions necessary for the therapeutic alliance.
- With the capacity to value one's own group, the individual in the final status, **Status 5:** Integrative Awareness, can empathize and collaborate with members of other oppressed

groups in working for social justice. At this point, alliances can be formed across the boundaries of difference to work for multiculturalism and health equity.

In learning about the development of social identity, our internalized views about what it means to be male or female, white or a person of color, a Muslim or other religious affiliate, able-bodied or disabled, or of any ethnic background are exposed for analysis, transformation, and confirmation. In learning about social identity, we also become aware of our membership in more than one social category. For example, a black female graduate student with mild hemiplegic cerebral palsy holds membership in the social categories of female gender, African American race, college-educated socioeconomic class, and disability. The degree to which she is privileged or oppressed by any one social category depends upon which social identity, or intersection of multiple social identities, is visible and salient in any given social context. In applying for a job with Maine Adaptive Sports, an agency that supports recreational and team sports for people in wheelchairs, her identity as a person with a disability tends to disappear as she organizes and coaches multiple sports, whereas her disability is a source of marginalization while living on a college campus. In being acutely aware of her difference as an African American woman living in Maine (a predominantly white state), she learns to downplay her urban African American heritage by acting white and middle-class in order to "fit in," and in this way she circumvents many potentially discriminating, and hurtful, situations. In a predominantly white community, her race is salient, so she acts to unmake race as a dominant social identity, thereby modifying racial inequality in her social interactions.[70]

Knowledge of social identity development affords us the opportunity to personalize the privilege of the dominant and the oppression of the marginalized. By making visible our own racial and other group identities, we learn how patients who hold differing group identities may perceive our positions of power and privilege, and we learn how those position of power and privilege may help or hinder engagement in a cross-cultural therapeutic alliance. As importantly, knowledge of social identity formation supports efforts to redirect our and our patients' ingroup (and implicit) biases toward a common ingroup identity that would support the collaborative processes of the therapeutic alliance.

"Understanding the dynamics of the therapeutic alliance, and understanding the dynamics of interracial interaction, can provide valuable insight into how the potential biases of both providers and patients can combine to contribute to racial disparities in health care and health status."[10,p482] With an understanding of power, privilege and marginalization, with an understanding of implicit biases, and with an understanding of social identity theories, health care practitioners can better direct the dialogue to overcome the barriers presented by differences in gender, class, age, religion, ethnicity, sexual orientation, and ablement. By engaging our patients and communities of difference in this dialogue, we can build the alliances needed to change the social systems that produce health disparities.

Working Within the Borderlands

"The 'development of voice' is not an act or offering that one individual is able to give to another; far too often [the dominant group in any society] assumes the condescending attitude that the 'oppressed' people need to be enlightened. Such an assumption only re-creates the unequal social structure where the powerful are capable of determining the parameters of reality for the powerless. Instead, I am suggesting that individuals develop their own voices by coming to terms with how the sociocultural forces that surround them have altered, silenced, or distorted their histories. Difference becomes central, norms are decentered, and dialogue remains a possibility. The consequence is that we dissolve boundaries and incorporate the idea of borderlands that we all inhabit. Our struggle is constantly to cross these borders and exist in tolerable discomfort with one another as we confront difference."[35,p10]

Empirical evidence provides a few practical solutions for reducing bias in the clinical environment. Researchers engaged in the study of power and privilege, racial biases, cultural competency, and health disparities uniformly recommend multicultural education for health care practitioners as a valued strategy in overcoming the cultural barriers that interfere in effective patient-practitioner relationships.[10,11,14,56,57,71] One researcher seemed to speak for many when stating that awareness of the problem of difference is the first step to eliminating it.[14] Other recommended solutions for the problem of difference include adopting professional organization policies in support of membership diversity, student diversity, inclusive professional services, and culturally competent practices.[14] The strongest recommendation from this body of literature is for health care providers to ally with the patient of difference in order to work together as partners in solving a common health problem. Building the mutuality inherent to the therapeutic alliance not only improves intervention outcomes but allows the practitioner to join with the patient of difference in obtaining a recognized, and valued, place in society—a place that honors cultural differences while providing equitable health care that does not vary in quality based on such personal characteristics as gender, age, religion, race, ethnicity, language, social class, sexual orientation, and ablement. As the preceding quote suggests, inviting the person of difference to join you in the borderland may produce a collective that becomes strong enough to promote social change.

CONCLUSION

Evidence based practice, a major organizing construct for the practice of physical therapy, posits that the therapeutic alliance supports quality therapeutic outcomes. Reviews of psychotherapy, psychology, counseling, and physical therapy research provide substantial evidence that the characteristics of the therapeutic alliance contribute to treatment success. Unfortunately, no research exists that delineates the essential processes for forming an alliance—for identifying the specific communication strategies and behavioral guidelines that would ensure that an alliance will develop.[22] Instead, some suggest that the therapeutic alliance is a creative process in which the therapist moves beyond the basic interpersonal skills to include interpersonal perception; anticipation of the patient's uniqueness; purposeful use of empathy, openness, and experimentation in the relationship; and revision of interpersonal patterns to adapt to successful, and not so successful, interactions.[72] Assuming that the therapeutic alliance is a creative process, this chapter has provided some ideas, supporting by empirical evidence, about how to communicate willingness and intent for developing the therapeutic alliance. Understanding processes of interacting across cultural differences offers well-intentioned health care practitioners the opportunity to provide the best care to the patient of difference and reduce the health disparities that plague the U.S. health care system.

The therapeutic alliance positions the patient as a co-creator in the development of a more culturally competent health care system. Inevitably, this type of relationship is political, leading to advocacy not only for the individual patient or client but also for changes in health care and other social systems. In assuming the responsibility for political advocacy as allies with our therapeutic partners, we become moral agents for social change. Some of us may accept this as part of our professional role; some may not. But by engaging in the respectful and difficult experiences of building therapeutic alliances with those who are different from us, we return to the basics of professional behaviors: practicing respect for the feelings, culture, and needs of those who seek physical therapy services; engaging in the complexities of our profession by thoughtfully pursuing evidence based practice in consideration of individualized needs; and, promoting a future that ensures and protects the equal right to health and wellness. Perhaps there is no way for the health care professional to escape the political when building therapeutic alliances with the people of difference we serve.

SELF-ASSESSMENT

1. **Being Put in One's Place:** People with disabilities are aware that they hold a minority status in a society that views ablement as a norm. This perceived social position enters the therapeutic alliance, often invisibly, producing inequalities in the perceived privileged status of the practitioner and of the patient. From this "less than" position, the patient or client may be oversensitive to your privileged position as a health care practitioner, leading to resistance or to "evening the score" by "putting you in your place." In treating the patient who is significantly different from you, have you ever experienced being "put in your place" as the patient:

- Makes a sexist remark about your gender?
- Suggests that you are poorly prepared to treat him or her because you are so young? Too old? Or, a woman?
- Disparagingly remarks upon someone else's color and you are a person of a different racial group?
- Undermines your knowledge with a dismissive comment about how college-educated people are "know-it-alls"?

    As this happened, did you consider that the patient may be unmaking your perceived privileged status by highlighting one of his or her perceived privileged social identities and demeaning one of your social identities? Such an unmaking of your privilege then puts the two of you on a more even basis so that the patient can feel more at ease with his or her perceived diminished status. Given a more equal social positioning, the patient may then more easily accept your services.

    If you accept that this power dynamic may have been functioning when you were "put in your place," how could you have responded in order to emphasize the equality of your therapeutic partnership with that patient or client?

2. **Thought for Consideration: Exploring the Patient's Cultural Values:** Kleinman[48] offers the following questions as part of his Explanatory Model:
    a. What do you call the problem?
    b. What do you think caused the problem?
    c. Why do you think it started when it did?
    d. What do you think the sickness does? How does it work?
    e. How severe is the sickness? Will it have a short or long course?

f. What kind of treatment do you think the patient should receive? What are the most important results you hope he/she receives from this treatment?

g. What are the chief problems the sickness has caused?

h. What do you fear most about the sickness?

Imagine how Sarah would introduce Kleinman's questions (for eliciting the patient's explanatory model) while in conversation. Would she introduce the questions as part of the interview or as part of a dialogue? Think of a patient exchange you have had and consider how you would have introduced these questions.

CONTINUED LEARNING

There are many excellent texts that explore the topics of this chapter. Select one of them from the Annotated Bibliography that follows, and after reviewing prepare an in-service presentation for your practice highlighting its implications for patient care.

Books that focus on the exploration of privilege and power differences:

• Johnson AG. *Privilege, Power, and Difference*, 2nd ed. Boston: McGraw Hill; 2006.

By directly challenging the beliefs supporting inequalities in our society, this sociologist author teaches how to critically appraise privilege and oppression. He then offers suggestions about how to turn the reader's beliefs about justice and equality into practice. This book is invaluable in teaching about the manifestations of social power.

• Pothier D, Devlin R., eds. *Critical Disability Theory: Essays in Philosophy, Politics, Policy, and Law*. Vancouver: UBC Press; 2006.

This book of essays by 23 scholars is for the reader who is concerned about the politics and consequent legal responses targeted at persons with disabilities. While written to question Canadian politics and law, the content applies to the United States in its use of critical theory as a political analytic tool to describe disability. This book is also valuable to the educator and student who wish to understand more about social injustice in regard to disability.

• Riddell S, Watson N., eds. *Disability, Culture and Identity*. New York: Pearson Education Limited, Prentice Hall; 2003.

This well-written book summarizes current research supporting disability studies. Studies exploring the culture of disability introduce concepts about the social construction of disability, disability identity, and the politics of disability and social justice. While written from the British viewpoint, it offers much to students and educators wanting to know more about the life experiences of people who are disempowered, and empowered, by disability.

• Fine M, Asch A., eds. *Women with Disabilities: Essays in Psychology, Culture and Politics (Health, Society, and Policy)*, reprinted. Philadelphia: Temple University Press; 1990.

While the research supporting this text is slightly outdated, its seminal collection of essays reveals the double jeopardy of gender and disability that women with disabilities face, and continue to face, in U.S. society.

- Smith BG, Hutchison B. *Gendering Disability*. New Brunswick, NJ: Rutgers University Press; 2004.

This text is for the scholar and activist interested in disability studies and gender studies. The scholarship presented here describes the complicated politics and practices that emerge from the intersection of gender and disability. The complexities of identity development and subsequent integration into society are revealed not only by the study of personal experiences but by the study of the arts, consumerism, and politics.

Books that focus on learning cross-cultural communication skills:
- Latanzi JB, Purnell LD. *Developing Cultural Competence in Physical Therapy Practice*. Philadelphia: F.A. Davis Company; 2006.

This book integrates Purnell's model for cultural competence into the practice of physical therapy for guiding the development of cross-cultural communication skills. The book then presents how to apply those skills in consideration of African American/black, Chinese, Latino, American Indian, Middle Eastern, and Jewish cultures. The last chapters discuss cultural competency in working with people with disabilities, veterans, those living in poverty and homelessness, and in pediatrics and geriatrics.

- Leavitt RL. *Cross-Cultural Rehabilitation: An International Perspective*. Philadelphia: W.B. Saunders; 1999.

This book brings an international perspective to the provision of rehabilitation services by presenting information on differing health beliefs and behaviors, religious attitudes toward disabilities, poverty, racial discrimination, and cross-cultural communication. Rehabilitation professionals working internationally will gain from the content describing appropriate assistive technology, orthotics, and prosthetics in less developed countries. The focus on community health services informs the discussion of culturally competent care in Guyana, Nicaragua, Botswana, South Africa, Mexico, Romania, American Indian nations, Palestine, Vietnam, Zimbabwe, and Jamaica.

- Lynch EW, Hanson MJ. *Developing Cross-Cultural Competence: A Guide for Working with Children and Their Families*, 3rd ed. Baltimore: Paul H. Brookes Publishing Company; 2004.

This text provides educational, psychological, and rehabilitation perspectives in presenting foundational content for the development of cross-cultural competence in serving families with young children. Specific chapters discuss the cultural perspectives of families with Anglo-European, American Indian, African American, Latino, Asian, Filipino, Hawaiian, Samoan, Middle Eastern, and South Asian roots.

- Satcher D, Pamies RJ. *Multicultural Medicine and Health Disparities*. New York: McGraw-Hill Medical Publishing Division; 2006.

Written by physicians, this book presents the challenges of the health disparities existing in the United States for disenfranchised groups defined by race, gender (women's health), age (children and geriatrics), and ethnic origin (immigrants). The authors also describe existing health disparities based on pathology. The text closes with chapters discussing health policy and health services that support culturally competent care.

- Stone JH. *Culture and Disability: Providing Culturally Competent Services.* Multicultural Aspects of Counseling Series 21. Thousand Oaks, CA: Sage Publications; 2005.

While the focus of this book is on the provision of services to the immigrant population with disabilities, it offers much about the process of providing rehabilitation services to people from differing cultures, whatever ethnic heritage they may have. Specific chapters address the cross-cultural rehabilitation of disabilities for immigrants coming from China, Jamaica, Korea, Haiti, Mexico, the Dominican Republic, and Vietnam.

REFERENCES

1. Davis CM. Letters and responses: More questions than answers. Phys Ther. 2002;82(3):289–292.
2. Rothstein JM. Letters and responses: Editor's response. Phys Ther. 2002;82(3):289–292.
3. Davis CM. *Patient Practitioner Interaction: An Experiential Manual for Developing the Art of Health Care*, 4th ed. Thorofare, NJ: Slack Incorporated; 2006.
4. Drench ME, Noonan AC, Sharby N, Ventura SH. *Psychosocial Aspects of Health Care*, 2nd ed. Upper Saddle River, NJ: Prentice Hall; 2006.
5. Purtilo R, Haddad A. *Health Professional and Patient Interaction*, 6th ed. Philadelphia: W.B. Saunders Company; 2002.
6. American Physical Therapy Association. *Normative Mode of Professional Physical Therapist Education, Version 4*. Alexandria, VA: American Physical Therapy Association; 2004.
7. Sackett DL. Evidence-based medicine: What it is and what it isn't. Brit Med J. 1996;312:71–72.
8. Sackett DL. Protection for human subjects in medical research. JAMA. 2000;283(18):2388.
9. Sackett DL, Parkes J. Teaching critical appraisal: No quick fixes. CMAJ. 1998;158(2):203–204.
10. Dovidio JF, Penner LA, Albrecht TL, Norton WE, Gaertner SL, Shelton JN. Disparities and distrust: The implications of psychological processes for understanding racial disparities in health and health care. Soc Sci & Med. 2008;67(3):478–486.
11. Gaertner SL, Dovidio JF. Understanding and addressing contemporary racism: From aversive racism to the common ingroup identity model. J Soc Issues. 2005;61(3):615–639.
12. Institutes of Medicine. Report brief: What health care providers need to know about racial and ethnic disparities in healthcare. Washington, D.C.; 2002.
13. Institutes of Medicine. Unequal treatment: Confronting racial and ethnic disparities in health care. In: Smedley BD, Stith AY, Nelson AR, et al., eds. Washington, D.C.; 2003.
14. Rudman LA. Social justice in our minds, homes, and society: The nature, causes, and consequences of implicit bias. Soc Justice Res. 2004;17(2):129–142.
15. Hall ET. *The Hidden Dimension*. New York: Doubleday; 1966.
16. Gabard DL, Martin MW. *Physical Therapy Ethics*. Philadelphia: F.A. Davis Company; 2003.
17. Noddings N. The cared-for. In: Gordon S, Benner P, Noddings N, eds. *Caregiving: Readings in Knowledge, Practice, Ethics, and Politics*. Philadelphia: University of Pennsylvania Press; 1996:21–39.
18. Crits-Christoph P, Gibbons MBC. Research developments on the therapeutic alliance in psychodynamic psychotherapy. Psych Inquiry. 2003;23(2):332.

19. Feller CP, Cottone RR. The importance of empathy in the therapeutic alliance. J Humanistic Counseling, Education & Development. Spring 2003;42(1):53–61.
20. Meissner WW. Therapeutic alliance: Theme and variations. Psychoan Psych. 2007;24(2):231–254.
21. Safran JD, Muran JC. Has the concept of the therapeutic alliance outlived its usefulness? Psychotherapy: Theory, Research, Practice, Training. 2006;43(3):286–291.
22. Castonguay LG, Constantino MJ, Holtforth MG. The working alliance: Where are we and where should we go? Psychotherapy: Theory, Research, Practice, Training. 2006;43(3):271–279.
23. Erskine RG, Moursund JP, Trautmann RL. Beyond Empathy: A Therapy of Contact-in-Relationship. Ann Arbor, MI: Taylor & Francis Group, Edwards Brothers; 1999.
24. Horvath AO, Symonds BD. Relation between working alliance and outcome in psychotherapy: A meta-analysis. J Counseling Psych. 1991;38:139–149.
25. Martin DJ, Garske JP, Davis MK. Relation of the therapeutic alliance with outcome and other variables: A meta-analytic review. J Consult & Clin Psych. 2000;68:438–450.
26. Lorish CD, Gale JR. Facilitating adherence to healthy lifestyle behavior changes in patients. In: Shepard KF, Jensen GM, eds. Handbook of Teaching for Physical Therapists, 2nd ed. Boston: Butterworth Heinemann; 2002:351–386.
27. Jensen GM, Gwyer J, Hack LM, Shepard KF. Expertise in Physical Therapy Practice, 2nd ed. Boston: Butterworth-Heinemann; 2006.
28. Jensen GM, Gwyer J, Shepard KF, Hack LM. Expert practice in physical therapy. Phys Ther. 2000;80:28–52.
29. Jensen GM, Lorish CD, Shepard KF. Understanding and influencing patient receptivity to change: The patient-practitioner collaborative model. In: Shepard KF, Jensen GM, eds. Handbook of Teaching for Physical Therapists, 2nd ed. Boston: Butterworth Heinemann; 2002:323–350.
30. Resnik L, Jensen GM. Using clinical outcomes to explore the theory of expert practice in physical therapy. Phys Ther. 2003;83(12):1090–1106.
31. Barr J, Threlkeld AJ. Patient-practitioner collaboration in clinical decision-making. Physiother Res Int. 2000;5(4):254.
32. Bezold C. The future of patient-centered care: Scenarios, visions, and audacious goals. J Alt & Comp Med. 2005;11:s-77–s-84.
33. Weston WW. Informed and shared decision-making: the crux of patient-centered care. CMAJ. 2001;165(4):438–439.
34. Chez RA, Jonas WB. Challenges and opportunities in achieving healing. J Alt & Comp Med. 2005;11:s3–s6.
35. Tierney WG. Building Communities of Difference: Higher Education in the Twenty-first Century. Westport, CT: Bergin & Garvey; 1993.
36. Johnson AG. Privilege, Power, and Difference, 2nd ed. Boston: McGraw Hill; 2006.
37. Tatum BD. Talking about race, learning about racism: The application of racial identity theory in the classroom. Harv Educ Rev. 1992;62(1):1–24.
38. Tatum BD. Examining racial and cultural thinking. Educ Leadership. 2000;57(8):54.
39. Tatum BD. Building a road to a diverse society. Chron Higher Educ. 2004;50(30):B6–B7.
40. Lynch EW, Hanson MJ. Developing Cross-Cultural Competence: A Guide for Working with Children and Their Families, 3rd ed. Baltimore: Paul H. Brookes Publishing Company; 2004.
41. Satcher D, Pamies RJ. Multicultural Medicine and Health Disparities. New York: McGraw-Hill Medical Publishing Division; 2006.
42. Kaplan SL. Outcome Measurement & Management: First Steps for the Practicing Clinician. Philadelphia: F.A. Davis Company; 2007.
43. Allan EJ, Gordon SP, Iverson SV. Rethinking practices of power: The discursive framing of leadership. Chron Higher Educ.
44. Sawicki J. Disciplining Foucault: Feminism, Power, and the Body. New York: Routledge; 1991.

45. Foucault M. *Power/Knowledge: Selected Interviews and Writings, 1972–1977.* Brighton, Sussex: Harvester Press; 1980.
46. Allen A. *The power of Feminist Theory: Domination, Resistance, Solidarity.* Boulder, CO: Westview Press; 1999.
47. McIntosh P. *White Privilege: Unpacking the Invisible Knapsack.* Wellesley, MA: Wellesley Center for Research on Women, 1988;163–168.
48. Kleinman A. *Patients and Healers in the Context of Culture.* Berkeley, CA: University of California Press; 1991.
49. Adams M, Bell LA, Griffin P. *Teaching for Diversity and Social Justice.* New York: Routledge; 1997.
50. Goodman DJ. *Promoting Diversity and Social Justice.* Thousand Oaks, CA: Sage Publications, Inc.; 2001.
51. Penner LA, Dovidio JF, Edmondson D, et al. The experience of discrimination and Black-White health disparities in medical care. J Back Psych. 2009;35(2):180–203.
52. Sue DW, Capodilupo CM, Torino GC, et al. Racial microaggressions in everyday life: Implications for clinical practice. Amer Psych. 2007;62(4):271–286.
53. Quillian L. Does unconscious racism exist? Soc Psych Quar. 2008;71(1):6–11.
54. Quillian L, Cook KS, Massey DS. New approaches to understanding racial prejudice and discrimination. Ann Rev Sociol. 2006;32(1):299–328.
55. Hall NR, Crisp RJ, Mein-woei S. Reducing implicit prejudice by blurring intergroup boundaries. Basic & App Soc Psych. 2009;31(3):244–254.
56. Helms JE. An update of Helms' White and people of color racial identity models. In: Ponterotto JG, Casas JM, Suzuki LA, Alexander CM, eds. *Handbook of Multicultural Counseling.* Thousand Oaks: Sage; 1995:181–198.
57. Lun J, Sinclair S, Whitchurch ER, Glenn C. (Why) do I think what you think? Epistemic social tuning and implicit prejudice. J Person & Soc Psych. 2007;93(6):957–972.
58. Helms JE. The conceptualization of racial identity and other "racial" constructs. In: Trickett EJ, Watts RJ, Birman D, eds. *Human Diversity.* San Francisco: Jossey-Bass Publishers; 1994:285–311.
59. Leach MM, Behrens JT, LaFleur NK. White racial identity and White racial consciousness: Similarities, differences, and recommendations. *J Multicult Couns & Develop.* April 2002;30:66–80.
60. Vinson TS, Neimeyer GJ. The relationship between racial identity development and multicultural counseling competency. J Multicult Couns & Develop. Jul 2000;28(3):177–192.
61. Cross WE, Jr. The Thomas and Cross models of psychological Nigrescence: A review. J Black Psych.1978;5:13–31.
62. Cross WE, Jr. The psychology of Nigrescence: Revising the Cross model. In: Ponterotto JG, Casas JM, Suzuki LA, Alexander CM, eds. *Handbook of Multicultural Counseling.* Thousand Oaks, CA: Sage; 1995:93–122.
63. Helms JE. Toward a model of White racial identity development. In: Helms JE, ed. *Black and White Racial Identity: Theory, Research, and Practice.* Westport, CT: Greenwood Press; 1990:49–65.
64. Phinney JS. Ethnic identity in adolescents and adults: Review of research. Psych Bull. 1990;108:499–514.
65. Verkuyten M. Ethnic group identification and group evaluation among minority and majority groups: Testing the multiculturalism hypothesis. J Person & Soc Psych. 2005;88(1):121–138.
66. Worrell F. The relationship between racial and ethnic identity in Black adolescents: The Cross Racial Identity Scale and the Multigroup Ethnic Identity Measure. Identity. 2006;6(4):293–315.
67. Gordon S. Making meaning of whiteness: A pedagogical approach for multicultural education. J Phys Ther Educ. 2005;19(1):21–27.
68. Sue DW, Sue D. *Counseling the Culturally Different: Theory and Practice,* 3rd ed. New York: Wiley, 1999.
69. Evans NJ, Forney DS, Guido-DiBrito F. *Student Development in College: Theory, Research and Practice.* San Francisco: Jossey-Bass Publishers; 1998.

70. Goar CD. Social identity theory and the reduction of inequality: Can cross-cutting categorization reduce inequality in mixed-race groups? Soc Behav and Person. 2007;35(4):537–550.
71. Correll J, Park B, Smith JA. Colorblind and multicultural prejudice reduction strategies in high-conflict situations. Group Proc & Intergroup Relat. 2008;11(4):471–491.
72. Anderson T, Ogles BM, Weis A. Creative use of interpersonal skills in building a therapeutic alliance. J Construct Psych. 1999;12(4):313.

chapter 7

The Patient Interview

John L. Coulehan, MD, FACP
Marian R. Block, MD, ABFP

A very good way to find out how another person is thinking or feeling is to ask him ... At this point, however, a difficulty arises. If I am to acquire information in this way about another person's experiences, I must understand what he says about them. And this would seem to imply that I attach the same meaning to his words as he does, but how, it may be asked, can I ever be sure it is so?

—AJ AYERS

•

❋ Mr. Ketterman's Case

Is it possible to do an effective interview with a patient like Mr. Ketterman, with advanced Alzheimer's disease? Will I be able to trust the information I receive from Mr. Ketterman's wife? How can I show respect, genuineness and active listening to a patient with Alzheimer's? *(See Appendix for Mr. Ketterman's health history.)*

INTRODUCTION

In this chapter, we consider the patient interview as an essential diagnostic tool in physical therapy. We sometimes look upon patient interviewing as a simple process, just a sequence of questions and answers about symptoms and disabilities. In this view, the therapist's role is simply to know the right questions to ask. The patient's role is to respond with clear and honest answers. When this does not happen, we tend to discount the medical history in favor of more "objective" clinical data.

However, any experienced clinician will tell you that this question-and-answer model is simplistic and self-defeating. It is not at all representative of successful clinician-patient interactions. Clinical interviewing is actually a complex interactive process that can produce highly reliable data about the patient's illness or injury, while at the same time building a therapist-patient relationship that facilitates cooperation and healing.[1-4] To accomplish this, the therapist must consider illness data in the context of the patient's personhood so that judgments about (or enhancements of) its objectivity can be made. Here we discuss three aspects of the interview as a diagnostic and relationship-building tool.

THE INTERVIEW AS A DIAGNOSTIC INSTRUMENT

The Interview as a Diagnostic Instrument

- Objectivity
- Precision
- Sensitivity and Specificity
- Reliability
- Skill

Physical therapy combines the science of healing with the art of caring. These two aspects of practice intersect in the patient interview. The information learned in the interview guides further testing, therefore providing a foundation for scientific assessment and clinical reasoning. The interview is also the primary source of information about patient beliefs, values, attitudes, and circumstances. Finally, the interview is an essential tool in relationship building. For example, good communication skills are highly correlated to patient satisfaction.[5,6] Given its importance in practice, we must approach the interview with the same scientific rigor that we use in learning and practicing other tests and measures.

Physical therapy is a practical science, the science of helping people manage, reduce, and alleviate their impairments and functional limitations. The physical therapist must strive to be objective, precise, sensitive, specific, and reliable when making observations about the patient's impairment. Here we discuss these terms as they relate to understanding and interpreting patient symptoms and impairments. We also examine interviewing skills as fundamental to the art, as well as to the science, of physical therapy.

Objectivity

What does it mean to be objective in clinical interviewing? Objectivity means striving to remove one's own beliefs, prejudices, and preconceptions from observations; it involves eliminating bias or systematic distortion from one's observations. Other words for objectivity are *accuracy* and *validity*. The data you obtain should correspond to the patient's expressed experience. If, for example, you start with a preconceived notion of the illness and you discard or minimize ill-fitting items, your objectivity is compromised. Lack of objectivity is not only unscientific and could lead to missed diagnoses; it is also likely to make patients feel ignored because you have not "heard" what they said. When patients feel ignored, they often respond by becoming less forthcoming and subsequently providing less information. Clinicians sometimes prematurely record their interpretation of patient statements rather than simply describe what the patient said. If you are treating a patient with a traumatic leg injury, you may interpret all of the symptoms as related to that injury, when in fact the muscular weakness the patient reports is a symptom of steroid myopathy—the patient is taking steroids for rheumatoid arthritis—and is actually the *cause* of the fall, rather than a *result* of it.

Patients, too, sometimes confuse their primary experience of symptoms with a later interpretation of that experience. This means that the physical therapist must be able to identify such an interpretation and distinguish it from primary symptom data. The therapist must skillfully direct the patient to report actual symptoms and limitations. This does not mean the interpretation should be ignored or discarded. It is important for you to acknowledge the patient's beliefs as legitimate, whether or not you agree with them. Such recognition of the patient's point of view helps generate the therapeutic alliance and allows you to maximize opportunities for engagement and education.

Precision

Precision is a characteristic of the scientific process that relates to the random distribution of observations around the "real" value. Precise observations cluster closely around the mean, whereas imprecise observations are widely scattered. In interviewing, the basic units of observation are words. As verbal measurements, words should be precise. They should be sufficiently detailed and unambiguous to contribute usefully to diagnostic reasoning. The good interviewer attempts to discover as precisely as possible the symptom complex actually experienced by the patient.

Whereas lack of objectivity suggests a systematic bias, lack of precision suggests a pattern of random error introduced by vagueness, poor listening, or lack of attention to detail. For example, if a patient complains of being tired, does "tired" mean that the patient feels short of breath, weak, unmotivated, or sleepy? Although the clinician may correctly register the patient's words, he or she may have no idea what the words are describing unless there is sufficient detail to distinguish among these and other options. To make this distinction, the next question might go something like:

- "What do you mean by tired?"
- "Can you tell me more about this tiredness?"
- "How would you describe this feeling without using the word 'tired'?"

Sensitivity and Specificity

Objectivity and precision are two criteria by which we judge health care data, including the clinical history. Two additional criteria are sensitivity and specificity. The sensitivity of a test expresses its ability to "pick up" real causes of the disease in question. The higher the test's sensitivity, the greater will be the percentage of cases accurately identified by the test. Specificity, on the other hand, refers to a test's ability to "rule out" disease in normal people. The higher the specificity, the greater is the likelihood that a negative test result identifies a person who does not have the disease. Few tests approach 100% sensitivity and specificity; certainly the interview will not yield such definitive information. Nonetheless, thinking of the interview in these terms helps us to maximize the usefulness of symptom data.

A symptom may be extremely sensitive (e.g., the great majority of patients with carpal tunnel syndrome experience numbness or tingling in the hand) but not in itself very specific (several medical conditions may cause numbness or tingling). Rarely, a symptom may have high sensitivity *and* specificity. The report of shaking the hand to get relief from nerve pain in the hand (the Flick Test) is both specific and sensitive in making the diagnosis of carpal tunnel syndrome. When this happens we call the symptom pathognomonic. These examples are somewhat artificial, though, because individual symptoms are rarely appropriate units on which to base decisions. In clinical practice we deal, rather, with symptom complexes, patterns, or stories. If you achieve mastery of common symptom complexes, your diagnostic interview may have high predictive value.[7] However, if you, the clinician, lack objectivity and precision, you will find it difficult to delineate symptom complexes well enough to assess their sensitivity and specificity.

It is important to consider the patient's whole story. A detailed reconstruction of the patient's illness, rather than isolated statements about symptoms—not just one symptom, but many; not just one point in time, but the whole story—will help you to make a better diagnosis.[8-10] A complete symptom complex may well be quite sensitive and specific; it may be adequate, in fact, to serve as the basis for diagnosis and therapy. Even when a thorough health history does not contain enough information to make a final diagnosis, it permits you to substantially narrow the range of possible problems and results in a small number of hypotheses to be ruled out, supported, or confirmed by physical examination and further studies. The well-conducted patient interview will usually yield a firm database on which to design an efficient diagnostic plan. To achieve this result, however, the clinician must approach the task objectively and precisely.

Reliability

Reliability, or reproducibility, is another important characteristic of scientific tests, including interviewing. A test is reliable when different observers are able to obtain the same results given the same condition or situation. With the clinical history, however, reproducibility is often tempered by several considerations about human nature and the interactive process.

Sometimes in caring for a hospitalized patient, three or four observers may obtain three or four different versions of the patient's story. Many of these differences may not be of great importance, but at times they will be crucial. This raises the issue of how reliable patients' reports are. If the story cannot be replicated, is it suspect? Apparent lack of reproducibility in history taking makes some clinicians question its value. However, when you consider the process more carefully, it becomes apparent that there are several good reasons why medical histories "evolve."

Why Medical Histories "Evolve"

Patients Learn to Tell a Good Story
Patients Recall New Information
Patients Have Beliefs about Their Illnesses
Patients Change Their Stories

Patients Learn to Tell a Good Story

Every patient comes to the hospital or the clinic with a personal story that includes various symptoms and concerns, but patients often do not have a point of reference indicating which of these are more or less important in explaining their condition. A severe headache may cause more pain than a sudden swelling of the left leg, even though the latter might actually have serious health implications (e.g., lymphatic obstruction by metastatic cancer), whereas the former may not be significant. Each time a patient relates the story, he or she learns, by virtue of questions asked and interviewer response, what items concern the interviewer most. The patient learns, in a sense, to "package" the story to make it more efficient or relevant or interesting to the clinician. Therefore, later observers may get a more clearly connected and flowing history, incorporating details more relevantly, than will the first interviewer.

Patients Recall New Information

A corollary to this educational process is that patients may also report symptoms that they had not mentioned originally. For example, the patient may not have reported falling from a bicycle 2 weeks earlier because he had forgotten it. Repetition and focusing may not only make the story more coherent but may also refresh the patient's memory or set the stage for a new connection. Therefore, later observers may record information that the patient neglected to mention earlier.

Patients Have Beliefs About Their Illnesses

Patients, especially those who are seriously or chronically ill or disabled, have usually organized their understanding of their condition in a way that makes sense to them before they see the clinician. They may have treated themselves or asked for advice from family or friends. They may have read health columns in newspapers, seen a commentator on TV, or searched the Internet for information. In addition, patients may have religious or cultural beliefs that frame their understanding of illness in general and their own condition in particular (see Chapter 6). In these ways, patients develop a framework for understanding their problems and what can or should be done about them. Consequently, they may tell their stories within a framework that makes them consistent with their beliefs and expectations. In such cases the primary data—perceived symptoms—are filtered through the patient's health belief system. Yet, in the process of being interviewed by several different clinicians focusing on strict health care hypotheses, a patient's beliefs about the data may change. When this happens, the narrative's elements—perceptions, symptoms, and attributions—may also change.

Patients Change Their Stories

Different observers may also record different histories because the patient simply and consciously changes the story. Clinicians often invoke this reason when they dislike the patient or cannot understand the narrative. The more the symptoms seem to be unrelated to the therapist's diagnostic test results, the more likely the therapist will consider these symptoms exaggerated or even imaginary and, therefore, susceptible to change from one interviewing session to another. Although some patients, of course, are careless or wish to mislead the clinician, this type of unreliability is a much less frequent cause of inconsistency than the cognitive factors described.

Skill

Most importantly for our purposes, interviewing skills also play a part in the reliability of the clinical history.[10] Skills that maximize objectivity and precision produce more accurate data and reduce false-positive (making a diagnosis that is not there) and false-negative (missing the diagnosis) rates. A skilled clinician who lets the patient tell his or her story and listens carefully is more likely to obtain an accurate picture than is a clinician who asks a list of questions by rote.[11,12] While skill bears a strong relationship to experience, it is also clear that an inexperienced student who has sufficient time to spend with a patient in a nonthreatening atmosphere may at times learn a lot more than a hurried clinical instructor.

ESTABLISHING A THERAPEUTIC RELATIONSHIP

The same techniques that help you achieve objectivity and precision in gathering data also facilitate your connection with the patient in a therapeutic relationship. The interdependence of science and art in clinical practice is much like the interdependence in most art forms, such as music or painting, which require both theory and execution as preconditions to producing something of beauty. Is there a contradiction between a "just get the facts" interview and an

---

Box 7.1 Active Listening Skills

You can connect with your patient through active listening. The following skills will help you to establish a therapeutic relationship.

- Choose a mutually comfortable setting.
- Remain quiet and attentive.
- Observe the patient respectfully as a whole person, and not just as a talker, or a diseased body, or a barrier to your lunch break.
- Allow the patient to tell the story with as few interruptions as possible.
- Listen for the primary symptom data.
- Assess the patient's words for accuracy and precision.
- Listen to the patient's inflection, tone, and pauses (paralanguage).
- Note discrepancies between what the patient says and how he or she says it, and discrepancies between the patient's words and gestures.
- Listen carefully for the patient's interpretation of the problem, for example, "I think I have a brain tumor."
- Do not confuse interpretation with description of symptoms.
- Avoid forming your own theory about the patient's illness until you obtain a precise description of the symptoms and a coherent narrative.

---

artful interview? No, when properly performed they are the same. You are unlikely to obtain a good history without utilizing active listening skills (Box 7.1). Active listening allows you to achieve objectivity and precision and is also the first step toward establishing a therapeutic relationship.

A patient's own words can best demonstrate how science and art go hand in hand, The following excerpt is part of an interview in which the patient describes how it feels to be listened to and understood:

Patient: Aw, I'm not usually able to talk to people like this. I don't really know you.

Clinician: That's true. I'm a total stranger.

Patient: And all of a sudden I have gone completely down the line and told you everything I could possibly think of to tell you. I've never been able to do that. I have very few people that I talk to personally or talk to about the way I feel … um … I talk to my family but there are only certain things that you can talk to your family about, and I have never had anyone I could talk to. I have always kept everything to myself. And now, all of a sudden, I've just flowed over like a broken toilet.

Clinician: Was it helpful?

Patient: Yes, because I just learned something else about myself. The funny thing is, I have said all these things to you, and most times talking to people, I always think before I talk. I have said everything I have said to you without thinking about it first, and without wondering what you are going to think about what I am saying to you. And I can honestly say that I have never done that with anyone.

Clinician: Uh huh.

Patient:	I ... um ... have, maybe, I have a lot of friends but I mean, I even, I even think before I say what I say to them because there's always a chance that someone misinterprets.
Clinician:	Well, I'm glad. Because I like to think it's helpful.
Patient:	It really is. I feel quite good about the whole thing.[4, p. 16–17]

This patient describes being able to say everything "without thinking about it first." He describes his ability to reveal uncensored data that are vital to the diagnostic process; he was able to do this because he wasn't "wondering what you are going to think about what I am saying to you." This is precisely the aim of competent clinical history taking.

"One thing that I think I've really improved on with practice is shutting up and listening, and that was real hard for me to do. It isn't really a problem getting the parents to tell you about the child. It's mostly just giving them the permission to tell you and acknowledging—honoring—what they say." Pediatric Physical Therapist Expert Practitioner, Jensen, et al. 2007.

THE INTERVIEW IN BUILDING A THERAPEUTIC RELATIONSHIP

Respect, genuineness, and empathy are three core qualities in clinical interviewing (Fig. 7-1).[4] When you first encounter these terms, they may seem to describe personality characteristics, rather than learnable and teachable skills. However, psychologists long ago discovered that each of these attributes can be analyzed into a set of microskills.[13, 14] In health care education we often use the term *competencies*.[15–17] Thus, for our purposes, respect, genuineness, and empathy are subcompetencies under the aegis of professionalism and interpersonal skills.

- Respect is the ability to accept the patient as he or she is.
- Genuineness is the ability to be congruent in your professional role.
- Empathy is the ability to understand the patient's experiences and feelings accurately; it also includes demonstrating that understanding to the patient.

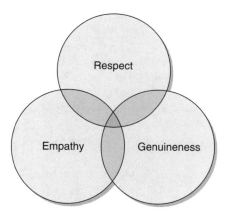

Figure 7-1 Core Qualities of a Clinician Interviewer.

Unfortunately, in clinical education we often evoke and praise these competencies in what we say to students (the explicit curriculum) but negate them in our behavior with patients (the hidden curriculum), so that the student gets mixed messages.[18–20]

Respect

You communicate respect by accepting a patient's traits and beliefs regardless of your personal feelings about them and by acknowledging a patient's emotions and behavior as a valid adaptation to their illness or life circumstances. Simply put, being respectful means being nonjudgmental.

Some patients have irritating habits, like smoking cigarettes, drinking too much, refusing to exercise, or even being antagonistic to their physical therapist. Other patients have beliefs about illness that try your patience; for example, the man with severe emphysema who explains that his illness was caused by a cold in 1966 that never got better and has nothing to do with his 100-pack-a-year smoking history. Another patient frustrates you with her devastating migratory pains that never disappear, despite a normal examination and negative diagnostic tests. Some patients are hostile, manipulative, arrogant, or deceptive. Many may be skeptical about the benefits of physical therapy. How do you respect such patients?

Respect requires you to separate your personal feelings about the patient's behavior or attitudes from your professional concern, assessing the patient's impairments and assisting him or her to overcome them. The patient who believes his emphysema has nothing to do with smoking may still be guided to give a reliable clinical narrative. Likewise, although a hostile patient may make you feel uncomfortable, you can still respect his or her reasons for being angry. Moreover, the emphysema patient's denial and the hostile patient's anger may be adaptations that help them cope with their illnesses. You should accept these feelings as aspects of the whole person, not reject them as threats to "truth" or to your ego. When patients act in ways that make you anxious or angry, they usually believe they have good reasons for doing so, although you may not understand those reasons. Box 7.2 presents a number of simple steps you can take to demonstrate respect.

Genuineness

Genuineness means not pretending to be somebody other than who you are; it means being yourself. The first time you encounter genuineness as a problem in the health professions may

---

Box 7.2 • How to Demonstrate Respect for Patients

- Introduce yourself clearly: "My name is John Smith; I'm a physical therapist."
- Do not use the patient's first name during an interview without permission: "May I call you John?"
- Explain your role: "I would like to spend about 30 minutes talking with you about your illness."
- Inquire about and arrange for the patient's comfort before getting started: "Is this a good time for you?"
- Continue to consider the patient's comfort during the course of your clinical evaluation: "Would you be more comfortable if I lowered the bed?"
- Warn the patient when you are about to do something unexpected or painful: "I'm going to check your nerve endings by touching you with this pin."
- Respond to your patient in a way that shows you have listened carefully to what he or she has said: "Let me see if I have the story straight."

be in your role as a student. If you are to be genuine, you must acknowledge who you are: a student. You should introduce yourself as such and, whenever appropriate, reaffirm your limited knowledge and limited responsibility in the patient's care. Physical therapists, physician assistants, nurse practitioners, and practicing physicians all experience situations in which patients ask for opinions or require procedures beyond the practitioner's capabilities. Even experienced clinicians need to call in consultants or refer patients to specialists. Genuineness requires you to be honest about your knowledge and abilities and to negotiate a plan for future care based on your capabilities.

Being genuine also means being yourself in another way, that is, being able to express your feelings while staying within the boundaries of a professional relationship. If a patient has experienced a recent loss, such as the death of a spouse, you should naturally respond with an affective statement such as "I am sorry to hear that. How has it been going for you?" However, adding personal details (e.g., you too have lost a spouse or parent) is usually inappropriate in a professional relationship. When patients tell jokes or make humorous comments, it is appropriate to respond genuinely, with a smile or laugh, rather than hiding behind a mask.[21] Demonstrating your interest in the patient as a person is another way of being genuine.

Sometimes, however, respect and genuineness may seem incompatible. Everyone has bad days, and you may happen to be at a low ebb yourself during your evaluation of the patient. You may be experiencing problems in your personal life, or eagerly anticipating a weekend trip. What is the role of genuineness in these situations? Should you hide your feelings, disguise your bad day, or express your emotions? Although genuineness means not pretending, it does not mean that you must share your inner feelings. This is a question of professionalism. It involves distinguishing your professional self (which includes compassion and empathy) from the vicissitudes, experiences, or interests that characterize your personal life, or self. The development of a set of core competencies in professionalism is an important part of physical therapy education. For example, the APTA Clinical Performance Instrument includes measures of professionalism.[22] This helps ensure that you gradually develop your professional self into a well-integrated instrument of healing. As a genuine professional, you acknowledge your distress and disappointment to the patient who persists in being late or missing appointments. However, you do not demonstrate your anger in a hostile or off-putting way. Rather, you might say, "I know it's hard for you to get here, but when you're late I can't give you the time and the care that you need." At the same time, you respect the patient when you attempt to understand his or her reasons for lateness, which may include chaotic lifestyle, young children at home, single parenting, difficult arrangements for transportation, and so forth.

Empathy

Empathy is a way of understanding another person's experience and how he or she feels about that experience.[23-25] As such, it should not be confused with sympathy, an emotion, or with compassion, a quality or virtue. Although in health care compassion may be our motivation for exercising empathy, empathy is not the same as compassion. This distinction may seem confusing because in ordinary conversation we sometimes employ these terms interchangeably.

Empathy is the ability to understand the patient's total communication, cognitive and affective: words, feelings, and gestures. To put it metaphorically, empathy means getting onto the patient's wavelength, figuring out where she is coming from, or walking a mile in his moccasins. Moreover, *clinical* empathy also requires us to let the patient know—by the manner in which we respond—that we have actually *heard* (i.e., understood) what he or she told us.[23]

When empathy is defined in this way, it should be clear that an interview conducted empathically is likely to yield more objective, precise, and reliable data than an interview in which little or no attempt is made to understand the patient.

Few health professionals deny the importance of empathy in clinical practice. However, many health professionals discount the value (or even the possibility) of *teaching* empathy as a clinical skill. They do this for one of two reasons. First, some practitioners believe that empathy is a characterological state; that is, some persons are naturally more or less empathic than others, a stable feature of identity (or even of "hard-wiring") that cannot be changed. This is at best a partial truth. While it is true that different people have different "talents" for empathy, it is also true that each person has the ability to develop and expand his or her own talent. This is analogous to one's natural talent for music, mathematics, or the visual arts. Not everyone has the ability to become a concert performer, but with appropriate training almost anyone can become a competent pianist.

Secondly, other practitioners believe that health care professionals do not need to be taught empathy because they "pick it up" with experience. These practitioners claim that interviewing skills, including empathy-building techniques, develop naturally as the trainee encounters diverse practice situations over a long time. Once again, this is a partial truth. Yes, it does take years of experience to master professional skills, but frequent repetition of poor techniques simply reinforces those techniques; it does not lead to improvement. Undirected experience is no guarantee of maturation in clinical empathy. Directed practice, on the other hand, is essential for mastering empathic interviewing skills.

Empathy as Process

It is useful to think of empathy as a positive feedback loop. You begin by listening carefully to what the patient tells you, including both cognitive and affective messages. When you think you understand, you respond by summarizing for the patient what you have heard. If you happen to be on the right wavelength, the patient will acknowledge that and be encouraged to reveal more of his or her thoughts and feelings, since you are such a good listener. If you do *not* get it right, but have still demonstrated your interest by checking back, the patient is likely to appreciate your attempt and feel comfortable enough to correct your impression, thereby giving you an opportunity to reassess and respond again. This process can be iterative, as in some cases you might check back several times to arrive at the most accurate characterization of the experience. Thus, achieving empathy is usually a conscious process and not a flash of intuition.

Levels of Responding

In social situations, we often ignore or minimize feelings. When people ask, "How are you?" or "How do you feel today?" they do not ordinarily expect you to tell them the truth about how lousy you feel. As a physical therapist, however, you do want to learn the details. When patients express them, you acknowledge their character and intensity, while indicating that you understand and accept them. Consider the following four levels of response you might have to a patient's self-revelation: "My back pain is killing me ... I can't walk, I can't sit, I can't do anything. It's just demoralizing. Sometimes when I go to bed I wish I'd just never wake up."

- *Ignoring Response:* You either do not hear what the patient has said, or act as though you do not hear. You avoid responding to either the cognitive or emotional content.
  - "And does the pain radiate anywhere?"

- *Minimizing Response:* You respond to the feelings and symptoms, but at a lower level than that associated with the patient's expressed concern.
  - "So your back pain is persistent."
- *Interchangeable Response:* You recognize the feelings and symptoms expressed by the patient and assess them accurately, and you feed back that awareness at the same level of intensity.
  - "So your back pain is constant and very disabling, and it sounds like you're getting really depressed about it."
- *Additive Response:* In an additive response, you recognize not only what the patient expresses openly but also what he or she feels but does not express.
  - "It sounds like the back pain has gotten so bad that you're afraid you won't be able to handle it, and you're scared of what you might do."

You should strive for interchangeable responses in clinical history taking and empathy building. When you respond interchangeably, patients will feel that you are "present" to them and trying to fully understand their problems. Two concise ways of responding interchangeably are through the use of mirrors and paraphrases. A mirror (or reflection) simply feeds back to the patient exactly what he or she said using the same words. A paraphrase is a restatement, in your own words, of what the patient told you.

Additive responses are frequently used when giving reassurance. Reassurance involves making an educated guess regarding what the patient is likely to be worried about and then attempting to alleviate those worries. The ability to give accurate additive responses develops over time with the clinician's experience of listening carefully to patients' stories and learning patterns of verbal and nonverbal cues. When we minimize the patient's concerns ("Oh, you'll see, everything will be all right") or make misleading statements about the patient's condition, we give *false reassurance*, which is dishonest and potentially alienates the patient. On the other hand, if we respond empathically, the patient is likely to appreciate our attempt and correct us, even if the additive response is not exactly on target.

Using Words Precisely

We must learn, or relearn, to use rich qualitative vocabulary when describing or assign the patient's mental and emotional state.

To increase your skill in responding appropriately, you need to pay careful attention to words used by both you and the patient. Professional education can sterilize your vocabulary. You become immersed in the language of health care, which, although precise in describing some features, like muscle physiology and function, remains rather vague about feelings, beliefs, and expectations. In clinical language, if we use adjectives and adverbs at all, they tend to be a few medicalized ones, such as *depressed* or *anxious*. These words are rather flat and generic. Patients, on the other hand, express themselves with a full spectrum of emotional language. Patients who describe their feeling as sad, gloomy, distraught, miserable, and overwhelmed, which might all be converted to "depressed" in medical thinking. Likewise, patients who are uneasy, worried, afraid, troubled, and terrified may all be translated into "anxious."[4, p. 37] Medical language lacks the ability to describe feelings, qualities, and emotions with precision. Thus, we must learn (or relearn) to use a rich qualitative vocabulary when describing or assessing the patient's mental and emotional state.

As physical therapists we may be inclined to describe pain or functional deficit using quantitative or visual analogue scales. However, patients more naturally tend to use analogies or comparisons to capture the intensity of their symptoms. The patient who describes the pain as being as severe as a kidney stone he or she once had is giving a precise description of the pain. This is certainly more understandable than the patient who says that the pain is 8 on a scale of 10. Without knowing a good deal about the patient, we may not have a reference point for the patient's 8, but we do know that renal colic is one of the most severe pains people experience.

This socialization into the language of health care can also present problems when you give patients information about their condition and treatment. The most obvious problem is that patients simply do not understand medical terms and are reluctant to ask. When you say "hemiplegia" rather than "weakness," or "paresthesias" rather than "pins-and-needles sensations," your patient probably will not know what you are talking about. They may ask for clarification one or two times, but if you continue using technical language in which not only the words but also the conceptual framework is foreign to them, they may simply withdraw in confusion. To ensure that your patient understands, you should translate clinical terms into plain English and present the whole problem in an understandable way.

The Challenge of Empathy

Despite your best efforts, some situations present unavoidable difficulties in understanding exactly what the patient means. Among these are technical problems, such as language barriers or skills, the patient's state of consciousness (coma, delirium, psychosis, dementia), educational level, or culture. With patients who do not speak your language or are demented, we ordinarily dismiss the possibility of a useful interview and seek information elsewhere. We may arrange for an interpreter or elicit information from a family member. Other challenges to acquiring accurate symptom data are subtler. The patient may understand English sufficiently to communicate but may only be able to express difficult concepts or feelings in their native language. It is useful early in the interview to detect problems that lead to faulty data collection.

NONVERBAL COMMUNICATION

Nonverbal communication is the process of transmitting information without words. It includes kinesics, that is, the way a person uses his or her body, such as facial expressions, eye contact, hand and arm gestures, posture, and movements of the legs and feet. Nonverbal communication also includes paralinguistics—verbal qualities such as tone, rhythm, pace, and vibrancy; speech errors; and pauses or silence. It is often through the nonverbal aspects of communication that we apprehend another's feelings. We recognize anger not so much by what a person says as by how it is said. Speech may slow down and become quieter in controlled anger, or the opposite may occur, with shouting and gestures such as pounding on a table. We can often tell when people lie unless they are experienced liars. They might look away, break eye contact, hesitate, or get "red in the face" (i.e., flush involuntarily). Common examples are hypomanic or anxious person's pressure of speech or the flat voice tone of a depressed patient. Patients who are seriously ill often sound weak; we may gauge a person's state of health by the quality and timbre of her or his voice ("She's been through a lot of surgery, but she really sounds strong").

During the clinical interview, you should be aware of your own nonverbal behavior as well. If you seem uninterested, averting your eyes or checking your watch, the patient will reasonably assume you are uninterested. Likewise, if you stand by the door rather than sit by the bed, patients may assume you are in a hurry and, respectful of your time, will gloss over critical data. Attention to your own nonverbal behavior requires self-awareness and discipline. It is particularly important to be conscious of how you handle distractions, such as telephone calls or interruptions by others. You need to demonstrate your focus on the patient by maintaining eye contact, attentive posture, and responsive attitude, despite such distractions.

Kinesics

Kinesics is the study of nonverbal behavior as it relates to movement, either of any part of the body or the body as a whole. This includes interpretation of body language, such as facial expressions and gestures. Although investigators have studied characteristic gestures and suggested generic interpretations for them, gestures should always be judged in context. Interpretation is easy when a gesture confirms the patient's statements or the clinician's hypothesis based on those statements. When the patient's gesture or facial expression implies a different message than the words, you should make an effort to ascertain which—the gesture or the words.

Other factors such as personal grooming, clothing, and odors (e.g., perspiration, alcohol, tobacco, perfume) also communicate information about the patient. If a patient who is normally careful about grooming comes in disheveled and unkempt, you are alerted to the possibility of a problem even before he or she begins to speak.

Paralanguage

When you listen to speech, you hear pauses, tone, and modulation as well as words. These features are called paralanguage. Likewise, the patient absorbs the pitch, pace, and rhythm of your conversation as well. Paralinguistic cues can contribute significantly to your understanding of the patient and to the patient's perception of you as a helping person.

Let us deal briefly with just one aspect of paralanguage, pauses. Why does a patient pause a moment before answering your question or before making her next statement? The functions of pausing include:

- Absolute recall time
- Language formation time
- Censorship of material
- Creating an effect (timing)
- Preparing to lie

People rarely need to pause before recalling a place, age, or date associated with a specific event. A person tends to remember the age at which a parent died but may have to think a moment before remembering a living parent's current age. It is easy to answer a yes/no question without pausing, even if giving the incorrect answer. If you ask, "Do you drink alcohol?" the yes or no answer has little meaning. Instead, you might ask, "How much alcohol do you usually drink in a day?" or "Tell me about your use of alcohol." To answer these questions requires thought and integration. Listen carefully. How much of a pause occurs before the answer? How much stumbling or backtracking do you notice?

In general, it is helpful to listen to the number, quality, and placement of pauses. Frequent long pauses associated with low-amplitude speech and a "dead" tone suggest clinical depression. Frequent pauses over factual answers suggest dementia or organic brain dysfunction. Pauses over answers in selected areas may indicate sensitive topics, with time required for censorship of material.

Responding to Nonverbal Communication

Even though the patient's use of nonverbal communication may be obvious to you, he or she is likely to be unaware of it. This does not mean that nonverbal messages are invalid; in fact, they may be more accurate than the verbal message, precisely because they are usually unintentional and uncensored. But how does nonverbal communication provide useful information in clinical practice?

Two features are especially useful. First, train yourself to observe inconsistencies or lack of congruence between verbal and nonverbal messages. When there is discrepancy, you should make an effort to ascertain which form of communication conveys the "real" message. Often the nonverbal message is more accurate than verbal statements. You may choose in some situations, especially early in the interview, to simply note a discrepancy and use it to help you steer the conversation or "tag" certain issues for follow-up at a later point. At other times you may gently confront the patient with your observations, "I noticed you were smiling when you told me about how much work you've been missing since the accident."

Second, you should also use the patient's nonverbal communication to modify your own verbal or nonverbal behavior, or both. If the patient seems tense, as evidenced by facial flushing or fidgeting, you might modify your voice tone and kinesics by speaking in a more soothing way and leaning forward to demonstrate your interest. If the patient appears angry, based on his voice tone, gestures, and guarded posture, you might indicate that he seems to be upset or angry, and ask what the problem is and if you can do anything to help.

CONCLUSION

"When your active listening results in symptom and patient data that are objective, precise, sensitive, specific, and reliable, you are practicing both the science and art of clinical interviewing."

The conversation between clinician and patient serves as the basis for diagnosis and treatment in physical therapy. To summarize our main points:

- Objectivity in clinician-patient interactions requires active listening.
- Jumping to premature interpretation of the patient's story compromises objectivity.
- Precision requires that the information we obtain be sufficiently detailed and unambiguous to contribute to clinical diagnosis and treatment.
- Sensitivity in an interview designates its ability to identify patients who suffer from an illness or medical condition.
- Specificity in an interview designates its ability to identify patients who are well.
- The use of good interviewing techniques will yield more reproducible (reliable) information about the patient and medical condition.
- We need also to be aware that for several reasons patient stories evolve with repeated telling.
- When your active listening results in symptom and patient data that are objective, precise, sensitive, specific, and reliable, you are practicing both the science and art of clinical interviewing.

- Respect, genuineness, and empathy are three fundamental skills of clinician-patient interactions:
  - Respect means being nonjudgmental.
  - Genuineness means being congruent, or being yourself, in your professional role.
  - Empathy means understanding exactly what the patient is saying and letting the patient know that you understand.
- To achieve empathy in the clinical encounter you should:
  - Strive for interchangeable responses.
  - Develop and use a good vocabulary of descriptive words.
  - Pay attention to, and consciously utilize, nonverbal communication

SELF-ASSESSMENT

1. How satisfied are you with the precision or objectivity of your patient interviewing skills? How often do you realize that you might have missed an important piece of information? What should you have asked your patient? What things do patients share with you in interviews that you find unhelpful? Why?
2. As a clinician we may form stronger therapeutic alliances with some patients than others. Is there a pattern to the types of interactions you have that are not as successful? What influences your ability to show respect, genuineness, and empathy?
3. Physical therapist's nonverbal communication includes therapeutic touch. How do you ensure that your verbal and nonverbal communication are congruent or additive in achieving your goals with your patients?

CONTINUED LEARNING

- Coulehan JL, Block MR. *The Medical Interview: Mastering Skills for Clinical Practice (Medical Interview)*, 5th ed. Philadelphia: F.A. Davis; 2006.

This is a widely respected text for teaching medical interviewing skills to a broad range of clinicians. Topics covered include understanding the patient's story through use of good communication skills, basic skills for interviewing, and challenges in the interactive process, such as telling bad news. Review this text and think about differences in the types of interviews done by different health practitioners.

1. Why are there differences?
2. Do different practitioners interview differently because of differences in the actual care provided? Or are they related to differences in education?
3. How can we learn from each other to improve our interview skills?

REFERENCES

1. Balint M. *The Doctor and His Patient and the Illness.* New York: International Universities Press; 1972.
2. Cassell EJ. *Talking with Patients. Volume 1, The Theory of Doctor-Patient Communication.* Cambridge, MA: MIT Press; 1985.
3. Cassell EJ. *Talking with Patients. Volume 2, Clinical Techniques.* Cambridge MA: MIT Press; 1985.

4. Coulehan JL, Block MR. *The Medical Interview. Mastering Skills for Clinical Practice*, 5th ed. Philadelphia: F.A. Davis; 2006.
5. Brown JB, Boles M, Mullooly JP, Levinson W. Effect of communication skills training on patient satisfaction. A randomized, controlled study. Ann Intern Med. 1999; 131:822–829.
6. Gross DA, Zyzanski SJ, Borawski EA, Cebul RD, Stange KC. Patient satisfaction with time spent with their physician. J Fam Pract. 1998;47:133–137.
7. Wall EM. The predictive value of selected components of medical history taking. J Am Board Fam Pract. 1997;10:66–67.
8. Charon R. Narrative medicine. A model for empathy, reflection, profession, and trust. JAMA. 2001;286:1897–1902.
9. Platt FW, Gaspar D, Coulehan JL, Fox L, Stewart M, Weston W, Smith RC, Adler A. Tell me about yourself: The patient-centered interview. Ann Intern Med. 2001;134:1079–1085.
10. Coulehan JL. Being a physician. In: Mengel MB, Holleman W. eds. *Fundamentals of Clinical Practice. A Textbook on the Patient, Doctor, and Society*, 2nd ed. New York: Plenum Medical Book Company; 2002, 73–98.
11. Novack DH, Suchman AL, Clark W, Epstein RM, Najberg E, Kaplan MD: Calibrating the physician. Personal awareness and effective patient care. JAMA. 1997;278:502–509.
12. Epstein RM. Mindful practice. JAMA. 1999;282:833–839.
13. Rogers C. *On Becoming a Person*. Boston: Houghton Mifflin; 1961.
14. Ivey AE, Authier J. *Microcounselling*. Springfield, IL: Charles C Thomas; 1978.
15. Accreditation Council for Graduate Medical Education, ACGME Outcomes Project, http://www.acgme.org/Outcome/ Accessed July 7, 2005.
16. American Association of Medical Colleges, Project Professionalism, Assessment, http://www.aamc.org/members/gea/professionalism.pdf Accessed July 7, 2005.
17. Epstein RM, Hundert EM. Defining and assessing professional competence. JAMA. 2002;287:226–235.
18. Hafferty FW, Franks R. The hidden curriculum, ethics teaching, and the structure of medical education. Acad Med. 1994;69:861–871.
19. Hunnert EM, Hafferty F, Christakis D. Characteristics of the informal curriculum and trainee's ethical choices. Acad Med. 1996;71:624–633.
20. Inui TS. *A Flag in the Wind: Educating for Professionalism in Medicine*. Washington, DC: Association of American Medical Colleges; 2003.
21. Berger J, Coulehan J, Belling C. Humor in the physician-patient encounter. Arch Intern Med. 2004;164:825–830.
22. The Development and Testing of APTA Clinical Performance Instruments. Task Force for the Development of Student Clinical Performance Instruments, APTA. Phys Ther 2002;82:329–353.
23. Coulchan JL, Platt FW, Frankl R, Salazar W, Lown B, Fox L. Let me see if I have this right: Words that build empathy. Ann Intern Med. 2001;135:221–227.
24. Frankel RM, Quill TE, McDaniel SH, eds. *The Biopsychosocial Approach: Past, Present, Future*. Rochester NY: University of Rochester Press; 2003.
25. Suchman AL, Markakis K, Beckman HB, Frankel R. A model of empathic communication in the medical interview. JAMA. 1997;277:678–682.

chapter 8

Learning About Patients' Perspectives: Qualitative Research

Kim Nixon-Cave, PT, PhD, PCS

By words we learn thoughts, and by thoughts we learn life.

—Jean Baptiste Girard

•

✳ Mr. Ketterman's Case

Mr. Ketterman's decision about his advanced directive means that he would not accept any end-of-life care. I would like to understand more about why he and his wife have made this decision, as it is very different from the one I would make.   *(See Appendix for Mr. Ketterman's health history.)*

INTRODUCTION

As we have discussed, evidence based practice requires that we both know and respect our patients' values as we make collaborative decisions with them about their health care. But, how do we learn about our patients and their values so as to facilitate the practitioner-patient partnership so essential to our practice? We can only do this through effective communication. The theories of communication and social interaction presented by Gordon in Chapter 6 provide us with a framework for this source of evidence for our health care decisions. In Chapter 7, Coulehan and Block presented a skilled method of interviewing patients so that we might uncover their strongly held values. This chapter will explore the components of evidence based practice (EBP) that focus on learning about patient values and preferences. It will also introduce qualitative research methods as a tool to achieve this goal.

Both our clinical wisdom from years of reflective practice and the research evidence can help us learn how to improve our knowledge of usual and unusual patient perspectives on health and illness. Adhering to the value for respecting our patients is necessary, but it is not sufficient to our goal of building a solid, trusting therapeutic relationship. We must be willing

117

to learn from the evidence about individual and group perspectives on recovery of function after disease or injury. Chapter 15 will introduce guidelines for determining the value of research evidence gained primarily from the traditional positivistic research paradigm; here we introduce an alternative research paradigm, the qualitative paradigm, which is uniquely suited to answering research questions that help us more deeply understand the patient's perspective. We will introduce the qualitative research paradigm first and then look at existing evidence developed with this approach as it relates to making patients true partners in the recovery or promotion of their health.

THE QUALITATIVE RESEARCH PARADIGM

Qualitative research paradigms offer a perspective that is different from the more familiar quantitative research designs. Quantitative research is linked to the philosophy of *logical positivism*, in which events are assumed to be limited to logical and controlled relationships between specific measurable variables. Therefore, the rationale for studying these relationships can be defined in advance, based on hypotheses that guide the methods of data collection. Accordingly, variables can be operationalized and assigned numerical values, independent of any historical, cultural, or social contexts within which the event is observed.[1] These assumptions apply well to most physical and many biological events. Many quality of life assessments, by virtue of their list of questions, are based on assumptions about measurable behaviors that reflect health status. By using a single rating scale for all subjects, investigators demonstrate the premise of quantitative research: that experience and clinical phenomena can be reduced to a set of specific questions and variables predetermined by the researcher.

The essence of the qualitative method, on the other hand, obliges the researcher to understand the person's perspective first. *Qualitative research* seeks to describe the complex nature of humans and how individuals perceive their own experiences within a specific social context.

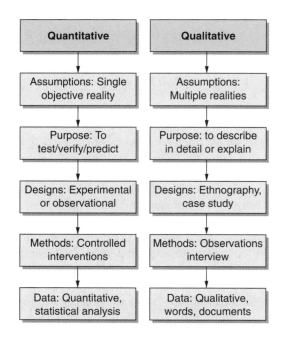

Figure 8-1 A Comparison of Quantitative and Qualitative Research Paradigms.

Qualitative methodology uses the subject's own words and narrative summaries of observable behavior to express data, rather than numerical data derived from predetermined rating systems. The qualitative approach emphasizes an understanding of human experience, exploring the nature of people's transactions with themselves, others, and their surroundings. Qualitative designs and methods also allow the study of many simultaneous variables contained in a phenomenon.

Questions that lend themselves to qualitative inquiry are generally broad, seeking to understand why something occurs, what certain experiences mean to a patient or client, or how the dynamics of an experience influence subsequent behaviors or decisions.[2] The purpose of qualitative inquiry is to examine such experiences using a holistic approach that is concerned with the true nature of "reality" as the participants understand it. Qualitative methodology has been a cornerstone of research in sociology and anthropology and has more recently received attention from clinical researchers.[3,4]

Qualitative research is not just a description of a particular situation. Instead, it uses specific research methods, in which the inquiry is tied to understanding, explanation, or the development of theory about an observed phenomenon. From such insightful description, relevant variables can be uncovered, and questions can then be posed to study quantitative aspects of those variables in controlled settings. Qualitative and quantitative aspects can also be combined within one study, to measure certain components of behavior and to see how such measurements relate to the nature of the actual experience.[5] Use of both qualitative and quantitative methods in the same study can increase the validity of the findings.[6]

PERSPECTIVES IN QUALITATIVE RESEARCH

There are a number of different approaches that clinicians will find in reading qualitative research. The most common of these include phenomenology, ethnography, and grounded theory.[7]

Phenomenology

The tradition known as *phenomenology* seeks to draw meaning from complex realities through careful analysis of first-person narrative materials.[8] These narratives are focused on a specific phenomenon; illness, physical disability and childbirth are examples of phenomena that have been explored by health professionals. The phenomenological perspective allows personal experiences to be seen through the individual's social context and therefore, allows the reader to gain a degree of empathy with the person reporting the experiences.[9]

Ethnography

A second common perspective, called *ethnography*, is the study of the attitudes, beliefs, and behaviors of a specific group of people within their own cultural milieu.[10] Ethnographic studies allow the reader to become immersed in the subjects' way of life to understand the cultural forces that shape behavior and feelings. Classic examples of ethnographic research are found in the well-known anthropological works of Margaret Mead.[11,12]

Grounded Theory

A third common approach is *grounded theory research*, which allows the reader to understand the development of theory from rich data about a phenomenon. In this approach the researcher collects, codes, and analyzes data simultaneously to identify relevant variables leading to the identification of theoretical concepts that are "grounded" in the observations.[13]

	Table 8.1	**A Comparison of Quantitative and Qualitative Research Paradigms**	
		Quantitative	**Qualitative**
Assumptions		Single objective reality	Multiple realities
Purpose		To test/verify/predict	To describe in detail or explain
Designs		Experimental or observational	Ethnography, case study
Methods		Controlled interventions	Observation, interview
Data		Quantitative, statistical analysis	Qualitative, words, documents

As data are collected and coded, each idea or theme is compared to others to determine where they agree or conflict. At any point in the study, if data do not support the theory, the data are not discarded, but the theory is refined so that it fits the existing data. As this process progresses, interrelationships emerge that lead to the development of theoretical frameworks. Studies using the grounded theory approach report the themes that the researchers identified, along with rich examples of the data that supported the development of the themes. These studies will also include the conceptual framework that drove the study as well as the revised framework or theory that arose from the data.

METHODS OF QUALITATIVE DATA COLLECTION

Because qualitative data can come from a wide variety of sources and take many different forms, the methods of data collection are also quite varied and somewhat different from the more familiar types of data collection used in quantitative research (Table 8.1). The most common forms of data collection are observation and interviews. Both of these types of data collection demonstrate one of the common aspects of qualitative research—the researcher is the primary research instrument. They also have the same end result—to generate rich deep descriptions of the phenomena being explored.

Observation

In *nonparticipant observation*, researchers use quiet and inconspicuous observation to identify people, interactions, the influence of sociocultural context, and even artifacts to acquire relevant data to answer the research question posed. The data from nonparticipant observation can be used to confirm or disconfirm findings from other types of data collection as well. Nonparticipant observation sessions can also be videotaped so that later the participants can discuss with the researcher what the participants were thinking while they observe their own behavior. This technique is used to capture the participant's reality while diminishing the sometimes distorting effects of recall.

The essence of qualitative research is that the individual's experience should be described as it is lived by that individual. Therefore, the researcher can embed him- or herself within the group, using a technique called *participant observation*. With this method, the researcher actually becomes a participant in the activities of the group under study so that observation of behaviors can be appreciated from the standpoint of those who are being observed. Although this technique, as with other research techniques, is inherently biased by the researcher's own preconceptions, it provides a mechanism for the researcher to describe the interactions of individuals within a social context and to analyze behaviors as a function of the subjects' personal realities. The researcher is in a position to recognize feelings and thoughts that emerge from the subjects' frame of reference. Participant-observer is a complex role, but one that is believed to enhance the validity of qualitative observations. [14]

Interviews

Interviews involve a form of direct contact between the researcher and the subjects within the subjects' natural environment. Interviews are used to gather information, with the researcher asking questions that probe the subjects' experiences and perceptions. Interviews are usually based on a predetermined script of open-ended questions, with opportunity for follow-up questions that are based on the participants' responses. In many studies, interviews are done with individual participants, sometimes with only one encounter and sometimes with multiple sessions. In other studies, interviews are done with groups of participants. The most well-known format for this type of interview is the *focus group*, which is generally conducted following a predetermined set of questions.[15] Interviews of individual participants for qualitative research may seem similar to the clinical interview, but it is important to remember a fundamental difference. Clinical interviews have as their primary focus arriving at a diagnostic decision; qualitative interviews are designed to bring about a better understanding of the phenomenon from the participant's perspective.[16]

Data Analysis and Interpretation

In contrast to quantitative research, qualitative data analysis is primarily an inductive process, with a constant interplay between data that represents the reality of the study participants and theoretical conceptualization of that reality. Therefore, the process of analysis is ongoing as data are collected. Because observational and interview responses are recorded as narratives, qualitative data are typically voluminous. Data are recorded through written memos or transcribed from audio- or videotapes. The specific techniques of data analysis can vary from purely narrative descriptions of observations to the creation of a coding system from which categories can be developed and, in a systematic way, patterns or themes developed from the mass of information that is available.[17]

Trustworthiness and Generalizability

Just as with all research, clinicians need to know whether they can trust the data and the analyses and whether they can apply the findings to their own patients and situations. (See Chapter 12 for a discussion of these concepts in terms of quantitative research.) Because the data sources are words rather than numbers, different terms are used to describe and determine the trustworthiness and generalizability of the data. Lincoln and Guba[18] have suggested the terms *credibility* and *truth value* to refer to internal validity or trustworthiness of the data analysis itself, *transferability* to refer to external validity or generalizability and *consistency* and *dependability* to refer to reliability or consistency of the data.

These concepts are typically examined in terms of judgments rather than numerical equivalency.[19] *Triangulation* refers to a process whereby concepts are confirmed using more than one source of data, or more than one data collection method, or more than one set of researchers. The concept actually originated as a technical term in surveying, to demonstrate how two visible points could be used to locate a third point. When a researcher has used triangulation, the reader can expect to find two or more types of data, such as information obtained from a participant's interview responses, by direct observation of group performance, and by analysis of written materials. If comparable conclusions are drawn from each method, the internal validity or credibility of the interpretation is considerably strengthened.

Because the researcher is the primary research instrument, there are many strategies for improving accuracy. They include the use of audit trails that provide a clear description of the thought processes used to interpret the data, the involvement of more than one investigator to confirm ideas, confirmation of conclusions with participants in the study through member checks, analysis until data saturation (no new themes identified) is reached, and searching for negative or disconfirming evidence.[20] Readers should expect to see examples of these processes in the reports of good qualitative research.

Sampling

Qualitative research has at its heart the understanding of human experiences and behaviors. Therefore, the selection of the people who provide the data for this research is a very important process. These people are typically termed *participants*, rather than *subjects*, since they participate in sharing their experiences, rather than subjecting themselves to an experimental intervention. In qualitative research these participants are selected in a *purposeful*, rather than random, way, as the investigator must locate subjects who will be effective informants and who will provide a rich source of information.[21]

Samples in qualitative research often seem quite small, especially in comparison to those of quantitative research. Since the premise of qualitative research is to understand human perceptions, enough participants are needed to allow the researcher to reach a point of saturation in the data, where no new information is obtained. On the other hand, samples that are too large will not permit the in-depth analysis that is the essence of qualitative inquiry. Sandelowski suggests that determining adequate sample size in qualitative research is a matter of judgment and experience in evaluating the quality of the information collected and the purpose of the research.[22]

Summary of Methods in Qualitative Research

Using qualitative methods to develop evidence for best practice allows clinicians "to study the complexity of human interactions and to understand the influence of contextual factors."[23, pg. 279] A naturalistic paradigm in developing evidence for clinical practice and the subsequent use of the evidence allows clinicians to appreciate the human experience in health and illness and the meaning an individual attributes to that experience. Use of qualitative research can address the gaps in the understanding of a phenomenon that quantitative methods cannot capture and provide a new perspective on the health care provided and the patient's view of the situation.[23]

We recognize that this brief introduction to qualitative analysis is by no means sufficient to demonstrate the scope of design and data collection and analysis methods that have been developed in qualitative research. We have provided some recommendations at the end of the chapter for further reading, particularly for those interested in using this approach for their own research.

USE OF QUALITATIVE RESEARCH IN EVIDENCE BASED PRACTICE

"Quantitative research, such as RCTs, can demonstrate that a[n] intervention leads to better control of behavior; qualitative research can provide an explanation and understanding of why it does it. It can bring to light the sometimes complex processes that underlie the positive results for why they remain absent."[24]

Qualitative research can enlighten us about all three aspects of evidence based practice: clinical judgment, patient values and circumstances, and evidence in the literature. Through these types of studies we can learn more about clinicians' and patients' participation in decision making; we can learn about patients' values and circumstances from their own perspectives; and we can also learn about ways that clinicians use (or do not use) the evidence from the literature.

Clinical Decision Making That Fully Engages Patient Values and Circumstances

✳ Case Example — Mrs. Stevenson

Mrs. Stevenson is a 76-year-old African American woman born in Mississippi living in a northeast urban environment. Mrs. Stevenson is the matriarch and the primary caregiver in her immediate and extended family, all of whom live in the same neighborhood. Mrs. Stevenson has a history of hypertension and type 2 diabetes. She was admitted to an acute rehab hospital and referred for physical therapy secondary to a diagnosis of a stroke. During the interview, the physical therapist assesses Mrs. Stevenson's goals for her rehabilitation. She appears apprehensive and is very brief and guarded in her responses to questions. At the end of the session Mrs. Stevenson indicates that she is skeptical and suspicious of the medical care she is receiving and indicates that she must return home immediately to care for her family.

Mazurek Melnyk and Fineout-Overbolt describe these three steps that health care practitioners can take to more fully engage the patient in evidence-based practice:

1. Value patient involvement in the clinical decision making.
2. Create time for assessment of patient preferences and values as part of the intake history in acute and primary care encounters.
3. Create patient information sheets about treatment plan options for common health care issues.[25]

A model that illustrates this perspective is the patient-practitioner collaborative model, which is an approach that can allow a positive therapeutic relationship to develop between the clinician and the patient. This approach invites patients to participate in the therapeutic process and helps the practitioner assess the patient's values, health beliefs, and preferences. Health care providers can fully engage the patient in evidence based decision making by demonstrating that they value the patient's involvement in the clinical decision making process. The patient-practitioner collaborative approach encourages this engagement. The process begins with mutual inquiry through an interview that explores the patient's values, preferences, health behaviors, and barriers to ideal care.[26] As we discussed in Chapter 7, clinicians can develop their interview skills so that patients will trust their clinicians and therefore share their experiences and preferences, leading to a partnership in the health care process.

As we have discussed in Section I, clinical decision making is a very complex process that has many opportunities for error. It is also a process that needs to be done collaboratively between the clinician and the patient. Even with the increasing access to information technology and the resultant increase in the knowledge available to the patient, patients still may not have the necessary information to make decisions in isolation. As clinicians, we must recognize the need to start the process of collaborative decision making by helping patients examine their own values and preferences and also help patients increase their health literacy, that is, their understanding of the information we share with them from the literature to support clinical decisions.

Numerous research studies have used qualitative approaches to explore and investigate methods of eliciting individual patients' preferences in the management of their disease or illness. Schulman-Green et al used a focus group approach to explore how older adults consider and discuss their life and health goals during clinical encounters and their willingness to participate in clinical decision making. This study may be helpful to clinicians to help with goal setting for the rehabilitation process when dealing with a patient like Mrs. Stevenson. Schulman-Green et al found that all participants were willing to discuss goals but varied in degree of participation. They concluded that in order to enhance goal setting clinicians need to address key barriers to discussing goals.[27]

Identifying patient values and preferences through the increased use of qualitative research and through improved interview skills is the first step. Next, we need to recognize that the roles and responsibilities that are chosen or assigned in the patient-provider relationship will affect the degree to which the patient is able to take part in deciding the choice of treatment.[28,29] The role chosen by or assigned to the patient will result in a collaborative, an active, or a passive role in clinical decision making.

There are several approaches that move us more toward an evidence-based practice based on a full respect for patient values and preferences, with a relationship where the patient has a collaborative or active role, rather than a passive one. Each of these approaches can be contrasted with what might be termed a traditional practice approach, one that identifies the health care provider's choices as primary, with the patient in a more passive role. We will review two overarching approaches here: ones that place the patient and family at the center of care and ones that focus on the exchange of information between the patient and the practitioner (shared decision making). Practitioners should examine these approaches and adapt them to best fit their specific practice and their patients' needs.

Patient- and Family-Centered Care

Patient- and family-centered care is defined by the Institute of Family Center Care as "an innovative approach to the planning, delivery, and evaluation of health care that is grounded in mutually beneficial partnerships among health care patients, families, and providers. Patient- and family-centered care applies to patients of all ages, and it may be practiced in any health care setting."[30] Patient- and family-centered care means remaining clearly focused on the well-being of individual patients.[31] Several concepts are identified as core for patient- and family-centered care, including:

- *Dignity and Respect.* Health care practitioners listen to and honor patient and family perspectives and choices. Patient and family knowledge, values, beliefs, and cultural backgrounds are incorporated into the planning and delivery of care.
- *Information Sharing.* Health care practitioners communicate and share complete and unbiased information with patients and families in ways that are affirming and useful. Patients and families receive timely, complete, and accurate information in order to effectively participate in care and decision making.

- *Participation.* Patients and families are encouraged and supported in participating in care and decision making at the level they choose.
- *Collaboration.* Patients and families are also included on an institution-wide basis. Health care leaders collaborate with patients and families in policy and program development, implementation, and evaluation; in health care facility design; and in professional education, as well as in the delivery of care.[30]

Shields et al conducted a literature search for a Cochrane systematic review of the use of patient- and family-centered care in pediatric hospitals. In their review, they suggested another definition of family-centered care: "family centred care is a way of caring for children and their families within health services which ensures that care is planned around the whole family, not just the individual child/person, and in which all the family members are recognized as care recipients."[32,p1318] The researchers included qualitative studies in their review and were able to identify three major themes related to the implementation of family-centered care arising from these qualitative studies. These themes were negotiation between staff and families, perception of roles by both staff and parents, and the cost of providing family-centered care. The themes are certainly important and warrant further research to fully examine their influence in family-centered care.[32]

While the concept of patient- and family-centered care is an approach that has become more widely used in care involving children, it is potentially useful for all age groups. In their systematic review, Shields et al found that the perceptions held by the clinicians and the patients influenced the delivery of family-centered care. Overall, the conclusion from this study was that further research is needed to generate evidence for appropriate family-centered care models because of the increased use of this approach in various practice settings.

Shared Decision Making

A second approach to inclusiveness of patients in decision making is the shared decision making approach. This has been described as a process by which patients are educated about their options, with the supporting evidence about potential outcomes, benefits, and harms, and then engaging them in deciding which choice is best for them, taking into account their preferences, values, and lifestyles.[33] The concept of shared decision making is to develop and implement strategies and processes that allow providers and patients to participate as equal partners in making decisions concerning health issues across the continuum of care.

Shared decision making is defined as "a particular process of decision making by the patient and clinician in which the patient:

- understands the risk or seriousness of the disease or condition to be prevented;
- understands the preventive service, including the risk, benefits, alternatives, and uncertainties;
- has weighed his or her values regarding the potential benefits and harms associated with the service; and
- has engaged in decision making at a level at which he or she desires and feels comfortable."

Thus, shared decision making goes beyond informed decision making by emphasizing that the decision process is joint and shared between the patient and provider.[34,p81]

Shared decision making is the collaboration between patients and caregivers to come to an agreement about a health care decision. This approach is especially useful when there is no clear "best" treatment option. The caregiver offers the patient information that will help the patient understand the likely outcomes of various options, think about what is personally important about the risks and benefits of each option, and participate in decisions about medical care.[35]

Shared decision making is important to consider in making clinical decisions because of the value judgment component. It also deals directly with the issues concerning informed consent. Patients' preferences are typically influenced by their values and beliefs, and clinicians cannot infer or assume what the patient's values are, nor can they assume what is the best decision for the patient. In many cases treatment decisions are difficult and usually there is not one right answer, so patients need to know the risks and benefits in order to make the best decision.

Patients can be more involved in treatment decisions, and risks and benefits of treatment options can be explained in more detail, without adversely affecting patient-based outcomes. Sharing decision making and communicating risk may be advocated on the basis of values and ethical principles even without evidence of health gain or improvement in patient-based outcomes, but the resources required to enhance these professional skills must also be taken into consideration.[36]

Protheroe et al investigated the impact of patients' preferences for the treatment of atrial fibrillation, by using individualized decision analysis that combined probability and utility assessments into a decision tree. The conclusion from looking at the outcome measures is that individualized decision analysis using a shared decision making model would lead to increased patient involvement and to fewer prescriptions of warfarin for elderly patients with atrial fibrillations in the study group.[37]

In an observational study, Montgomery, Harding, and Fahey investigated the impact of shared decision making, especially patient preferences, on the treatment recommendations for hypertension. The authors discussed the improved patient knowledge, comfort, and participation in decision making and the impact on the treatment selection. They noted that using a shared decision-making model affected whether the patients would be recommended for antihypertensive medication or not.[38] These types of qualitative studies may provide the evidence that may assist in addressing Mrs. Stevenson's preferences and concerns about her care.

Mrs. Stevenson (see case example) is in a patient age group that may not fully participate in clinical decision making and that may be difficult to engage in setting goals for their health care. Her apprehension and guarded response could be related to her perceptions of a lack of autonomy and competency to actively participate. Moser et al conducted a qualitative study using an interview approach for patients with type 2 diabetes mellitus to investigate which concepts of autonomy people used in a shared decision making setting. Several themes emerged, indicating that "autonomy is a multidimensional, dynamic and complex construct." The authors' conclusion indicates that further research is needed to investigate which type of decision making processes patients need, based on their diagnosis and/or illness.[39,p417]

Schulman-Green et al used focus groups in a qualitative study to understand how older adults discuss their life and health goals during the clinical encounter. Several themes emerged from this interview form. Although all participants were willing to discuss their goals, the degree of participation varied. Reasons for nonparticipation included goal setting not being a high priority for patients, patients focusing more on symptoms than goals, mutual perception of disinterest by both patient and clinician, and the presumption by clinicians that all patients' goals were the same.[40]

Learning About Patients' Values Through Qualitative Research

Another way that qualitative research can assist in practicing fully from an evidence based perspective is by helping us see patients' perception of what is called the "lived life."

Qualitative designs are especially suited to allowing expression of the actual experiences of people in particular circumstances. By applying the methods and analyses of qualitative research, we can move beyond the anecdote, as powerful and moving as that may be, to see the common themes that occur in certain circumstances, thereby giving us the opportunity to better understand the situations of others. The literature is full of such examples. We will offer a few of them here and have included others in a reference list at the end of the chapter for further reading.

Some studies are focused on having a disease or living with a disability. For example, Schmid and Rittman conducted interviews with people who had expressed some concern about falls as a post-stroke consequence. They learned that these patients were concerned that falls could lead to physical limitations, increased dependence, and further fear of falling and that these concerns were common among these patients.[41] Although this study included only males, it can still help us understand whether this is an unspoken concern of Mrs. Stevenson.

The following are two more examples demonstrating the breadth of qualitative work that explicates the lives of our patients.

1. A study by Carpenter explored the experience of a spinal cord injury (SCI). The work demonstrated that education about living with SCI provided by health care professionals did not match the lived experience of those with the injury, suggesting the need to transform educational approaches.[42] The qualitative investigation helped to uncover the meaning of SCI to those who experience it and how it affects their behavior, emotions, body image, self-esteem, and interactions.
2. A study by Dickie et al used interviews focused on a critical incident (a "good" sensory experience and a "bad" sensory experience) to learn how parents viewed the sensory experiences of their children with autism as compared to parents of children not diagnosed with autism. They found that parents of both groups of children identified the negative aspects of some sounds and of food-related events and the positive aspects of movement, although parents with children with autism reported more extreme reactions.[43]

Other studies focus on whether outcome tools actually measure things that are important to patients with the disease, impairment, or disability. For example, Hamilton et al conducted a qualitative study to better identify the coping strategies of African American women with cancer. They developed a survey tool based on the data from in-depth interviews that could be used as an outcome measure and identified several coping strategies that reflect the cultural and social influences on this group, including the need to be strong for others and the role of church as a support mechanism.[44] The disease state experienced by these women is not the same as Mrs. Stevenson's, but we might still learn something that can help improve our interactions with her by understanding the health needs and perceptions of women similar to her culturally and socially.

Many such studies help us refine our instruments so that they accurately reflect what patients are experiencing. Two of these are described next.

1. Monninkhof and colleagues used in-depth home interviews of patients with chronic obstructive pulmonary disease (COPD) to better understand the importance of self-management in COPD. The data obtained explained how and why standardized health related quality-of-life scales failed to accurately capture the patient's experience. In

particular, standardized measures failed to identify the importance of certain aspects of well-being, namely, self-confidence, feeling safe, and social isolation.[45]

2. Gooberman-Hill et al used focus group interviews to expand on reports of pain by patients with chronic joint pain. Using standardized tools for assessing pain, the Hip Disability and Osteoarthritis Outcome Score and the Knee Injury and Osteoarthritis Outcome Score, they asked participants to identify aspects of their pain that might affect the accuracy of these tools as measures. Patients reported that certain aspects were not specifically identified on the standardized tools but affected their responses to the items. These included intermittent and variable pain, pain elsewhere in the body influencing the experience of joint pain, pain inextricable from function, and adaptation and avoidance strategies modifying the experience of pain. The authors recommended that clinicians assess these aspects of pain in addition to using the standardized tools.[46]

Qualitative research can also help clinicians understand the impact on patients of selected interventions and recognize reasons why patients may not always accept clinicians' recommendations, especially ones that require behavioral change. Malpass, Andrews, and Turner used in-depth interviews to identify the best way to help patients with type II diabetes understand and accept the need to make changes in both diet and activity level. Their results showed that patients were better able to make both types of changes when they were explained together and understood the interaction of the two behavioral changes.[47] Because of her stroke, Mrs. Stevenson may not be able to make all the behavioral changes needed to manage her diabetes, but the results of this study may still help us understand the type of information we need to provide to her so that she can be as fully engaged as possible in managing her disease.

Much research has been done to examine the ability and willingness of patients to cooperate with interventions, especially ones, like so many of those in physical therapy, that require behavioral change. Some examples follow.

• Sabiston et al used interviews to learn about overweight women's perceptions of a program that involved vigorous exercise. They were able to identify three distinct groups, each of whom responded differently to the activity in terms of their self-perceptions: women who consistently struggled with negative self-perceptions, women who consistently experienced positive self-perceptions, and women who began with negative self-perceptions and developed more positive self-images. The groupings appeared to be related to the ability of the women to see exercise as beneficial to health and well-being, as distinct from concerns about body appearance.[48]

• Galantino and colleagues used focus groups, nonparticipant observation, and journals to gather data that demonstrated the use of exercise groups resulted in positive physical changes, enhanced psychological coping, and improved social interactions for a group of people living with acquired immunodeficiency syndrome (AIDS).[49]

Qualitative Research and an Understanding of the Clinician's Willingness to Use Evidence in Practice

Qualitative research can help us understand our patients' behavior; it can also help us understand our own behavior. As we will discuss in more depth in Section III, much guidance is available for making the best recommendations to our patients, but, as we discuss in Section IV, clinicians do not always accept the recommendations made in the literature or make the required changes in their behavior. From evidence explicating the beliefs and perceptions of clinicians about information found in the literature, we can better understand the reasons for this seemingly incongruent behavior.

Salbach et al conducted in-depth interviews with physical therapists about the nature of their clinical questions and the sources of their information when choosing rehabilitation interventions for stroke patients in the management of walking. They found that therapists were most likely to consult with peers rather than the literature. Therapists cited difficulty with technology in accessing information and also indicated that appraisal of the literature was a challenging task. These types of perceptions and problems can keep therapists from identifying the most effective interventions available to help patients like Mrs. Stevenson.[50]

Very similar results were found by Schreiber et al in their study of school-based pediatric physical therapists' perceptions of evidence based practice. All participants viewed it favorably, but they also cited as barriers difficulties with accessing and analyzing literature and relied on peers and supervisors for assistance in making clinical decisions rather than evidence in the literature.[51] A study by Hutchinson and Johnston of nurses in Australia echoed these results. Interviews designed to understand the development of clinical management tools to guide care showed that while the nurses assumed responsibility for this activity, they were more likely to use personal experience and knowledge arising from direct patient care than information from the literature.[52]

ROLE OF QUALITATIVE RESEARCH

As we discuss in Chapter 10, defining the clinical question is the important first part of providing evidence-based care for patients. Both quantitative and qualitative research can answer many of the same questions, but the central issue is what the best approach is to a full exploration of the issues or phenomena that answer the question.

Here are two studies, one qualitative and one quantitative, that appear to address a similar clinical question: What role do parents play in the motor development of their children? Nixon-Cave used qualitative methods to understand the influence of the family's cultural and ethnic beliefs on the motor development of infants from three ethnic groups: African American, Hispanic/Latino and Anglo European. The study, focused on the environmental/cultural influences, including maternal childrearing practices and behaviors, demonstrated that parents do indeed have different expectations of motor development, what constitutes normality, and what their role is in fostering normal development.[53] This is consistent with the purpose of the qualitative study—to understand a phenomenon, the experience of an individual, a process and the outcome, and to answer questions like why and how and to describe experience using both inductive and deductive approaches.

A second study by Kolobe of Mexican American mothers is a quantitative study of the relationship between maternal childrearing practices and behaviors and the developmental status of Mexican American infants. This study used standardized surveys with forced-choice responses along with outcome measures of infant development to identify through statistical analysis the relationships between certain aspects of childrearing and infant development. A quantitative study, it sought to identify clear, specific outcomes—objective, measurable outcomes that could predict cause-effect relationships and could be generalized to a larger population.[54] This approach attempts to answer how many, how much, and what questions. These two studies complement each other and are very good examples of studies that provide different types of data around similar, but not identical, questions. The two approaches used—in-depth interviews in one and standardized surveys in the other—could easily be combined in what is termed the mixed methods approach to make sure no evidence is missed. What must always be the first consideration is what type of data best answer the clinical question.

CONCLUSION

An outcome of integrating the patient's values into practice allows for a positive patient-therapist relationship that is focused on patients and their needs. This relationship is enhanced by considering the patient's values and preferences through a mutual inquiry process, finding common ground to negotiate care and a plan for intervention through teaching and problem solving.

In light of the increasing adoption of evidence-based practice (EBP), it is crucial for the clinician to be able to identify the patient's values and preferences and therefore seek evidence from research approaches that address these issues. In this chapter, we reviewed the concept of EBP and introduced qualitative research methods, which appears to be an approach that is well suited to fully understanding the patient's preferences and values.

SELF-ASSESSMENT

1. Think back to your last two or three patients. Identify at least one question about each patient that will help you better understand their values and perspectives.
2. Using these questions, think about how you might structure some qualitative data collection to help answer each question.
3. Describe the value of qualitative research to one of your colleagues who is familiar only with the quantitative paradigm.

CONTINUED LEARNING

There are some excellent texts that describe qualitative research. Several are referenced in this chapter:

- Morse JM, Swanson MN, Kuzel A, eds. *The Nature of Qualitative Evidence.*
- Hammell KW, Carpenter C. *Qualitative Research in Evidence-Based Rehabilitation.*
- Creswell JW. *Qualitative Inquiry and Research Design: Choosing Among Five Traditions.*
- Moustakas C. *Phenomenological Research Methods.*
- Denzin N, Lincoln Y. *Handbook of Qualitative Research,* 2nd ed.
- Fetterman DM. *Ethnography: Step by Step.*
- Strauss A, Corbin J. *Basics of Qualitative Research: Grounded Theory Procedures and Techniques.*
- Patton MQ. *Qualitative Research and Evaluation Methods,* 3rd ed.

1. Identify a research question that you have had about patient care.
2. Using one of these texts, design a qualitative study that will help answer your question.

REFERENCES

1. Leininger MM. *Qualitative Research Methods in Nursing.* Orlando, FL: Grune & Stratton; 1985.
2. Sofaer S. Qualitative methods: What are they and why use them? Health Services Research. 1999;34:1101–1108.
3. Morse JM, Swanson MN, Kuzel A, eds. *The Nature of Qualitative Evidence.* Thousand Oaks, CA: Sage; 2001.
4. Hammell KW, Carpenter C. *Qualitative Research in Evidence-Based Rehabilitation.* Philadelphia: Churchill Livingston; 2004.
5. Goering PN, Streiner DL. Reconcilable differences: The marriage of qualitative and quantitative methods. Can J Psych. 1996;41:491–497.
6. Morgan D. Practical strategies for combining qualitative and quantitative methods: Applications to health research. Qual Health Res. 1998;8:362–372.
7. Creswell JW. *Qualitative Inquiry and Research Design: Choosing Among Five Traditions.* Thousand Oaks, CA: Sage; 1998.
8. Moustakas C. *Phenomenological Research Methods.* Thousand Oaks, CA: Sage; 1994.
9. Gubrium JF, Holstein JA. Analyzing interpretive practice. In: Denzin N, Lincoln Y, eds. *Handbook of Qualitative Research,* 2nd ed. Thousand Oaks, CA: Sage; 2000.
10. Fetterman DM. *Ethnography: Step by Step.* Newbury Park, CA: Sage; 1989.
11. Mead M. *Coming of Age in Samoa.* New York: Morrow; 1928.
12. Mead M. Ethnological aspects of aging. Psychosomatics 1967:8(Suppl);33–37.
13. Strauss A, Corbin J. *Basics of Qualitative Research: Grounded Theory Procedures and Techniques.* Thousand Oaks, CA: Sage; 1990.
14. Kielhofner G. Qualitative research, part two. Methodological approaches and relevance of occupational therapy. Occ Ther J Res. 1982;2:150.
15. Kreuger RA, Casey MA. *Focus Groups,* 3rd ed. Thousand Oaks, CA: Sage; 2000.
16. Britten N. Qualitative research: Qualitative interviews in medical research. BMJ 1995;311:251–253.
17. Santasier AM. Factors that influenced individuals from ethnically diverse groups to become physical therapists. Diss. Philadelphia: Temple University; 2004.
18. Lincoln YA, Guba EG. *Naturalistic Inquiry.* Thousand Oaks, CA: Sage; 1985.
19. Brink PJ. Issues in reliability and validity. In: Morse JM, ed. *Qualitative Nursing Research: A Contemporary Dialogue.* Rockville, MD: Aspen, 1989; 151–168.
20. DePoy E, Gitlin N. *Introduction to Research: Multiple Strategies for Health and Human Services.* St. Louis: Mosby; 1993.
21. Patton MQ. *Qualitative Research and Evaluation Methods,* 3rd ed. Thousand Oaks, CA: Sage; 2002.
22. Sandelowski MM. Sample size in qualitative research. Res Nurs Health 1995;18:179–183.
23. Jack SM. Utility of qualitative research findings in evidence-based public health practice. Pub Health Nurs. 23(3);277–283.
24. Grypdonck MHK. Qualitative health research in the era of evidence-based practice. Qual Health Res.2006;16(10):1371–1385.
25. Mazurek Melnyk, B, Fineout-Overbolt, E. *Evidence Based Practice in Nursing and Healthcare.* Philadelphia: Lippincott Williams and Williams; 2005.
26. Lorish CD, Gale JR. Facilitating adherence to healthy lifestyle behavior changes in patients. In: Shepard KF, Jensen GM. *Handbook of Teaching for Physical Therapists,* 2nd ed. Boston: Butterworth Heinemann; 2002.
27. Schulman-Green D, Naik AD, McCorkle, R, Bradley EH, Bogardus ST. Goal setting as a shared decision making strategy among clinicians and their older patients. Pat Educ and Counsel. 2006;63(1/2):145–151.
28. Wirtz V, Cribb A, Barber N. Patient-doctor decision making about treatment within the consultation—A critical analysis of models. Soc Sci and Med. 2006;62(1):116–124.
29. vanZwieten MCB, Willems DL, Knegt LK, Leschot NJ. Communication with patients during the prenatal testing procedure. An explorative qualitative study. Pat Educ and Counsel. 2006;63(1–2):161–168.

30. Institute for Family-Centered Care. http://www.familycenteredcare.org/faq.html Accessed August 29, 2009.
31. Stewart M. Towards a global definition of patient centred care. BMJ 2001; 322(7284):444–445.
32. Shields L, Pratt J, Hunter J. Family centred care: A review of qualitative studies. J Clin Nurs. 2006;10:1317–1323.
33. Patient Preferences in Health Care Decision Making. http://people.dbmi.columbia.edu/~cmr7001/sdm/html/shared_decision_making.htm Accessed March 27, 2011.
34. Kaplan RM. Shared medical decision making: A new tool for preventive medicine. Am J Prevent Med. 2004;26(1):81–83.
35. Woolf SH. Shared decision making: The case for letting patients decide which choice is best. J Fam Pract. 1997;45(3):205–208.
36. Edwards A, Elwyn G, Hood K, Atwell C, Robling M, Houstin H, Kinnersley P, Russell I. Study Steering Group. Patient-based outcome results from a cluster randomized trial of shared decision making skill development and use of risk communication aids in general practice. Fam Pract. 2004;21(4):347–354.
37. Protheroe J, Fahey T, Montgomery AA, Peters TJ. The impact of patients' preferences on the treatment of atrial fibrillation: Observational study of patient based decision analysis. BMJ 2000;320:1380–1384.
38. Montgomery AA, Harding J, Fahey T. Shared decision making in hypertension: The impact of patient preferences on treatment choice. Fam. Pract. 2001;18:309–313.
39. Moser A, van der Bruggen H, Widdershoven G. Competency in shaping one's life: Autonomy of people with type 2 diabetes mellitus in a nurse-led, shared-care setting; a qualitative study. Int J Nurs Studies. 2006;May;43(4):417–427.
40. Schulman-Green D, Naik AD, McCorkle, R, Bradley EH, Bogardus ST. Goal setting as a shared decision making strategy among clinicians and their older patients. Pat Educ and Couns. 2006;63(1/2):145–151.
41. Schmid AA, Rittman M. Consequences of poststroke falls: Activity limitation, increased dependence, and the development of fear of falling. Am J Occ Ther. 2009: 63:310–316.
42. Carpenter C. The experience of spinal cord injury: The individual's perspective— Implications for rehabilitation practice. Phys Ther. 1994;74(7):614–628.
43. Dickie VA, Baranek GT, Schultz B, Watson LR, McComish CS. Parent reports of sensory experiences of preschool children with and without autism: A qualitative study. Am J Occ Ther. 2009;63:172–181.
44. Hamilton JB, Stweart BJ, Crandell JL, Lynn MR. Development of the Ways of Helping Questionnaire: A measure of preferred coping strategies for older African American cancer survivors. Res in Nurs & Health. 2009;32:243–259.
45. Monninkof E, van der Aa M, van der Valk P, van der Palen J, Zielhuis G, Koning K, Pieterse, M. A qualitative evaluation of comprehensive self-management programmme for COPD patients: Effectiveness from the patients' perspective. Pat Educ and Counsel. 2004;55:177–184.
46. Gooberman-Hill R, French M, Dieppe P, Hawker G. Expressing pain and fatigue: A new method of analysis to explore differences in osteoarthritis experience. Arth & Rheum (Arthritis Care & Research). 2009, March 15;61(3):353–360.
47. Malpass A, Andrews R, Turner KM. Patients with type 2 diabetes experiences of making multiple lifestyle changes: A qualitative study. Pat Educ and Counsel. 2009;74:258–263.
48. Sabiston CM, McDonough MH, Sedgwick A, Crocker PRE. Muscle gains and emotional strains: Conflicting experiences of change among overweight women participating in an exercise intervention program. Qual Health Res. 2009;19:466–480.
49. Galantino ML, Shepard K, Krafft L, Laperriere A, Ducette J, Sorbello A, Barnish M, Concoluci D, Farrar, JT. The effect of group aerobic exercise and T'ai Chi on functional outcomes and quality of life for persons living with acquired immunodeficiency syndrome. Alt and Complement Med. 2005;11:1085–1092.
50. Salbach NM, Guilcher SJT, Jaglal SB, Davis DA. Factors influencing information seeking by physical therapists providing stroke management. Phys Ther. 2009;89:556–568.

51. Schreiber J, Stern P, Marchett G, Provident I, Turocy PS. School-based pediatric physical therapists' perspectives on evidence-based practice. Pediatr Phys Ther. 2008;20: 292–302.
52. Hutchinson AM, Johnston L. An observational study of health professionals' use of evidence to inform the development of clinical management tools. J Clin Nurs. 2008;17:2203–2211.
53. Nixon-Cave KA. Influence of the family's cultural/ethnic beliefs and behaviors as well as the environment on the motor development of infants 12–18 months of age in 3 ethnic groups: African-American, Hispanic/Latino and Anglo-European. Diss Philadelphia: Temple University; 2001.
54. Kolobe THA. Childrearing practices and developmental expectations for Mexican-American mothers and the developmental status of their infants. Phys Ther. 2004;84:439–453.

chapter 9

The Health Care System and Patient Circumstances

Michael P. Johnson, PT, PhD, OCS

"Everyone in a complex system has a slightly different interpretation. The more interpretations we gather, the easier it becomes to gain a sense of the whole."

—Margaret J. Wheatley

•

* Mr. Ketterman's Case

I know that Mr. and Mrs. Ketterman have had to pay for their assisted living facility themselves, and that a physical therapist comes into the facility to see many of the residents. They are confused about what services Mr. Ketterman is eligible for under his Medicare insurance and what he is entitled to from the facility. They are also trying to decide if he should be admitted to a nursing home. They would like my advice about the best way to get him the services he needs, at the lowest cost to them. *(See Appendix for Mr. Ketterman's health history.)*

INTRODUCTION

Sociologists suggest that disease, and therefore health, are fundamentally impacted by access to resources, which allow the ability to avoid risk or minimize the effects of disease once it has occurred.[1] It is important to recognize that the ability to access services can be modified by financial, social, and cultural factors.[2-6] Andersen[7] developed a behavioral model that has been used over the years to understand why patients use health services and what factors impact their ability to access these services. In his initial model, proposed in the 1960s,[8] he described three factors that primarily impact a patient's access to care:

1. predisposing characteristics, such as age, race/ethnicity, gender, education level, and health beliefs;
2. enabling resources, such as income level, insurance coverage, proximity to services, and having a regular source of care; and
3. need, such as health and functional status (Fig. 9-1).

135

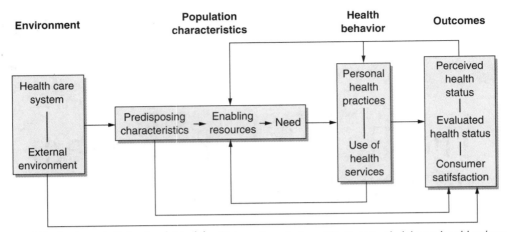

Figure 9-1 Andersen's Behavioral Model. *(Redrawn from: Andersen RM. Revisiting the behavioral model and access to medical care: Does it matter? J Health Soc Behav. 1995;36:1–10.)*

There is ample evidence in the current literature to support that many of these factors do, in fact, impact the patient's circumstance regarding access to health care.[9-23] Later, Andersen recognized that in addition to these three factors there were other things that impacted the patient's use of services, such as the external environment (physical—air/water quality, food supply—politics and the economy) and the health care system (health policies and resources).[7]

The United States (U.S.) health care system consists of a large and complex collection of federal, state, and local government organizations, private entities, and practitioners, all of whom provide or pay for a wide array of health care services. The United States is the only large industrialized country in the world that does not have a single-payer system providing health care to all of its citizens. Instead, we have developed a payment system in which employers and local, state, and federal government programs finance most health care delivery through a variety of health benefits programs. In addition, individual patients pay for a portion of their health care costs directly. Providers (physicians, hospitals, etc.) and payers (insurance companies, health plans, etc.) alike function within a health care market where they compete for beneficiaries and patients.

The delivery of health care services occurs in a variety of settings, including acute care hospitals, skilled nursing facilities, community health centers, and the patient's own home, to name a few. The setting in which a patient receive services is determined by a number of factors, such as injury acuity, disease specificity (e.g., cancer), age, etc. These are intended to reflect the patient's needs related to care but are often influenced by additional factors unrelated to need, such as insurance coverage, proximity to health care facilities, and the availability of providers.[8]

The number of Americans involved in the organization, delivery, and payment for health care services in this country is large and makes up over 11% of the total U.S. workforce.[24] The workforce is diverse and has been historically organized in a hierarchical fashion, with physicians most often serving as the primary decision makers. Physicians have held that authority within health care for nearly a century and, therefore, the delivery system has been structured largely to meet their needs.[25] As our health care system evolves, physicians still play a significant role in determining a patient's need for health services and directing how and where that care will occur. Many others health professions, however, such as nursing, physical therapy, pharmacy, psychology, and others, have been growing and expanding their knowledge and skill over this same time period.[26,27] As a result, there are now many health care practitioners who provide similar services and are involved in making care decisions for and with their patients.[28,29] While recommendations have been made for greater patient input into their own care,[30,31] the historically authoritative role of health professionals continues to have a significant impact on how, where, and under what circumstances patients receive care.

Many aspects of the U.S. health care system either aid or impede a patient's ability to access high-quality care. Access to care is not assured by simply having specific health services available; rather, access is defined as the "freedom or ability to obtain or make use of [those services]."[32] Andersen modified his initial behavioral model in order to acknowledge the impact that the health care system had on access to care.[7] In order to begin to appreciate the circumstances that impact a patient, one must have a basic understanding of health policy. By definition, the term *policy* means "a definite course or method of action selected from among alternatives and in light of given conditions to guide and determine present and future decisions."[32] Public health policy refers to any course of action, influenced largely by the need for health care, that helps determine the decisions related to the financing and delivery of health care services in this country. One example would be creation of the Medicare program, which provided a structure for financing health care for all citizens aged 65 years and older.[33]

Given the myriad of people and organizations who are involved in determining, setting, and modifying health policies, we can begin to understand how and why this "system" became so complex. Ours is the most heavily regulated health care system in the world.[34] As a result, patients (and practitioners) must navigate through a labyrinth of rules and regulations, mostly crafted by those who pay for health care, in an attempt to meet their health needs.

This chapter will provide an overview of the U.S. health care system, including

- systems for the delivery of services,
- resources for providing and improving care,
- the health care market's influence on service delivery, and
- regulations defining the rules by which care can be rendered (Fig. 9-2).

As well, we will review of health services research and examples of specific patient circumstances, which are known to influence the care they receive. It is expected that by understanding the issues patients must contend with in an effort to maintain or improve their health and well-being, health care practitioners will be better prepared to care for patients and their families, including advocating more effectively for their health needs.

OVERVIEW OF THE HEALTH CARE SYSTEM

As we begin to look at the U.S. health care system and patient circumstances related to maintaining and improving their health, we must first ask ourselves what is it we mean by "health"? The Merriam-Webster Online dictionary defines health simply as "freedom from physical disease or pain."[32] However, the World Health Organization (WHO) defines health in broader terms as "the state of complete physical, mental and social well-being and not merely the absence of disease or infirmity."[35] This definition is accepted within the United States[36]; it recognizes that health is a multifaceted issue, with intersecting anatomical, physiological, psychological, and social factors impacting the patient. In this context, health and well-being

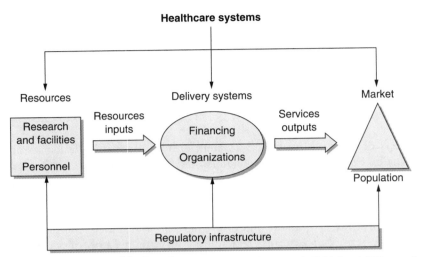

Figure 9-2 Overview of the Health Care System. *(Adapted from: Kissick W. Medicine's Dilemmas: Infinite Need Versus Finite Resources. New Haven, CT: Yale University Press; 1994.)*

are also affected by cultural influences, as well as the external environment and the health care system itself.

Let's look at the following two case examples in order to get a sense of how we might gauge someone's "health."

✳ Case Example — Mrs. Alexander

Mrs. Alexander is a 78-year-old retired seamstress with severe arthritis, non-insulin-dependent diabetes mellitus, and cardiovascular disease. She has had the same primary care physician for the last 15 years, who has managed her diseases with medication and recommendations for activity modification. She is able to live in her own home with some assistance from her daughter, who lives nearby. Although Mrs. Alexander needs assistance for some activities of daily living (ADLs), she can prepare her own meals, attend a weekly bridge club with her friends, and participate in family and community events.

✳ Case Example — Mr. Tomba

Mr. Tomba is a 42-year-old male who has a history of low back pain, works for a landscape company, and receives no health benefits. He has been diagnosed as prediabetic but manages his health without regular medical visits or health education. Two weeks ago, Mr. Tomba strained his low back at work and has been in constant pain. He is able to continue working but cannot tolerate performing ADLs at home (such as mowing the lawn, cleaning the gutters) after work due to pain. He has stopped participating in family activities and has missed the last two of his son's baseball games.

Discussion Questions
- So, which of these two patients has less disease?
- Which has more functional limitations?
- Which patient would you classify as having better "health"?

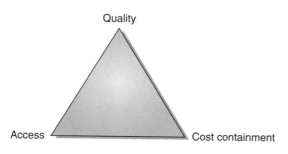

Figure 9-3 The Iron Triangle of Health Care as Defined by Kissick. *(Redrawn from: Kissick W. Medicine's Dilemmas: Infinite Need Versus Finite Resources. New Haven, CT: Yale University Press; 1994.)*

Kissick's Model: The Iron Triangle of Health Care

In 1994, William Kissick[37] described a model referred to as the "Iron Triangle of Health Care" in an effort to clarify the factors that influence health policy decisions and thus the health care system. This model represents the inextricable link between competing issues of access, cost containment, and quality in health care.

Kissick suggests that, much like the angles of an equilateral triangle, altering any one of these elements requires a change in one or both of the others (Fig. 9-3). This suggested balance among these key elements within our health care system begins to inform our understanding of the competing tensions between access to and the cost and quality of health services that can occur. Because one or more of these three elements primarily shape nearly every health care debate, the model is helpful when attempting to understand the U.S. system. It is important for physical therapists to have an understanding of how health policies are derived because they can significantly impact the patient's circumstances related to cost, quality, and access to care.

Over the past 100 years, the U.S. health care system has evolved through periods that have focused on each element of Kissick's Iron Triangle. Quality of care was the primary concern at the turn of the last century (1890s to1920s), resulting in advancements in public health such as immunizations and the use of quarantines to control large-scale disease epidemics as well as medical education and state licensure laws to improve the training and practice of health professionals.[25] Access to care was the focus from the 1920s to1960s; it was accomplished through two primary mechanisms, payment and infrastructure development. Payment for health services moved from a being a direct responsibility of the patient to being handled by employers through development of employer-based health insurance in the late 1920s[25] and the federal government through development of Medicare and Medicaid programs in 1965.[38] Last, containing the rising costs of health care has been a major focus since the 1970s.[30,39–41] The tension across the elements of Kissick's Iron Triangle can still be felt as we continue to search for the right balance within our system.

Elements of the Health Care System

In the following sections, we will explore four distinct aspects of the U.S. health care system:

1. resources,
2. the delivery system,
3. the regulatory infrastructure, and
4. health care markets (see Fig. 9-2).

In particular, we will examine how these elements of the health care system impact the patients' circumstances when it comes to receiving the care they need.

Resources: Personnel

Our health care system relies on multiple resources for providing evidence-based care. These resources include:

- an educated, highly skilled workforce to provide services,
- health care facilities that provide a place for patients to receive services, and
- research infrastructure and funding to expand knowledge and understanding of disease and disability.

All of these resources (people, places, and knowledge) are important components of the system we have created, and their availability directly impacts a patient's circumstance related to care. The quality of health professionals, the accessibility of health care facilities (i.e., hospitals, health centers, etc.), and the availability of knowledge and information all help shape the patient's experience.

Health care in the United States today is based primarily upon the "medical model" of care. This model is built upon the cultural authority and autonomy of physicians over patient care, with a strong reliance on science and technology. Since the turn of the last century, physicians have held a position of authority over the delivery of health care and many related services. This authority was gained through a confluence of events in the late 1800s and early 1900s, which included the development of state boards of medicine and subsequent licensure requirements within the states, elevation of academic standards within medical schools, and effective utilization of professional representation and advocacy through the American Medical Association. In large part, these events lead to physicians gaining nearly complete authority over health care, control that continued largely unabated until the latter part of the 20th century.[25]

The U.S. Department of Labor reports that there are over 500,000 medical physicians in this country (Box 9.1).[24] The majority of physicians practice in specialty areas, with the rest

Box 9.1   Number of Physicians in the United States

Primary Care:	
Family and General Practitioners	109,400
Internists, General	48,700
Obstetricians and Gynecologists	22,520
Pediatricians, General	28,930
	209,550
Speciality Care:	
Psychiatrists	24,300
Anesthesiologists	29,890
Surgeons	51,900
All Other Physicians	208,960
	315,050
Total Physicians	524,500

Data from the National Occupational Employment and Wage Estimates, Healthcare Practitioner and Technical Occupations. U.S. Department of Labor, 2008. (http://www.bls.gov/oes/current/oes_nat.htm#b29-0000; accessed March 28, 2011.)

Box 9.2 Number of Other Health Professionals in the United States

Health Care Professionals:

Dieticians / Nutritionists	51,230
Pharmacists	239,920
Physician Assistants	62,960
Registered Nurses	2,417,150
Audiologists	10,910
Occupational Therapists	88,570
Physical Therapists	156,100
Speech-Language Pathologists	98,690
	3,125,530
Health Technicians / Support Personnel:	5,724,170
Grand Total:	8,849,700

Data from the National Occupational Employment and Wage Estimates, Healthcare Practitioner and Technical Occupations. U.S. Department of Labor, 2008. (http://www.bls.gov/oes/current/oes_nat.htm#b29-0000; accessed March 28, 2011.)

serving as primary care providers. Over the past decade the emphasis on specialty care in medicine has resulted in a relative decrease in the number of primary care physicians. As a result, other health professionals, such as certified registered nurse practitioners (CRNP) and physician assistants (PA), have a growing presence in primary care. These two provider groups are considered to be part of a larger group of health professionals, including physicians, known as primary care providers (PCP).

In the past 10 to 20 years, such health professionals as nurses, physical therapists, and pharmacists have begun to assume a greater role within the health care delivery system. Box 9.2 gives a sense of the variety and number of other health professionals who have become integral to health care delivery in this country.[24] This growth resulted, in part, from a sense of increased need for providers and from the concept of using health teams, with "physician extenders," as a way to increase access and decrease costs.[25] Over the past 25 to 30 years, advances in science and technology have required new skill sets and knowledge from all health care providers, so there has been a concomitant growth in the expertise of these other health professionals, whose academic requirements for graduation from their accredited programs have been consistently elevated in response to a changing health care environment.[42–44] Today, significantly more people are utilizing nonphysician clinicians for certain types of care, such as preventive services.[28]

The Institutes of Medicine (IOM) recently recommended improvements in the quality of care in this country, including changing the existing model of health care delivery.[45] It recommended transitioning away from an autonomous physician model and instead moving toward a collaborative, multidisciplinary team model in which nonphysician providers play a more central role. Within this team model, the IOM notes that the "individual who serves as the [team] leader may not be ... associated with a particular discipline, such as medicine."[30]

True multidisciplinary practice will require the collaboration and interdependence of all providers with a shared focus on efficient, accessible, quality patient care. The IOM specifically noted the "importance of collaborative work both for clinical care and for improvement efforts."[30] Multidisciplinary collaboration models have been shown to be effective in improving the care of patients with chronic conditions[46] and when providing preventive services.[47] However, the availability of these types of multidisciplinary teams to help manage the myriad of health problems in the aged and those with chronic disease is limited.[48]

Physical therapists, originating as physician extenders, typically function under the medical model of care (emphasizing the management of disease), particularly as it involves the use of scientific knowledge and evidence to promote quality practice. However, they are educated in a rehabilitation model of care, which is built upon

1. a collaborative, team approach for the enhancement of efficient, quality patient care;
2. a focus not only on disease and illness but also a strong emphasis on wellness and prevention; and
3. a paradigm of health management that is broader than disease management and endeavors to look at the whole person.

The concept of health management uses medical and social models of functioning to provide a framework within which health is part of a process. This process encompasses health conditions and their impact on the components of bodily function and structure, activities an individual undertakes, and the individual's participation life situations. Therefore, physical therapists are prepared to work interdependently, as members of health care teams, functioning collaboratively within the health care system and remaining patient-centered when it comes to care delivery.[26]

✳ Case Example — Mrs. Kimble

Mrs. Kimble is a 74-year-old female who lives alone and was recently hospitalized secondary to a fall and resultant intertrochanteric hip fracture. She had an ORIF four days ago and has been receiving inpatient physical therapy services. Mrs. Kimble is now ready for discharge from the hospital.

Discussion Questions
- What factors determine where she will be transferred for the next level of care?
- What role does Mrs. Kimble have in determining who provides her physical therapy care and where she will receive those services?
- Who does or should decide what is best for this patient regarding the next setting where she receives further physical therapy?

Resources: Facilities and Research Infrastructure

In addition to a highly educated and skilled health care workforce, other resources are necessary for the delivery of quality care, including facilities in which to deliver a wide range of health services and good scientific evidence regarding the diagnosis and treatment of disease and dysfunction. Infrastructure development was undertaken to make sure there were adequate facilities (hospitals, health centers, etc.) and knowledge (via research) to allow for the delivery of high-quality health services.

In 1930, the federal government passed legislation to provide public funding for medical research.[25] Eventually, the National Institutes of Health (NIH) was created, one of the largest agencies funding the development of health-related research in the United States. Today, the NIH supports basic science, clinical, and health services research. The Foundation for Physical

Therapy Research, although not of the size and impact of the NIH, is designed to focus completely on research in these three areas that helps to promote the needs of patients cared for by physical therapists.

Shortly after initiating the NIH, the federal government pledged to assist "states, counties, health districts, and other political subdivisions of the states in establishing and maintaining adequate public-health services" via Title VI of the Social Security Act.[49] In 1946, the Hospital Survey and Construction Act (known as the Hill-Burton Act) provided federal funding to construct community hospitals across the country.[50] This effort ultimately resulted in the array of facilities available today, ranging from small community clinics and hospitals to large, complex, tertiary care facilities, under a variety of forms of ownership, including publicly traded companies, religious groups, community boards, and governmental units.[51] As a result of these and other initiatives, Americans have expanded resources for care through improved evidence based knowledge for providers and the construction of facilities across the country where patients can receive services.

Delivery System

The ability to provide services requires a delivery system that integrates the resources (people, places, and knowledge) to do the job and the finances to pay for it. In most industrialized countries, the central government plays the primary role in resource management and funding for health care, with some variation across countries. Examining the systems in Great Britain, Canada, and the United States can be very helpful in identifying the unique features of our system and putting them into context.

The British National Health Service (NHS) plays the largest governmental role in health care funding; nearly 90% of funding comes from the government and the rest from private sources (voluntary insurance, out-of-pocket payment). The Canadian system is somewhere in between the British and the U.S. systems, with nearly 70% percent paid by governmental sources (~30% federal and ~40% provincial) and the rest by private sources (voluntary insurance, out-of-pocket payment). Of the three, otherwise similar countries, the U.S. government plays the smallest role in health care funding, with the federal and state governments (primarily through Medicare and Medicaid) providing approximately 40%, private insurance (provided largely by employers) nearly 30%, and the final 30% percent coming directly from patients in the form of out-of-pocket expenses.

The funding of the British NHS and its authority over the types of services offered and how they are provided are very centralized. In contrast, control in the U.S. system is very decentralized in terms of determining the types of services offered and how (and by whom) they are provided. The U.S. physician's level of autonomy in decision making is very high, a result, in part, of a historically well-organized and politically active medical profession.[25] Private funding for health care is under less centralized control, but the insurance industry is closely regulated by the states (solvency, fiduciary requirements, mandated benefits). The financial control of publicly funded government programs such as Medicare and Medicaid is very centralized, but they are much less so regarding organization (eligibility, types of services, e.g., state control of Medicaid).

The greatest focus of the NHS is on primary care and is therefore designed to address the health of the population as a whole. This is consistent with its viewpoint, which emphasizes the good of society and is more in keeping with a public health perspective. The emphasis is on primary care for *everyone*, which sacrifices (perhaps) timely specialty care. Each patient is attached to a general practitioner (GP). The GP (who is not directly employed by the government, but rather is an independent contractor with a Family Health Services Authority) acts as a gatekeeper for all specialty and hospital care. The control of care is at the level of the GP, yet it exists within very prescribed government-mandated guidelines.

One of the criticisms of the NHS (by Americans more so than the British) is the long waiting periods for specialty care such as elective surgery (e.g., joint replacements, etc.) Within the United States, the emphasis has long been on specialty care. Americans pride themselves on having the best health care in the world, and by this they typically mean specialty care (e.g., cardiac surgery, total joint replacements, liver transplants). The U.S. system is based on a strong foundation of autonomy and is designed with a focus on the individual patient. Specialty care, however, is expensive. When managed care organization took a dominant role in the U.S. health system during the push for cost containment in the 1990s, it emphasized primary care over specialty care and used PCPs as "gatekeepers" (much like the NHS).

The Canadian system falls in between the British and American systems with its strong emphasis on primary care (much more so than in the United States) through a government-funded system. However, the private sector functions more like that of the United States, allowing those who can afford it greater options for specialty care. The Canadian system is a hybrid, with everyone covered for primary care as well as individual options (based on means, not need) for other types and amounts of services.

We can see how a nation chooses to organize its health system and, philosophically, how choices are made between approaches that focus on populations (public health model) versus individuals (medical model) can impact the patient's circumstances. Within the United States, in a system that focuses on the individual and allows high levels of decision making autonomy to physicians and other providers, the provider can exert a great degree of control over some aspects of the patient's circumstances. In addition, health insurance coverage and health benefits plans, which are responsible for reimbursing providers for the services they render, also impact the patient's circumstances.[52–54] Historically, health care payment mechanisms arose from both the public and private sectors. Employer-based health insurance started in the late 1920s,[25] and Title V of the Social Security Act of 1935[49] included funding for "services for promoting the health of mothers and children, especially in rural areas and in areas suffering from severe economic distress."

The next section of this chapter will briefly review some of the primary programs responsible for paying the health care bill in the United States. They are divided into

1. federally funded programs,
2. programs funded by both state and federal governments, and
3. private insurance programs.

Federally Funded Programs

Medicare The Medicare program[55–60] was created in 1965 through an amendment to the Social Security Act (Title XVIII of the Social Security Act of 1965, 42 U.S.C. § 1395 et seq.).[38] It provided a mechanism to increase access to health care for older Americans.[61,62] Medicare consists of a compulsory hospital insurance program under Social Security (Part A) and a government-funded voluntary insurance program to cover payment for physician services (Part B). Medicare Part A covers the costs of inpatient hospitalization. The Hospital Insurance (HI) Trust Fund for Part A, a form of social insurance based on the same concept as Social Security, is funded through mandatory employee contributions, with an associated employer match, from all working Americans.[55] Enrollment is based upon age. People are automatically eligible once they reach 65 years of age.

Medicare Part B was developed as a voluntary, supplemental insurance program to help pay for physician services. It has since been extended to a variety of outpatient services, including physical therapy. Participation in this aspect of the program is voluntary for both beneficiaries and providers; however, most do choose to participate.[33] If patients choose to enroll, they contribute to the Supplemental Medical Insurance (SMI) Trust Fund through voluntary payroll deductions and a 75/25 funding match from the government.[58,59] Medicare payment was, and still is, based upon the private insurance model present in the 1960s—fee for service—which reimbursed providers on the basis of the amount of services provided. As well, the payment model was based primarily on the management of acute disease.[59]

The proportion of the population over 65 is expected to increase from 13.3% to 18.5% between 2010 and 2025.[3] While Medicare insures one in every seven Americans today, it is predicted that by 2030 it will insure more than one in every five Americans.[57] Medicare recently added a prescription drug benefit (Medicare Part D) in 2003.[63] Medicare does not cover long-term care, resulting in a significant portion of the cost of long-term care borne by the public through Medicaid.[64]

Discussions of the strengths and weaknesses of the Medicare program are ubiquitous in policy literature and the popular press. Overall, however, many would agree that Medicare has successfully accomplished what it was set out to do: provide access to medical care through a defined set of benefits available to all Americans aged 65 and older.[58,60,65,66]

Other Federal Programs There are many other programs funded through federal dollars that provide either payment for services or direct services. They include the Federal Employees Health Benefits Program, which is offered to all federal employees, retirees, and their survivors.[67,72] Other programs, which also provide direct services, include the Indian health service, the health services of the Department of Veteran Affairs, and the health care services and insurance for military personnel and their dependents.

Programs with Dual (State and Federal) Oversight

Medicaid The Medicaid program was created in 1965 through an amendment (Title XIX) to the Social Security Act.[38] Unlike Medicare, the Medicaid program is administered by the states and paid for in part by both the state and federal governments. This shared financial partnership was, and remains, a unique feature of Medicaid. Through it, the states retain more local control over services provided to beneficiaries deemed eligible through means testing while receiving matching funds from the federal government to pay for a variety of services.

A welfare program jointly administered by the state and federal government, Medicaid originally provided services to the "deserving" poor, who typically included the aged, blind, disabled, and dependent children. More recently, Medicaid has been expanded to include pregnant mothers and infants, a greater number of children, poor Medicare recipients (as a form of supplement,which pays largely for long-term, nursing home care), and finally a much greater number of those with disabilities. Medicaid provides funding for some federally mandated benefits such as inpatient hospital services, outpatient hospital services, rural health clinics, laboratory and x-ray services, screenings, diagnosis and treatment of children, physician services, family planning services, and nursing services. However, the states have the discretion to cover other services as well (e.g., prescription drugs, complementary medicine, physical therapy, etc.).

In 1984, Congress mandated Medicaid coverage for pregnant women and children from birth to 5 years of age. Over the years, eligibility has expanded to provide coverage for more low-income women and children. The state children's health insurance program (sCHIP), created by the Balanced Budget Act (BBA) of 1997,[42] covers children whose family income is too high for Medicaid eligibility and it has become, along with Medicaid, the primary mechanism of health insurance for poor children across the country.[69,70] In 2006, sCHIP provided coverage for 6 million children, while Medicaid covered 28 million.[71] Unlike Medicaid, in which the federal government will match a certain percentage of each dollar the states elect to spend on health care, the sCHIP program is funded with a fixed amount of grant money (block grants).[70]

Workers' Compensation Worker's compensation provides benefits to injured workers that help to cover lost wages and medical expenses resulting from an injury that was sustained while on the job. The program was created in the early 1900s by the Federal Employment Compensation Act (FECA), 5 U.S.C. §§ 8101–8193.[72] It is a form of no-fault insurance that is regulated by the states and administered through the Office of Workman's Compensation Programs within the U.S. Department of Labor. The purpose of workers' compensation was to provide all civilian employees a guaranteed safety net against a loss of income due to work-related injuries. Previously, workers would have to sue their employers and assume the burden of proving that the employer was at fault for the injury (e.g., unsafe work environment, etc.). Employers were willing to embrace the workers' compensation program because it limited their liability from injury claims. Workers' compensation is thus considered the first program of social insurance to provide health benefits to Americans. Some believe that it paved the way for other forms of social insurance, such as unemployment insurance, Social Security Disability Insurance (SSDI), and eventually, in 1965, the Medicare and Medicaid programs.[38]

Private Insurance

Fee-for-Service World War II brought about price and wage freezes along with a shortage of available workers in the 1940s.[25] Companies struggled for a way in which to attract and keep a good quality workforce. Since salaries could not be adjusted, companies looked to benefits, such as health insurance, to attract employees. Thus began the link between employment and health insurance in the United States. Shortly after the end of the war, a large percentage of the workforce was covered by employer-based health insurance. The link was strengthened as labor unions used benefits, such as health insurance, in their continued negotiations with company management.[25] Government intervention, in the form of tax credits for these benefits, has continued to help maintain the link, as have employee expectations that these benefits would be provided as part of compensation for their labor.

Managed Care HMOs began in this country in the 1970s with the passage of the HMO Act in 1973. Interest in HMOs, at that time, arose from the perception of a health care "crisis" fueled by escalating costs. Managed care organizations address cost control, in part, through controlling access. Shifts in social attitudes toward viewing health care as a right, meaning everyone should have access and input, prompted further concern over cost containment. Federally qualified HMOs, unlike traditional insurance companies, regulated strictly by the states (via the McCarran-Ferguson Act), had to provide a rating scale for charges based on the community (versus experience) and allow a 30-day open enrollment period to all individuals (regardless of their health) annually. These additional requirements made HMOs the most heavily regulated form of third-party insurance. Although initially it had limited success, due in part to legislative restraints, the concept of managed care (HMOs, POS plans, and PPOs) has come to permeate and dominate the payer environment in health care. More than 80% of all Americans receive health care insurance under some form of managed care.

Impact of Rising Health Care Costs

As a result of double-digit increases in health care expenses for employers, particularly from the late 1970s to the early 1990s (and again beginning to increase as a result of an end to the cost containment effect of managed care), employers have seen health benefits for employees becoming a larger and larger burden on their "bottom line." To remain competitive and viable in the marketplace, employers have adopted a number of strategies to reduce their costs. They have

1. switched to lower-cost managed care options for employees,
2. turned to self-insurance (more likely in larger companies), and
3. begun to shift more and more of the expense for health care onto employees.

As well, companies have induced employees to opt for single coverage versus the more expensive option of family coverage (for those employees with families). The effect of cost shifting has been seen in a number of forms:

1. the capping of total employer benefit contributions, thus requiring employers to choose which benefits they want and how much extra they are willing (or able) to pay for benefits beyond the cap;
2. requiring employees pay more for health care benefits;
3. requiring higher co-pays and deductibles for indemnity and PPO plans; and
4. covering the employee only and not families.

These strategies of cost shifting to employees have had a direct effect on the number of uninsured persons in this country.[73] Employees who can no longer afford their health insurance benefit choose to opt out for other benefits or employees choose coverage for themselves, but not for family members. Many of these people earn too much money to be eligible for Medicaid or other assistance. Thus the system of employer-based health coverage, which is still the primary source of health insurance for the working population (18 to 64 years), has led us to a dependence on the employer as the market player who bears the burden for this group. The result of some employers' inability to afford these benefits for their employees and remain viable in the marketplace has forced some tough choices (particularly for small businesses—fewer than 50 employees—which employ the greatest number of Americans). Thus the numbers of workers and their families without the benefit of health insurance have increased, a circumstance that has had a drastic impact on them.

Markets

The health care market is unlike the typical economic market model in which there are consumers (households) who demand goods and services and producers (firms) who supply those goods and services. The interplay between supply and demand helps determine pricing. The supply curve signals trends and relationships in the market with regard to product pricing. It describes the amount of supply of a product or service and the demand for that product or service in relation to price (Fig. 9-4). According to traditional market forces, if the supply increases and the demand decreases, the price will decrease to stimulate demand in order to improve profits. If demand rises and supplies are low, the price will rise to decrease demand.

True economic markets have two key players, consumers (households) and producers (firms). The health care market has four distinct players:

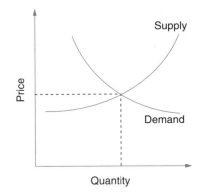

Figure 9-4 The Supply and Demand Curve.

- households, who consume health services and pay, directly (self-pay) or indirectly (insurance), for those services;
- providers (like firms), who deliver services and get paid for them; providers also play a large role in determining the type and amount of services a patient will receive;
- insurers, who reimburse the provider for services rendered; and
- employers, who pay the insurer to provide coverage for their employees.[37]

If we look at health care, therefore, we see that the economic model of supply and demand does not apply. For example, the price of cardiac bypass surgery is closely regulated and is in fact relatively "fixed" by the third-party insurer. Therefore, to improve profits, one must increase the supply and the demand at the same time. Since payment is provided by a third-party insurer, the patient has no incentive not to have the procedure (if indicated by the physician) and the physician has little incentive not to perform a lot of these surgeries.

Moral hazard is defined as "the possibility of loss to an insurance company arising from the character or circumstances of the insured."[32] The fact that a cardiac bypass surgery may be insured against and utilization of the procedure can be controlled (increased or decreased) gives rise to the temptation to use the insurance. In this example of cardiac bypass surgery, moral hazard is likely to flatten the supply curve such that a direct correlation between supply and demand is created. As more cardiac bypass surgical units become available, more surgeries will be performed. In large part, physicians determine the demand as well as the supply. They have gained much of their control over the health care market through the regulatory mechanisms of state licensure requirements and increased academic standards/requirements. They therefore control access to health services via referral and are then also the primary provider of many of those services.

Physical therapists are also in a position to determine the amount of services a patient receives, usually within the confines of an insurance company's defined therapy benefit. The physical therapist often decides how many visits patients should receive to effectively address their problem. While the *Guide to Physical Therapist Practice*[74] helps provide parameters, there is limited evidence regarding the appropriate dosage of physical therapy services within an episode of care. Up until out-of-pocket co-payments by consumers of therapists' services were required, patients had little incentive, other than time and effort, for not complying with the recommended plan of care. With the advent of out-of-pocket co-payments, which can range from $5 to $60, patients as consumers of physical therapists' services are becoming more involved in decisions regarding the amount of care they need.

We can begin to appreciate the circumstance of the 19-year-old college volleyball player, Ms. Tyler (see Case Example). As a result of insurance regulations that have limited where she can receive her care, as well as the $30 co-pay for each visit, she and her parents (as consumers) are demanding more input into the plan of care. Ms. Tyler and her parents have requested a course of therapy that requires only two to four visits per month, despite the surgeon's recommended 2 to 3 visits per week for 6 to 8 weeks. This means maximum out-of-pocket costs of $720 for 24 visits, which does not include the cost of travel or account for time getting to and from therapy. The impact of these changes within the health care system are requiring physical therapists and other providers to consider their patient's circumstances more closely as they make recommendations for care.

✳ Case Example — Ms. Tyler

Ms. Tyler is a 19-year-old college volleyball player who recently sustained a Grade III ACL tear. She underwent reconstructive surgery 4 weeks ago and received initial physical therapy at a clinic near the university. Ms. Tyler has returned home for summer vacation and her surgeon wants her receiving outpatient physical therapy 2 to 3 times per week for the next 6 to 8 weeks. She lives in a rural area and needs to travel 40 minutes to get to the only physical therapy clinic that accepts her insurance. Her co-pay for each visit is $30. Ms. Tyler and her parents have requested a course of therapy that requires only 2 to 4 visits per month.

Discussion Questions
- Are the family's decisions based upon the need for care?
- Is their request unreasonable?
- Could you deliver quality care to this patient if you complied with her request?

As we can see, the health care market is very different from a true economic market; as such, it affects a patient's circumstances. Employers, insurers, and providers make decisions about care delivery and payment that are not always based on issues that are directly related to patient need. As a result, patients are being forced to become more active "consumers" regarding services that address their health needs.

Regulatory Infrastructure

As we have shown, a wide variety of delivery systems provide both insurance and direct services in the United States. Compounding this complexity are the detailed regulatory systems that govern each of these systems.

The clinical practice environment in the United States is one of the most heavily regulated of any health care system in the world.[34] As a result, "[t]here is now an accumulation of bad feeling between the regulated and the regulators in the Federal Government."[61] For example, Medicare payment policies for providers were at the outset relatively unobtrusive, reflecting the balance of power between the federal government and provider groups. Over the past 40 years, policy makers have created specific programs that have resulted in greater regulation of hospitals and physicians. Therefore, one wonders how increasing regulation has affected providers' behavior and their willingness to comply with externally imposed guidelines and rules. As noted by Cohodes, "... health professionals have demonstrated that they can outmaneuver, outspend, and overcome virtually any regulatory tactic."[65] The resulting animosity between federal regulators and health care providers affects the environment in which patients receive care. These tensions undoubtedly impact patient access to the care they need.

It is of particular interest to note that physicians' historical unwillingness to tolerate the intrusion of public regulatory involvement in medicine appears to have contributed to an erosion of trust and faith in the profession, which has in turn promoted greater societal tolerance of government regulation in health care.[34] Much of the regulation in health care centers on control over how services are paid for (payer), who can deliver those services (provider), and how patient rights, privacy, and access are protected (consumers).

Payment for health care was initially based on the costs incurred in delivering the services. Those costs were determined by providers (e.g., physicians and hospitals). But as the health care costs began to escalate rapidly, starting in the 1970s, payers developed policies to contain them. For example, policies developed for use within the Medicare program shifted payment from a cost to a prospective basis, in which payment was determined prior to the delivery of care based on certain factors, such as the patient's diagnosis.[61] Diagnostic related groups (DRGs), implemented in the early 1980s, were applied to Medicare Part A payments to hospitals. Outpatient (Part B) services, however, continued to be reimbursed on a cost basis. Hospitals were paid a set amount per patient based on the patient's primary diagnosis. This policy served as an incentive for hospitals to decrease both the length of stay and thus the costs of inpatient care.

In 1992, Resource Based Relative Value Scales (RBRVS) were introduced for Medicare Part B payments to physicians and other health care providers.[75,76] This resulted in creation of the Medicare Physician Fee Schedule (MPFS), a form of prospective payment, based on a relative value recommendation for common procedures (CPT codes). The determination of relative value for a procedure was based upon three distinct components:

1. physician expense (time, effort, and skill),
2. practice expense (medical equipment, office space, etc.), and
3. liability insurance premiums.[55,75,76]

Much like the prospective payment system for inpatient Part A services (DRG), the MPFS was introduced to create financial incentives for more efficient delivery of health care services.

In 1973, in an effort to provide an alternative to centralized government financing of health care with its fee-for-service model, the Health Maintenance Organization (HMO) Act was passed.[25] HMOs manage the care of a voluntarily enrolled population and control costs through predetermined fixed payments (capitation) to participating providers (physicians, hospitals).[36] Capitated payments shift more of the risk from HMOs to physicians and physician group practices,[77] and, given a fixed amount per patient, provide an incentive for physicians to manage and limit their patients' use of health care services. HMOs attempted to manage the care of their beneficiaries by relying on primary care physicians to play the role of gatekeeper.[77,78] They expected physicians to control utilization of services by more closely monitoring and controlling their patients' access to specialty care. With the total payment fixed, more services result in increased costs and therefore decrease provider profits.[78] The financial risk of managing health care utilization thus came to rest much more squarely on physicians.[77–79] Private insurance programs, including HMOs, also often limit the number of visits (e.g., 24 visits) or days (e.g., 60 days) of services for a given problem. These "defined benefits" allow the payer to predict and control costs; however, they can impact a patient's access to care that may be needed beyond the defined limit. Payment regulations such as DRGs, the MPFS, capitation, and defined benefits allow the payer rather than the person providing the services (physician, physical therapist) to determine the amount to be paid for services. All insurance companies and health benefits programs use these and a variety of other regulations to contain costs while simultaneously attempting to provide their beneficiaries or members access to quality care.

The practice of health care (i.e., who can provide what types of services) is also strictly regulated, primarily through state licensure and educational accreditation and standards. Originally established by the health professions, these regulations were intended to promote a highly educated workforce and to tightly control entry. As mentioned earlier, nearly 100 years ago the medical profession encouraged the establishment of state boards and subsequent state licensure requirements and raised academic standards within medical schools. These regulatory efforts were intended not only to increase the quality of medical school graduates but to control the quantity of physicians allowed to practice. As a result, through much of the 20th century the medical profession exercised significant authority over health care decision making.[25] Similarly, licensure requirements and closely regulated academic standards have been used by many other health professions as a way to elevate their standing within the U.S. health care system, to ensure a quality workforce, and also to increase their own autonomy in clinical decision making.[26,27]

It is important to point out that while the professions directly control the national academic standards within their individual educational programs, licensure is regulated by a legislatively appointed state board. Each state has jurisdiction over licensure requirements and definitions of scope of practice, with the result that there is variation from state to state in the range of activities allowed within a professional practice. The purpose of state licensure boards is to protect the public from unqualified practitioners. This is primarily achieved by requiring the passing of an examination to gain a license to practice within that state and by establishing a description of the scope of practice for each profession, known as a practice act.

An example of how this situation pertains to physical therapy in terms of direct access[80] may help illustrate the discussion. The majority of state practice acts allow for some form of direct access to physical therapy without a physician referral for evaluation and/or treatment; however, there is much variation across the states. Some states allow a patient to see a physical therapist for any condition that would appear to benefit from such services; other states allow access without a referral only to patients with neuromusculoskeletal conditions. A few state practice acts still require a physician referral for access to services. These variations are not related to third-party payment systems; rather, they are state mandates about how practice should occur. In the case of states that require a referral, patients who are uninsured would still need a physician referral in order to receive pro bono physical therapy services. Thus we can see how regulations designed to ensure a quality workforce can have a direct impact on the patient's circumstances in terms of the quality of care and their access to it.

Lastly, there are many regulations that fall under the rubric of patient protection. Examples of these include the following:

- the Health Insurance Portability and Accountability Act (HIPAA), which ensures that a patient's health information is protected,
- the Americans with Disabilities Act (ADA), designed to ensure that citizens with disabilities are not discriminated against based upon their disability, and
- the Emergency Medical Treatment and Active Labor Act (EMTALA), which requires all hospitals, both private and public, that have an Emergency Department (ED) to accept any patient regardless of legal status, citizenship, or ability to pay and to provide interventions to stabilize the patient's condition.

EMTALA, also referred to as the "Patient Dumping Act," was passed in 1986 to prohibit the practice of transferring patients with unstable medical conditions to another hospital ED. The practice of "dumping" patients had been used to avoid having to treat patients who could not pay for care.[80]

We can see that health care regulations are designed for many purposes. Some are created in the best interests of the patient (consumer), such as licensure, HIPAA, and EMTALA; others benefit the payer (capitation, DRGs) or the health provider (licensure and practice acts). All of the regulations that impact health care delivery contribute to the complexity of our system. This complexity affects both health providers and patients by creating circumstances where determining who has access to what type and how much care can become difficult. Regulations are used as a way to balance costs, quality, and access to care; however, as the next section will discuss, there are many competitors for the billions of dollars spent on health care services each year.

✳ Case Example — Mr. Martinez

Mr. Martinez is an 81-year-old man who has hypertension and insulin-dependent diabetes mellitus. He was admitted to an inpatient rehabilitation facility (IRF) for treatment following a left transtibial amputation 2 weeks ago that was secondary to complications of his diabetes. He has a large, extended family and would prefer to get his physical therapy at home where Medicare will cover home health services. The physician feels that he needs rehabilitation in an intensive inpatient environment to achieve a good outcome.

Discussion Question
- What role should Mr. Martinez and his family have in determining what type of care he needs?

As can be seen from the preceding description of its resources, delivery systems, regulatory systems, and markets, the U.S. health care system is a complex entity. This makes it difficult to understand, control, and improve the system.

HEALTH SERVICES RESEARCH

Most health care practitioners are familiar with the concept of evidence-based practice and recognize the value of scientific clinical and bench research, but many are unaware of health services research and its potential to impact patient care. According to the Agency for Health Care Research and Quality (AHRQ), "health services research examines how people get access to health care, how much care costs, and what happens to patients as a result of this care. The main goals of health services research are to identify the most effective ways to organize, manage, finance, and deliver high quality care; reduce medical errors; and improve patient safety."[82]

Health services research examines a multitude of factors that impact patients' circumstances regarding access to and the cost and quality of health services. This is an important area for further study because we know that in many cases there is good evidence available to support certain treatments or methods of practice, yet for a variety of reasons clinicians often fail to use the best evidence in practice. Some of these reasons are a matter of individual provider choice; others are due to failures in the system of care delivery. Exploration of the multiple factors impacting the delivery of health care includes (but is not limited to) such areas as utilization, coverage, quality measurement and improvement, health disparities, cost-effectiveness, and workforce. In order to be more effective advocates for patients and clients, practicing physical therapists would benefit from an increased awareness of this type of research.[83]

PATIENT CIRCUMSTANCES AND ACCESS TO CARE

This section will focus on examples in the literature related to those predisposing, enabling, and need factors, as described by Andersen,[7] that illustrate how patients' circumstances will have a direct impact on their ability to access care. A number of physical therapist researchers,[9–13,15,16,84] as well as others,[17–23] have explored numerous elements of service delivery and access related to these factors. A full description of all the research related to these factors is beyond the scope of this chapter, but examples from a few key areas—insurance coverage, geography, socioeconomic status, and race and ethnicity—will provide a good understanding of the contribution of health services research.

Insurance Coverage

The lack of health insurance is a growing problem.[45,54,73,85] The U.S. Census Bureau, in August 2007, estimated that 46.6 million Americans were without health insurance, representing nearly 16% of the entire U.S. population.[86] Eight out of ten people who are uninsured come from working families, and nearly 60% of uninsured adults have been without coverage for at least 2 years.[73] Research has shown that the uninsured

- use fewer preventative and screening services,
- are sicker when diagnosed, and
- have poorer health outcomes.[73]

Simply having health insurance, however, does not necessarily guarantee equal access to care.[9–11,22,84,87] A recent study examining the relationship between primary care services and insurance type revealed unequal access to and quality of primary care services.[87] Adults less than 65 years of age who had private insurance were able to obtain better primary care services than those with public insurance (i.e., Medicare, Medicaid, etc.). Americans with fee-for-service insurance experience better access and improved quality of care as measured by the length of time that the person has a relationship with a PCP and the degree to which their overall care is coordinated with other health care providers.

Numerous authors have also described differences among patients related to rehabilitation services, including physical therapy, based on insurance type.[9–11,22,84,87] These differences occurred in a number of areas, including physician referral for physical therapy, access to rehabilitation services, and amount of rehabilitation services. Freburger and colleagues, examining factors relating to physician referral to physical therapy, noted that reimbursement type influenced the likelihood of referral.[10] Patients with musculoskeletal conditions who visited a primary care physician were less likely to be referred for physical therapy if they had Medicaid or a managed care plan compared to those with private insurance or a non-managed care plan.

Johnson et al[14] found that Medicare beneficiaries were nearly two-thirds less likely (65%) to access outpatient rehabilitation services than patients with insurances other than Medicare. This disparity is particularly interesting given that older adults (65 years or older) have higher levels of self-reported functional limitation, which represents a potential need for rehabilitation services.[8,11] Many factors may have contributed to this finding, but it is consistent with previous research.[3,11] Carter et al,[11] using Medical Expenditure Panel Survey (MEPS) data from 1996 to 2000, found that people with musculoskeletal conditions who had public insurance (not including CHAMPUS/VA) were 34% less likely to receive outpatient physical therapy services.

Wodchis et al examined the impact of payer incentives on the receipt of rehabilitation services and reported that patients with more generous payers, such as Medicare, received more care than patients with less generous insurance plans.[23] Although this report appears to balance the findings in some of the previous literature, these authors were examining PPS in skilled nursing facilities where treatment was targeted to profitability levels. PPS was associated with increased likelihood of therapy among Medicare patients, but they received less rehabilitation therapy time.

Geography

There is ample evidence of significant geographic variation in the utilization of health services in this country.[20,88–90] This variation appeared true, across all settings, for Medicare beneficiaries utilizing Part B rehabilitation services from 1998 to 2000. People in the Northeast had higher rates of utilization than those in other parts of the country.[18] In their study of community-based older adults, Freburger and Holmes found variation in access to physical therapy services by census division. Those Medicare beneficiaries in the East South Central division were over 35% less likely, and those in the Pacific division were 1.35 times more likely, to have access to services compared to beneficiaries in the South Atlantic division.[16]

Carter et al, using combined data from the 1996 to 2000 MEPS, found regional variation in access to outpatient physical therapy services among U.S. adults with musculoskeletal conditions.[11] Adults in all other regions were between 24% and 45% less likely to receive services than their counterparts in the Northeast. Like Freburger and Holmes,[16] Carter et al found access was worst in the South. What we do not know is whether the utilization of physical therapy services was appropriate in the Northeast. Perhaps patients who live in the South were using the correct amount of therapy services based on need, and their northern counterparts were overutilizing services. Because there is no clear method of determining the true need for therapy services or the exact dosage required for a given functional limitation or disability, geographic variation may be impacted by cultural differences or other factors in addition to patient need.

Socioeconomic Status

Socioeconomic status (SES) has been defined as a "broad concept that refers to the placement of persons, families, households, and census tracts or other aggregates with respect to the capacity to create or consume goods that are valued in society."[91] Factors related to SES that impact health include education, income, occupation, accumulated wealth, and neighborhood or geographic region (county, state, etc.).[91–94] Many consider SES a fundamental cause of disease and, consequently, health.[1,4,95] People of lower SES tend to be in poor health[96] in large part, it is believed, due to health disparities resulting from unequal distribution of education and income.[97,98]

Health and income in the United States have a parallel relationship. Income inequality in this country is greater than in other rich nations and the resulting health disparities impact mortality and morbidity.[99] The impact of income inequality on health in the United States is supported by the findings of several health service researchers[3,101]; the disparity exists because the market has a larger role to play in the allocation of health care resources.[99] Since the market also plays a central role in the allocation of high-quality education, he concludes that health care "utilization in the United States tends to be related to the ability to pay."[99] Freburger and Holmes, for example, examined characteristics of people who used physical therapy and factors associated with its use and noted that factors other than need were related to actual use.[9] They reported that people with high income were twice as likely to receive physical therapy services as those with low income. Number of years of education was also positively correlated with the likelihood of receiving services, as was having supplemental private insurance.

Education must also be considered along with income when examining the relationship between SES and health. Education, in particular, is the most commonly used measure of SES because it has less connection to disease in adulthood than does income or occupation.[91] Additionally, education reflects noneconomic social characteristics such as lifestyle and behavior.[91,93,99] Numerous authors suggest that education plays a pivotal role in determining health outcomes among older patients.[97,98,100] In the study by Johnson et al for the 4-year period between 1997 to 2000, people with lower education levels were less likely to access outpatient rehabilitation services.[14] This finding was consistent with previous studies, which observed that those receiving services tended to have higher levels of education.[11–13,16] Carter et al found that among patients of all ages diagnosed with a musculoskeletal condition, those with lower levels of education were nearly 30% less likely to receive outpatient physical therapy services.[11] These findings suggests that education is a key SES indicator[91,93,99] of access to outpatient rehabilitation, including physical therapy services.

Race and Ethnicity

There is ample evidence that individuals experience disparities in access to and utilization of health care services based on their race and/or ethnicity.[20,21,96,102–106] Race is defined as "a class or kind of people unified by shared interests, habits, or characteristics"; ethnicity means "of or relating to large groups of people classed according to common racial, national, tribal, religious, linguistic, or cultural origin or background."[32] For over 40 years, race and/or ethnicity classifications have been used to collect data for a variety of purposes. Used for research related to disparities, these groupings were based on the needs of federal agencies rather than a specific desire by individuals within the groups.[107] As such, race and ethnicity are largely social rather than biological constructs. Therefore, when examining causation health disparities among different racial/ethnic groups need to be considered in light of other underlying issues of culture and community.[93,95]

In a longitudinal study of access to ambulatory health services from 1977 to 1997, Weinick et al[104] reported that whites were more likely to use ambulatory services than blacks and Hispanic Americans. When the authors took into account other key factors, such as insurance status and income levels, that could explain some of these differences, race/ethnicity remained a strong determinant of who was most likely to use ambulatory health services. Recently, Skinner et al[108] found that race was the primary determinant among Medicare patients who received a total knee arthroplasty. Black men and Asian women were significantly less likely to have surgery than their white counterparts. Dunlop and colleagues found similar disparities among blacks and Hispanics receiving joint arthroplasty,[109] as well as their use of outpatient surgical interventions in general.[103]

Research supports the existence of similar disparities in the receipt of rehabilitation services, including physical therapy.[9,12,21,110–113] As early as 1992, Mayer-Oakes and colleagues reported in a study of community-dwelling elders that the use of physical and occupational therapy

(PT/OT) was lower among minority group members than among nonminority members.[110] These authors initially surveyed men and women who were 65 and older regarding demographic characteristics, health and disability status, and use of preventative health services. A follow-up survey 12 months later then examined their use of PT/OT services in the previous year; it found that nonwhites were significantly less likely to receive services despite indicators of need, such as increased disability or lower health status.

Several researchers reported disparities in the receipt of physical therapy services after hip fractures.[111–113] Harada et al reported that blacks were 30% less likely to receive physical therapy services after hip fracture than whites[112]; Hoenig et al reported that black patients were more likely to receive low-intensity physical therapy services compared with nonblack patients.[113] In these two studies, therefore, white patients who sustained a hip fracture were more likely to receive physical therapy services and generally received a higher intensity of services (i.e., number of visits, length of treatment, etc.) to address the functional limitations associated with their injury. In contrast, Freburger and Holmes found that in a population of community-based older persons, African Americans had more physical therapy visits and higher costs, perhaps because there were associated, unmeasured, comorbid medical conditions.[9] Examining a separate population of disabled elderly individuals, White-Means et al found that whites tended to receive more physical therapy services than blacks.[21] However, this difference varied depending on the patient's diagnosis. White patients with musculoskeletal conditions were more likely to receive therapy services than blacks, but black patients with a diagnosis of stroke were more likely to receive therapy than whites. These findings suggest that some of the health disparities present among racial and ethnic groups may be due to differences in the prevalence of certain diseases across these groups.

Update on Health Care Reform

To the surprise of many, the United States adopted health care reform legislation in 2010. However, the actual impact of this legislation, the Patient Protection and Affordable Care Act (PPACA), remains to be seen due to the scope of the legislation, its staged implementation, and the continued attempts to repeal all or part of it. Because of these uncertainties, we provide here a basic overview of the legislation, with some useful resources for monitoring its impact on health care and physical therapy over time.

As citizens and health care practitioners, and perhaps as business owners and managers, we have many reasons to be interested in health care reform. Depending on which hat we are wearing, we may have different views of the same provisions at the same time! To help you learn more about health care reform as it is implemented, we have identified a list of useful resources (Box 9.3).

CONCLUSION

Equipped as they are with an understanding of the many factors that can impact patients' circumstances, health care providers are well positioned to assist them in meeting their health needs. Through an understanding of the relationships among access, quality, and cost of care, physical therapists can better appreciate the current state of health care in this country. From a position of knowledge, physical therapists will be even better suited and prepared to advocate for effective health policy changes that will ultimately improve the circumstances of all patients who have the need for physical therapy and other health care services.

Box 9.3   Health Care Reform Resources

1. American Physical Therapy Association

Resources available at www.apta.org/HealthCareReform

- A Physical Therapy Perspective on Health Care Reform
- Role of the Physical Therapist in National Health Care Reform
- APTA Summaries of Health Care Reform Rules & Regulations
- APTA Summary of the Patient Protection and Affordable Care Act
- APTA Summary of Key Provisions of the Patient Protection and Affordable Care Act
- APTA Summary of the Health Care and Education Affordability Reconciliation Act
- Health Care Reform: Issue in Focus Series (www.apta.org/IssueinFocus/)

The Issues in Focus series is a great resource for understanding how certain health care issues or practice settings may be affected by the Health Care Reform bill. These documents also provide information on when these new laws take effect, as well as who will be implementing them. Examples of topics include:

- Home Health Care
- Skilled Nursing Facilities
- Accountable Care Organizations
- Comparative Effectiveness Research
- Disability
- Health Disparities
- Health Information Technology
- Medicaid Expansion
- Prevention: Annual Wellness Visit and Personal Prevention Plan
- Quality Improvement and Initiatives
  - Rehabilitation as an Essential Benefit
  - Self-referral
  - Workforce Initiatives

2. CMS Health Reform Resource Center (www.cms.gov/Center/healthreform.asp)

The Department of Health and Human Services has been entrusted with the responsibility for implementing many major provisions of the historic health reform bill, the Patient Protection and Affordable Care Act (hereafter "Affordable Care Act"), which the president signed into law on March 23, 2010. This bill was further improved by the Health Care and Education Affordability Reconciliation Act of 2010, which the president signed into law on March 30, 2010. The Centers for Medicare & Medicaid Services is dedicated to helping the department implement many of the provisions of the legislation that address Medicare, Medicaid, and the Children's Health Insurance Program (CHIP). Additional information on the implementation of the Affordable Care Act can be found on the Regulations and Guidance page of the Office of Consumer Information and Insurance Oversight (OCIIO).

3. Kaiser Family Foundation Health Reform Source (healthreform.kff.org/)

Resources include:

- The Basics: Confused by health care reform? Get basic information here to help you understand the new law.

(Continued on p 158)

Box 9.3 Health Care Reform Resources—cont'd

- Research and Analysis: A gateway to in-depth reports on health reform as implementation proceeds.
- Public Opinion: A roundup of surveys from the Kaiser Family Foundation and others assessing public attitudes and experiences over time related to the health reform law.
- The States: Get a state-by-state view of health care reform implementation and news.
- Topics: Explore a variety of health reform-related topics.
- The Scan: A roundup of studies and developments related to health reform.
- Quick Links: Quiz, Timeline, Document Finder, etc.

4. Kaiser Family Foundation's animated short on health care reform (/healthreform.kff.org/the-animation.aspx)

An entertaining but highly informative presentation on health care reform. Quite suitable to share with patients.

SELF-ASSESSMENT

1. Based on five patients you have treated or observed, identify how each of the elements of the health care system, (resources, delivery system, market, and the regulatory infrastructure) affects your ability to provide appropriate care for each patient and the impact each of these elements has on the patient's likelihood of maximal recovery.
2. Choose another country and compare and contrast the elements (resources, delivery system, market, and the regulatory infrastructure) of that country's health care system to those of the U.S. system. What are the benefits of that country's system, including outcomes, compared to the those of the United States? Can aspects of that system be implemented here?

CONTINUED LEARNING

- Each issue of the *New England Journal of Medicine* (NEJM) has several articles analyzing contemporary issues in the U.S. health care system.

1. Choose a recent issue and describe how the issues identified in the articles apply to physical therapy practice.

- Identify two or three legislative issues in a state or the federal legislature that have an impact on the health care system.

1. Review the issues carefully to determine how they will differentially impact the three aspects of the iron triangle: access, cost, and quality.

REFERENCES

1. Link BG, Phelan J. Social conditions as fundamental causes of disease. J Health Soc Behav. 1995;Spec No:80–94.
2. Lynch JW, Kaplan GA, Shema SJ. Cumulative impact of sustained economic hardship on physical, cognitive, psychological, and social functioning. N Engl J Med. 1997;337:1889–1895.

3. Chen AY, Escarce JJ. Quantifying income-related inequality in healthcare delivery in the United States. Med Care 2004;42:38–47.
4. Fiscella K. Socioeconomic status disparities in healthcare outcomes: Selection bias or biased treatment? Med Care. 2004;42:939–942.
5. McIntosh MA. The cost of healthcare to Americans. JONAS Healthc Law Ethics Regul. 2002;4:78–89.
6. Bailey EJ. Sociocultural factors and health care-seeking behavior among black Americans. J Natl Med Assoc. 1987;79:389–392.
7. Andersen RM. Revisiting the behavioral model and access to medical care: Does it matter? J Health Soc Behav. 1995;36:1–10.
8. Andersen RE. *Behavioral Model of Families' Use of Health Services*. Chicago, IL: University of Chicago; 1968.
9. Freburger JK, Carey TS, Holmes GM. Physician referrals to physical therapists for the treatment of spine disorders. Spine J. 2005;5:530–541.
10. Freburger JK, Holmes GM, Carey TS. Physician referrals to physical therapy for the treatment of musculoskeletal conditions. Arch Phys Med Rehabil. 2003;84:1839–1849.
11. Carter SK, Rizzo JA. Use of outpatient physical therapy services by people with musculoskeletal conditions. Phys Ther. 2007;87:1–16.
12. Jette A, Davis K. A comparison of hospital-based and private outpatient physical therapy practices. Phys Ther. 1991;71:366–75; discussion 76–81.
13. Jette AM, Smith K, Haley SM, Davis KD. Physical therapy episodes of care for patients with low back pain. Phys Ther. 1994;74:101–110; discussion 10–15.
14. Johnson MP, Valdmanis V, Hack L, Maritz CA, Metraux S. The Influence of Health Policy on Utilization of Outpatient Rehabilitation Services by Medicare Patients with Musculoskeletal Conditions. Diss. Philadelphia: University of the Sciences in Philadelphia; 2009.
15. Freburger JK, Carey TS, Holmes GM. Management of back and neck pain: Who seeks care from physical therapists? Phys Ther. 2005;85:872–886.
16. Freburger JK, Holmes GM. Physical therapy use by community-based older people. Phys Ther. 2005;85:19–33.
17. Dunlop DD, Manheim LM, Song J, Chang RW. Health care utilization among older adults with arthritis. Arthritis Rheum. 2003;49:164–171.
18. Olshin JM, Ciolek DE, Hwang W. Study and report on outpatient therapy utilization: Physical therapy, occupational therapy, and speech-language pathology services billed to Medicare Part B in all settings in 1998, 1999, and 2000. AdvanceMed. 2002;Report No.: 500-99-0009.
19. Maxwell S, Baseggio C, Storeygard M. Part B therapy services under Medicare in 1998–2000: Impact of extending fee schedule payments and coverage limits. Urban Institute;2001; Report No.: 500-95-0055.
20. Skinner J, Weinstein JN, Sporer SM, Wennberg JE. Racial, ethnic, and geographic disparities in rates of knee arthroplasty among Medicare patients. N Engl J Med. 2003;349:1350–1359.
21. White-Means SI. Racial patterns in disabled elderly persons' use of medical services. J Gerontol B Psychol Sci Soc Sci. 2000;55:S76–89.
22. Wodchis WP. Physical rehabilitation following Medicare prospective payment for skilled nursing facilities. Health Serv Res. 2004;39:1299–1318.
23. Wodchis WP, Fries BE, Pollack H. Payer incentives and physical rehabilitation therapy for nonelderly institutional long-term care residents: Evidence from Michigan and Ontario. Arch Phys Med Rehabil. 2004;85:210–217.
24. National Occupational Employment and Wage Estimates, Healthcare Practitioner and Technical Occupations. U.S. Department of Labor, 2008. http://www.bls.gov/oes/current/oes_nat.htm#b29-0000 Accessed March 28, 2011.
25. Starr P. *The Social Transformation of American Medicine*. New York: Basic Books; 1982.
26. Johnson MP, Abrams SL. Historical perspectives of autonomy within the medical profession: Considerations for 21st century physical therapy practice. J Orthop Sports Phys Ther. 2005;35:628–636.

27. Cooper RA, Henderson T, Dietrich CL. Roles of nonphysician clinicians as autonomous providers of patient care. JAMA. 1998;280:795–802.
28. Druss BG, Marcus SC, Olfson M, Tanielian T, Pincus HA. Trends in care by nonphysician clinicians in the United States. N Engl J Med. 2003;348:130–137.
29. Cooper RA. Health care workforce for the twenty-first century: The impact of nonphysician clinicians. Annu Rev Med. 2001;52:51–61.
30. Institute of Medicine. *Crossing the Quality Chasm: A New Health System for the 21st Century.* Washington, DC: Institute of Medicine; 2001.
31. Institute of Medicine. *Rewarding Provider Performance: Aligning Incentives in Medicare.* Washington, DC: Institute of Medicine, National Academy Press; 2007.
32. Merriam-Webster Online Dictionary. Merriam-Webster, 2011. www.Merriam-Webster.com Accessed March 28, 2011.
33. Kulesher RR. Medicare—The development of publicly financed health insurance: Medicare's impact on the nation's health care system. The Health Care Manager. 2005;24:320–329.
34. Brown LD. Political evolution of federal health care regulation. Health Aff (Millwood). 1992:17–37.
35. WHO, Definition of Health. World Health Organization, 2009. http://www.who.int/about/definition/en/ Accessed March 28, 2011.
36. AcademyHealth. Glossary of terms commonly used in health care. AcademyHealth, 2004. http://www.academyhealth.org/publications/glossary.pdf Accessed March 28, 2011.
37. Kissick W. *Medicine's Dilemmas: Infinite Need Versus Finite Resources.* New Haven, CT: Yale University Press; 1994.
38. Social Security Act, Title XVIII and XIX—Health Insurance of the Aged and the Poor. In: 42 USC § 1395; 1965.
39. Institute of Medicine. *To Err is Human: Building a Safer Health System.* Washington, DC: National Academy Press; 2000.
40. Iglehart JK. The American health care system—expenditures. N Engl J Med. 1999;340:70–76.
41. Reinhardt UE, Hussey PS, Anderson GF. U.S. health care spending in an international context. Health Aff (Millwood). 2004;23:10–25.
42. H.R. 2015, Balanced Budget Act of 1997. In: Medicare and Medicaid Provisions as incorporated into Title IV of PL 105–33, enacted August 5, 1997.
43. Mrtek RG. Pharmaceutical education in these United States—An interpretive historical essay of the twentieth century. Am J Pharm Educ. 1976;40:339–365.
44. Edwardson SR. Matching standards and needs in doctoral education in nursing. J Prof Nurs. 2004;20:40–46.
45. Institute of Medicine. *Coverage Matters: Insurance and Health Care.* Washington, DC: National Academies Press; 2001.
46. Wagner EH. The role of patient care teams in chronic disease management. BMJ. 2000;320:569–572.
47. Glasgow RE, Orleans CT, Wagner EH. Does the chronic care model serve also as a template for improving prevention? Milbank Q. 2001;79:579–612, iv–v.
48. Tinetti ME, Fried T. The end of the disease era. Am J Med. 2004;116:179–185.
49. The Social Security Act. In: 42 USC Chap 7 § 401. United States: Title 42—The Public Health and Welfare; 1935.
50. Hospital Survey and Construction Act. In: 42 USC Supp 291. United States; 1946.
51. Bureau of Primary Health Care. About Health Centers. U.S. Department of Health and Human Services, Health Resources and Services Administration, 2011. http://bphc.hrsa.gov/about/ Accessed March 28, 2011.
52. Fuchs VR. What's ahead for health insurance in the United States? N Engl J Med. 2002;346:1822–1824.
53. Hair LP. Clinton, health care, and the crystal ball. With the Democrats back in power, where do we go from here? J Health Care Mark. 1996;16:6–13.
54. Strunk BC, Reschovsky JD. Trends in U.S. health insurance coverage, 2001–2003. Track Rep. 2004:1–5.

55. Iglehart JK. The American health care system—Medicare. N Engl J Med. 1999;340:327–32.
56. Moon M. Will the care be there? Vulnerable beneficiaries and Medicare reform. Health Aff (Millwood). 1999;18:107–117.
57. Moon M. Medicare. N Engl J Med. 2001;344:928–931.
58. Moon M, Davis K. Preserving and strengthening Medicare. Health Aff (Millwood). 1995;14:31–46.
59. Wilensky GR. Medicare reform—Now is the time. N Engl J Med. 2001;345:458–462.
60. Wilensky GR, Newhouse JP. Medicare: What's right? What's wrong? What's next? Health Aff (Millwood). 1999;18:92–106.
61. Gluck MG, Reno V. *Reflections on Implementing Medicare*. Wasington, DC: National Academy of Social Insurance; 2001, January 2001.
62. Iglehart JK. The Centers for Medicare and Medicaid Services. N Engl J Med. 2001;345:1920–1924.
63. Medicare Prescription Drug, Improvement, and Modernization Act. In: 2003:1–416.
64. Iglehart JK. The dilemma of Medicaid. N Engl J Med. 2003;348:2140–2148.
65. Cohodes DR. Pragmatism and health care reform. Health Aff (Millwood). 1994;13:264–273.
66. Brook RH. Perspectives on Medicare: Medicare quality and getting older—A personal essay. Health Aff (Millwood). 1995;14:73–81.
67. Florence CS, Thorpe KE. How does the employer contribution for the federal employees health benefits program influence plan selection? Health Aff (Millwood). 2003;22:211–218.
68. Federal Employees Health Benefits Program (FEBPH). Office of Personnel Management. http://www.opm.gov/insure/health/ Accessed March 28, 2011.
69. Tannewald R. Implications of the Balanced Budget Act of 1997 for the "devolution revolution." Inquiry. 1998;28:23–48.
70. Cuttler L, Kenney GM. State Children's Health Insurance Program and pediatrics: Background, policy challenges, and role in child health care delivery. Arch Pediatr Adolesc Med. 2007;161:630–633.
71. Kaiser Family Foundation. *Medicaid and the Uninsured: State Children's Health Insurance Program (sCHIP) at a Glance*. Washington, DC: Henry J. Kaiser Family Foundation; 2007.
72. Federal Employment Compensation Act. In: 5 USC Chapter 81 United States; 1993.
73. Kaiser Family Foundation. *The Uninsured: A Primer—Key Facts About Americans Without Health Insurance*. Washington, DC: The Henry J. Kaiser Family Foundation; 2006.
74. American Physical Therapy Association. *The Guide to Physical Therapist Practice*, 2nd ed. Phys Ther. 2001;81:9–744.
75. Hsiao WC, Braun P, Becker ER, et al. Results and impacts of the Resource-Based Relative Value Scale. Med Care. 1992;30:NS61–79.
76. Hsiao WC, Braun P, Dunn D, Becker ER. Resource-based relative values. An overview. JAMA. 1988;260:2347–2353.
77. Sleeper S, Wholey DR, Hamer R, Schwartz S, Inoferio V. Trust me: Technical and institutional determinants of health maintenance organizations shifting risk to physicians. J Health Soc Behav. 1998;39:189–200.
78. Clancy CM, Hillner BE. Physicians as gatekeepers: The impact of financial incentives. Arch Intern Med. 1989;149:917–920.
79. Hellinger FJ. The impact of financial incentives on physician behavior in managed care plans: A review of the evidence. Med Care Res and Rev. 1996;53:294–314.
80. Direct access to physical therapists' services: Is yours a direct access state? American Physical Therapy Association; 2005. www.apta.org Accessed March 28, 2011.
81. Emergency Medical Treatment and Active Labor Act (EMTALA). In: 42 USC § 1395dd. United States; 1986.
82. What is HSR? AcademyHealth. http://www.academyhealth.org/About/content.cfm?ItemNumber=831&navItemNumber=514 Accessed March 28, 2011.

83. Resnick L, Johnson MP. Health services research: A review of domains relative to rehabilitation. HPA Resource/HPA J. 2006;6:J1–J8.
84. Johnson MP, Metraux S. The prevalence of musculoskeletal conditions among the U.S. population: Considerations for physical therapists. HPA Resource/HPA J. 2009; in press.
85. Tieman J. Unsure about the uninsured. With the nation's uninsured population up another 3.2%, politicians spin the news, while hospitals wait for solutions. Mod Healthc. 2004;34:6–7, 16.
86. DeNavas-Walt C, Proctor BD, Lee CH. Income, Poverty, and Health Insurance Coverage in the United States: 2006. Current Population Reports P60–233. Washington, DC: U.S. Department of Commerce, Economics and Statistics Administration; 2007, August.
87. Shi L. Type of health insurance and the quality of primary care experience. Am J Public Health. 2000;90:1848–1855.
88. Fisher ES, Wennberg DE, Stukel TA, Gottlieb DJ, Lucas FL, Pinder EL. The implications of regional variations in Medicare spending. Part 1: The content, quality, and accessibility of care. Ann Intern Med. 2003;138:273–287.
89. Wennberg DE. Variation in the delivery of health care: The stakes are high. Ann Intern Med. 1998;128:866–868.
90. Stearns SC, Slifkin RT, Edin HM. Access to care for rural Medicare beneficiaries. J Rural Health. 2000;16:31–42.
91. Shavers VL. Measurement of socioeconomic status in health disparities research. J Natl Med Assoc. 2007;99:1013–1023.
92. Pollack CE, Chideya S, Cubbin C, Williams B, Dekker M, Braveman P. Should health studies measure wealth? A systematic review. Am J Prev Med. 2007;33:250–264.
93. Braveman PA, Cubbin C, Egerter S, et al. Socioeconomic status in health research: One size does not fit all. JAMA. 2005;294:2879–2888.
94. Isaacs SL, Schroeder SA. Class—The ignored determinant of the nation's health. N Engl J Med. 2004;351:1137–1142.
95. Fiscella K, Williams DR. Health disparities based on socioeconomic inequities: Implications for urban health care. Acad Med. 2004;79:1139–1147.
96. Institute of Medicine. Unequal Treatment: Confronting Racial and Ethnic Disparities in Health Care. Washington, DC: Institute of Medicine; 2003.
97. Guralnik JM, Land KC, Blazer D, Fillenbaum GG, Branch LG. Educational status and active life expectancy among older blacks and whites. N Engl J Med. 1993;329:110–116.
98. Guralnik JM, Leveille SG. Race, ethnicity, and health outcomes—Unraveling the mediating role of socioeconomic status. Am J Public Health. 1997;87:728–730.
99. Marmot M. The influence of income on health: Views of an epidemiologist. Health Aff (Millwood). 2002;21:31–46.
100. Norris JC, van der Laan MJ, Lane S, Anderson JN, Block G. Nonlinearity in demographic and behavioral determinants of morbidity. Health Serv Res. 2003;38:1791–1818.
101. Smith JP. Healthy bodies and thick wallets: The dual relation between health and economic status. J Econ Perspect. 1999;13:144–166.
102. Hannan EL. The continuing quest for measuring and improving access to necessary care. JAMA. 2000;284:2374–2376.
103. Dunlop DD, Manheim LM, Song J, Chang RW. Gender and ethnic/racial disparities in health care utilization among older adults. J Gerontol B Psychol Sci Soc Sci. 2002;57:S221–233.
104. Weinick RM, Zuvekas SH, Cohen JW. Racial and ethnic differences in access to and use of health care services, 1977 to 1996. Med Care Res Rev. 2000;57 Suppl 1:36–54.
105. Kaiser Family Foundation. Medicare and Minority Americans. Washington, DC: The Henry J. Kaiser Family Foundation; 1999.
106. Castillo RC, MacKenzie EJ, Webb LX, Bosse MJ, Avery J. Use and perceived need of physical therapy following severe lower-extremity trauma. Arch Phys Med Rehabil. 2005;86:1722–1728.

107. Standards for the Classification of Federal Data on Race and Ethnicity. White House; Office of Management and Budget, 1995. http://www.whitehouse.gov/omb/fedreg_race-ethnicity Accessed March 28, 2011.
108. Skinner J, Zhou W, Weinstein J. The influence of income and race on total knee arthroplasty in the United States. J Bone Joint Surg Am. 2006;88:2159–2166.
109. Dunlop DD, Song J, Manheim LM, Chang RW. Racial disparities in joint replacement use among older adults. Med Care. 2003;41:288–298.
110. Mayer-Oakes SA, Hoenig H, Atchison KA, Lubben JE, De Jong F, Schweitzer SO. Patient-related predictors of rehabilitation use for community-dwelling older Americans. J Am Geriatr Soc. 1992;40:336–342.
111. Buchanan JL, Rumpel JD, Hoenig H. Charges for outpatient rehabilitation: Growth and differences in provider types. Arch Phys Med Rehabil. 1996;77:320–328.
112. Harada ND, Chun A, Chiu V, Pakalniskis A. Patterns of rehabilitation utilization after hip fracture in acute hospitals and skilled nursing facilities. Med Care. 2000;38:1119–1130.
113. Hoenig H, Rubenstein L, Kahn K. Rehabilitation after hip fracture—Equal opportunity for all? Arch Phys Med Rehabil. 1996;77:58–63.

Analyzing the Evidence in the Literature

The third element in the effective integration of evidence-based principles into physical therapist practice is the use of scientifically derived evidence. Over the past two decades, studies suggest that health-care practitioners have difficulty changing their methods of practice from those they were taught in school and in enhancing their knowledge with newly developed scientific findings. Accessing and evaluating the quality of scientific evidence has become a challenge for busy practitioners. Each year brings new and better tools to help clinicians integrate evidence into their clinical practice.

Although there are numerous excellent textbooks available for physical therapists with an in-depth approach to accessing and evaluating scientific evidence, this section of our text will present a broader perspective on integrating evidence. We are strongly influenced in our framework for this section by the work of R. Brian Haynes, who has recommended a hierarchical model for organizing information of value to clinicians in making clinical decisions.[1,2] The pyramidal format (Fig. 1) is based on the relative value of various sources of evidence to clinicians. It is not based on the strength of the original evidence, such as the pyramid found in Chapter 11 of this section, but is based upon the value-added aspects that come with filtered and enhanced sources of evidence. Haynes' evidence pyramid acknowledges the value to the clinician when evidence from single studies has undergone secondary review and synthesis by experts.

Haynes recommends that clinicians work from the top down in this model, trying first to obtain the most limited but the most valuable of the evidence-based information sources available to them. In presenting the chapters in this section, we will work from the bottom of the pyramid, which is more familiar to most and where the volume of available resources is greatest, and then move upward.

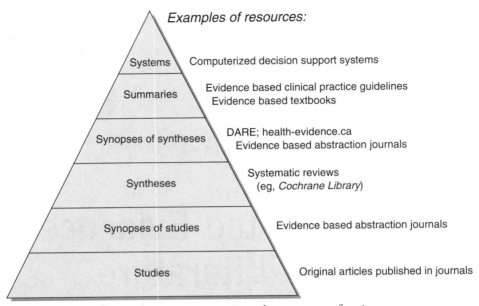

Figure 1 Types of research to answer questions about aspects of patient management. *(From DiCenso, Bayley L., Haynes RB, Accessing pre-appraised evidence: fine-tuning the 5S Model into a 6S model. Evid Based Nurs 2009;12:99–101.)*

Chapter 10 sets out the first step in using any source of evidence, asking a sound clinical question that is based on the needs of patients and the judgment of the clinician. These questions guide the search for new knowledge about the diagnosis, prognosis, or treatment of patients. Knowing what you are looking for in the evidence will enhance the likelihood that the evidence you find will fit your purpose. In Chapter 11, Connie Schard discusses current resources and methods to access unfiltered evidence contained in original scientific studies. The chapter also describes access to databases of filtered syntheses, synopses, and summaries. Chapter 12 reviews the value of original experimental research by highlighting the methodological and statistical principles that represent high-quality research. Chapter 13 provides a set of questions to use in assessing individual studies for their utility in guiding care. In Chapter 14 we address a variety of evidence resources both in physical therapy and medicine that are *synopses of* original studies and discuss the strengths of each type of synopsis. In Chapter 15, Alison Hallam, an experienced physical therapist reviewer for the Cochrane Collection, moves up the pyramid to *syntheses* in the form of systematic reviews or meta-analyses, discussing how the clinician might read and evaluate this very useful form of evidence for practice. She also includes a discussion of the *synopses of syntheses*. In Chapter 16, we describe Haynes's recommendation to produce *summaries* as evidence that integrates data on a specific topic from the previous four levels of the model, often in the form of practice guidelines. This chapter also provides a discussion of how evidence from physical therapy practice can be integrated with scientific evidence in point-of-care *systems*, which can be integrated into electronic record systems.

By exploring each of these sources of evidences, we provide many tools with which to find and assess the evidence that is available to help you improve care for your patients.

References

1. Haynes RB. Of studies, syntheses, synopses, summaries, and systems: The "5S" evolution of information services for evidence-based healthcare decisions. Evid Based Med. 2006;11:162–164.
2. DiCenso A, Bayley L, Haynes RB. Accessing pre-appraised evidence: Fine-tuning the 5S model into a 6S model. Evid Based Nurs. 2009;12:99–101.

chapter 10

Asking Clinical Questions

The art and science of asking questions is the source of all knowledge.

—THOMAS BERGER

•

✳ Mr. Ketterman's Case

Mr. Ketterman presents us with many questions. Some might be:

1. How will the new diagnosis of congestive heart failure affect Mr. Ketterman's prognosis?
2. What side effects can I expect from the medications that have been prescribed for Mr. Ketterman?
3. Can I, as a physical therapist, identify interventions that can be used in the presence of these diseases to improve his function?
4. Can I alter the course of either disease with my interventions?

How can a busy clinician find answers to these questions that reflect the most up-to-date evidence?   *(See Appendix for Mr. Ketterman's health history.)*

INTRODUCTION

We have always had questions like these about patients like Mr. Ketterman. In the past, we have turned to a variety of sources for answers, including:

- Tradition: *This is the way it's always been done.* Tradition has been handed to us by our academic and clinical teachers as well as by role models and mentors.
- Authority: *This is the way I'm told to do it.* Again, our teachers sometimes tell us to do things in certain ways. We may also be told to do them in a certain way by our clinical supervisors or employers.
- Trial and error: *This seems to work before, let's see if it will work now.* Sometimes we try to organize the responses to our trial and error to learn from them, but often trial and error just happens as we search for solutions in our practice. As we learned in Section I, our memories of what worked may not be very reliable.

None of these sources is very satisfactory as a way to really improve patient care. Instead, it would be much better to build decisions on the research that has been done about care. In the past, this task was quite daunting due to the vast amount of information and a lack of a framework for assessing the information. But the principles of evidence based practice provide an organized and systematic way to ask and answer these kinds of questions.

Asking the Question

The very first step of evidence based practice is to convert clinical questions like the ones about Mr. Ketterman into questions whose answers can be sought in the literature. The first step in that process is to recognize that different kinds of questions will be answered in different ways. The first two questions, those about Mr. Ketterman's diagnosis, are what have been called *background* questions.

Background Questions

Background questions focus on learning more about the typical course or natural history of a pathology or trauma. Background questions also focus on the typical management of a patient problem and the typical responses to this management. Clinicians tend to ask background questions when they are new to a particular patient population. For students and new graduates this can be almost all the time, since they have not yet had a chance to become familiar with the course of disease or disability across a patient's life or episode of care. Clinicians who have experience with a particular patient population may also want to ask background questions to identify new knowledge, such as advances in what is known about etiology, life expectancy, or changes in typical management. But an experienced clinician can also ask background questions when faced with a patient from a population that is unfamiliar.

Foreground Questions

Once clinicians have an understanding of the typical course of events, they can begin to ask more specific questions having to do with the particular care being provided to this patient. These are called *foreground* questions. Questions 4 and 5 in Mr. Ketterman's case study are examples of foreground questions. These are questions asked to help choose tests and measures for diagnosis and prognosis or to choose interventions. Foreground questions apply both to management of known problems and to prevention and wellness. All clinicians need to ask foreground questions all the time since the evidence about the better choices in care is constantly changing. But they can't stop and ask questions about everything they do. As discussed in Section I, clinicians need to use clinical judgment to identify those topics that matter most. So, clinicians can focus foreground questions on patient issues that represent a significant portion of care, on aspects of care that pose an increased risk for the patient, or on aspects where they know the evidence is changing rapidly.

Figure 10-1 shows the relationship between background and foreground information. As clinicians gain in experience and knowledge about particular patient issues, their background questions about exactly what the problem is will diminish, to be replaced by increasing foreground questions to help them improve their diagnostic ability or intervention choices. The two triangles extend out beyond each other to show that even when the questions are primarily of one type, there are still questions of the other type.

Clarifying whether the question is background or foreground can immediately lead to determining how and where to search for answers. Background information is more typically found in textbooks and clinical updates; foreground information is more typically found in the evidence from research. In either case, we want to ask the best question that we can in order to find the best answers. Generally, this means being as precise as possible, without

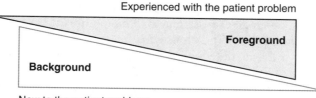

Figure 10-1 Types of Clinical Questions Typically Generated by Clinicians Based on Their Familiarity with the Topic.

being so specific that no answers can be found. The questions arise from the patient in front of the clinician and therefore will almost always be quite specific as they are first formulated. What is happening to *this* patient? How can I help *this* patient improve? But, of course, that is not how the literature is organized. So the question must be changed to something like: What *typically* happens to patients like this one? What *typically* helps patients like this one improve?

Structure of Clinical Questions

Because it is the structure of the question that will lead to the answers, crafting the best questions possible is key. Many people working in the evidence based practice world recommend a particular format for formulating foreground questions about interventions, known as PICO questions.[1,2] A PICO question has four parts: the **P**roblem or **P**opulation being addressed, the **I**ntervention being considered, a **C**omparison intervention, and the **O**utcome that is of interest.

In formulating a specific PICO question, the **P** (problem or population) can be first developed by considering the patient's chief complaint or by generalizing the patient's condition to a larger population. In Mr. Ketterman's case, it would be: *In patients with congestive heart failure. . . .* As you develop the P in your question it is helpful to ask:

- How could you describe a group with a similar problem?
- How you would describe the patient to a colleague?
- What are the important characteristics of this patient?
  - Disease or health status
  - Age, race, sex, previous ailments, current medications
- Should these characteristics be considered as I search for evidence?

As the answers to these questions become more specific, the P part of the PICO question might become: *In patients over 65 with congestive heart failure. . . .* You might be tempted to ask: *In white male patients over 65 with congestive heart failure who take Lasix to control their disease and who also have hypothyroidism. . . .* But by providing this much detail, it becomes almost impossible to find relevant research, so you must strike a balance between precision and too much detail.

The second part of the PICO question concerns information sought about the **I**ntervention. It's really important to recognize that this is based on the plan for the patient. If what you really want to ask is *What can I do for this patient?*, then you should consider this a background question and become more familiar with the specific options available for the patient's care and then focus a PICO question on one particular option. The options in a PICO are generally about interventions, but PICO questions can be asked about diagnostic or prognostic tests as well. In Mr. Ketterman's case, you might want to ask about the value of *exercise* for him. But simply asking about all exercise may well be too broad. You might focus on *aerobic exercise* or *strengthening exercises*. The choice we make will most likely be related to the outcome(s) in which we are interested, as we will discuss below. Avoid search terms that are actually practice-specific but not used by researchers in describing their work. For example, physical therapists use "short arc quads" to describe a specific type of exercise, but this is not a searchable term in most databases. As is discussed in Chapter 11, many databases of health care research are organized using Medical Subject Headings (MeSH) terms. It is useful to spend some time with each database to learn the keywords or terms used by that database to organize the articles included in it.

The next part of the PICO question is the **C**omparison intervention to be explored. Many times clinicians need to make a choice between two different interventions. For example, they often wonder whether a new intervention might be superior to the existing one. In this case, the existing one becomes the comparison. Or they might want to consider two different approaches to reaching the same outcome. As with the primary intervention, the comparison intervention should be specific. In Mr. Ketterman's case, we may actually need to choose between aerobic and strengthening exercises and therefore want to understand the ability of each type of exercise to reach a certain outcome in patients like Mr. Ketterman. Choosing several multiple comparison interventions will most likely result in a less effective computer search, so comparisons are usually limited to one. The Comparison is the only component in the PICO question that can be omitted, as clinicians sometimes choose to look at the Intervention without exploring alternatives, and in some cases, there may not be an alternative. When there is no comparison of interest, the question is sometimes called a three-part question, that is, one that identifies:

1. the patient population,
2. the intervention in question, and
3. the outcomes of interest.

The final part to the PICO question is the **O**utcome of interest. The outcome specifies the result(s) of what the clinician plans to accomplish, improve, or affect and should be measurable. The outcomes may consist of things such as relieving or eliminating specific symptoms at the impairment level or improving or maintaining function. Specific outcomes will yield better search results and allow you to find the studies that focus on the actual outcomes that matter for your patient. When defining the outcome, a term such as *more effective* is not specific enough; rather, you should describe *how* the intervention is more effective. For example, you could say more effective in increasing flexibility or in decreasing contractures.

So, we might ask a question like this to help us in treating Mr. Ketterman: In patients with Alzheimer's Disease with functional limitations related to deconditioning **(P)**, will an impairment-based exercise program for endurance **(I)** versus a planned increase in daily activities **(C)** be more effective in restoring function **(O)**?

Questions About Diagnosis, Prognosis, and Outcomes

The examples used so far in developing sound clinical questions have all been related to choosing interventions for patients, but clinicians usually have questions across the patient care management model. In the areas of diagnosis, prognosis, and outcomes, they most often ask questions about whether a specific test or tool is the best available to help make a particular clinical decision. In Mr. Ketterman's case, we might want to know the best available tests to monitor Mr. Ketterman's ongoing cardiac status to use in his home, or what test will best help determine the progress made in his care. Both the PICO and the three-part question format can be used to help formulate these questions. The P remains the same—we always specify the patient problem or population of interest. Intervention and Comparison are used to refer not only to treatment intervention but to tests and measures. The Outcomes are framed in terms of the ability of the test to answer the clinical question. For example, we might ask an impairment-based diagnosis question such as: In patients with congestive heart failure is the 6-minute walk test a valid measure of impaired aerobic capacity? Or we might ask a prognosis question such as: In patients with Alzheimer's Disease and gait limitations, does the Berg balance test accurately predict the risk of falls?

> In patients with multiple sclerosis, does strengthening exercise versus aerobic exercise better improve walking speed?
> In patients with low back pain, does manipulation versus manipulation with exercise better reduce time to return to employment?
> In clients with a need to improve activity performance, does exercise versus exercise with imagery better improve ability to conduct the task?
> In patients over 75 years, do strengthening exercise versus flexibility exercise better improve ability to maintain activity of daily living (ADL) levels?

Choosing the Answers

Once the question is clear, the next step in identifying the evidence needed to guide care is to decide what kind of resources will provide the necessary answers. Chapter 11 provides much more detail about how and where to seek answers. Chapter 12 will provide guidance on how to assess the literature once it is found. This chapter will focus on the type of literature we would want to find if we could.

Trustworthiness of Sources of Evidence

It is important to consider the varying levels of trustworthiness of the many sources of literature. Trustworthiness of the research that makes up the evidence can be described from a design or statistical point of view (see Chapter 12), but here we mean simply, what do I know about the sources that present the evidence to me? The materials considered to have the highest level of trustworthiness are those articles that have been subjected to masked peer review. This means that experts in the field have reviewed the authors' report of their research methods and findings and have found them acceptable for publication, without knowing who the authors were. Many journals are now adding to trustworthiness by requiring authors to indicate if they had any monetary support from entities related to the research question being studied. At the other end of the continuum would be claims made by manufacturers or sellers of a product. We are all familiar with the claims made in advertising for things like diet supplements that rely on testimonials that may not even come from actual people, but are just advertising claims. Between these two extremes of trustworthiness are a host of sources for information. Figure 10-2 lists some of these sources in declining order of trustworthiness. Unfortunately, as the potential trustworthiness declines, the ease of access increases.

As you search for information, there are many questions to ask, including:

- Is the material a report of research or is it opinion?
- What are the credentials and the motivations of the authors?
- What are the credentials and the motivations of the publishers?

When at all possible begin your search for answers with peer-reviewed information.

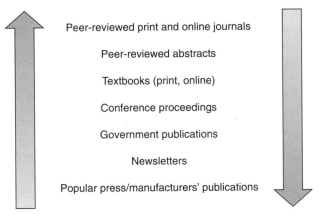

Ease of access increases

Peer-reviewed print and online journals

Peer-reviewed abstracts

Textbooks (print, online)

Conference proceedings

Government publications

Newsletters

Popular press/manufacturers' publications

Trustworthiness increases

Figure 10-2 Trustworthiness of Various Sources of Information.

Types of Peer-Reviewed Research

One important factor to consider is the type of research needed to answer specific kinds of questions. This factor is so important that some people say the question format should be PICO**D**, where the D stands for *design*.[3] There are two overarching types of research design that can be explored to find answers to questions. One type of research is termed *quantitative* research, primarily because it uses numbers to measure the activity being studied. But sometimes, we really need to understand the underlying phenomenon, and for that we turn to *qualitative* research, which typically uses words to describe what is being studied.

But these two types of research also have a more fundamental distinction than simply whether they use words or numbers. Quantitative research is also known as positivistic research since it is rooted in the concept that there is one certain or positive answer for a question and that by careful construction of experiments, one truthful answer can be found. Qualitative research is also known as phenomenology, because it is based on the belief that any given phenomenon, especially a human phenomenon, has many aspects, all valid and all truthful to the person experiencing the phenomenon. (See Chapter 8 for a description of qualitative research and ways to assess its trustworthiness, and Chapter 12 for a deeper description of quantitative research.) In health care clinicians often need to learn from both types of research.

Many questions can best be answered by various forms of quantitative research (Fig. 10-3). Questions about the accuracy of diagnostic tests can best be answered by seeking studies that

The most useful sources of research evidence

To improve:	are:
• Diagnosis	⟶ • Cross-sectional studies
• Prognosis	⟶ • Longitudinal studies
• Intervention	⟶ • Experimental studies

Figure 10-3 Sources of Information About Evidence.

are *cross-sectional*. These are studies that include subjects who are known to have a variety of diagnoses that all possess some similarities and among which we want to differentiate. The researchers then administer the test to see if it was able to correctly differentiate patients with different diagnoses.

If the question is about the tests used to help us make prognostic decisions about patients, clinicians would want to find reports of studies that are *longitudinal* in nature. The only way to tell if a test accurately predicts a future event is to follow patients for an extended period after the test has been administered to see if the test results were correct.

Questions about the usefulness of an intervention are answered by studies that are *experimental*. These types of studies use controlled trials to compare the results of a given intervention for the experimental group against the results in a control group that did not receive the intervention. The many aspects of experimental research that need to be considered in assessing literature will be discussed in much greater depth in Chapter 12, but it is important to recognize these major differences in types of studies as you search out literature to help improve care. There is also an increased emphasis on using well-designed descriptive research to understand interventions. These designs allow the gathering of data from actual clinical practice, when structured experiments may not be possible. These approaches are also discussed in detail in Chapter 12.

All of these types of studies—cross-sectional, longitudinal, and experimental—are quantitative or positivistic. But sometimes questions concern what it actually means to a person to live with a particular disease or level of disability or why a person might choose to accept or reject a particular intervention against the advice of the therapist. In this case, the clinician would turn to qualitative or phenomenological research, as it allows exploration of the perceptions and beliefs (see Fig. 10-3 and Chapters 8 and 12).

Types of Evidence

As we discussed in the introduction, evidence in the literature comes in many forms, as shown in Figure 10-3.

Single Study

The individual *study* is the most easily identified type of evidence used to help answer questions. When first beginning the work of seeking answers to questions, clinicians sometimes assume that somewhere out there will be *the* study that exactly answers their specific question about a specific patient. They also may assume that the study will be perfectly designed so that they can have complete faith in its results and that the results of the study are so powerful that they can have no doubt about what the results mean for the patient. But as the searcher progresses, it is soon found that this perfect study is ephemeral and elusive, always somewhere just out of grasp. Individual studies, no matter how well done, can seldom meet all of the desired qualities. This means studies must be analyzed carefully to determine their value in answering a particular question with a particular patient; in other words, are their results trustworthy (can we believe them) and generalizable (can we apply them to this specific patient)? Chapter 12 will cover this in some detail. Despite the difficulties in seeking answers study by study, this remains the most common way to find evidence, since individual studies are by far the most prevalent source of evidence. In fact, the sheer volume of individual studies can sometimes make a search seem endless. Chapter 11 suggests ways of searching with greater focus to help sift through the volume.

As Haynes has discussed,[4,5] if the information from these individual studies can be combined into more integrative forms of evidence, the job of the clinician becomes easier. He has

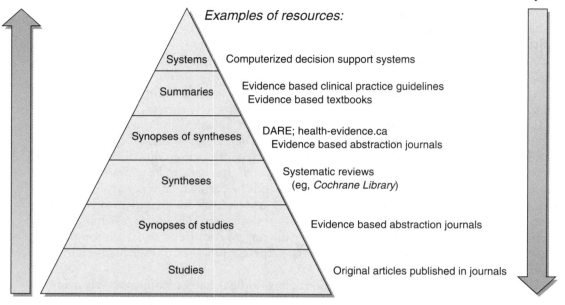

Availability increases

Examples of resources:

Systems — Computerized decision support systems

Summaries — Evidence based clinical practice guidelines / Evidence based textbooks

Synopses of syntheses — DARE; health-evidence.ca / Evidence based abstraction journals

Syntheses — Systematic reviews (eg, *Cochrane Library*)

Synopses of studies — Evidence based abstraction journals

Studies — Original articles published in journals

Utility increases

Figure 10-4 Types of Research to Answer Questions About Aspects of Patient Management. *(Adapted from DiCenso A, Bayley L, Haynes RB. Accessing pre-appraised evidence: Fine-tuning the 5S model into a 6S model. Evid Based Nurs. 2009;12:99–101.)*

described six levels of organization of evidence (Fig. 10-4), beginning with the *single study*. (Assessing single studies for their value in answering questions is covered in Chapter 12.) As mentioned, searching for answers single study by single study poses several problems, including their sheer numbers and the rigor needed to determine their usefulness. But for clinicians, one of the biggest problems may be that single studies tend to focus on only a single aspect of patient management, while the clinician must balance all of the patent's diagnostic and intervention needs at once.

Synopsis

The next level Haynes identifies in describing sources of information about evidence is the *synopsis*. A synopsis provides information about choices that can be determined from single studies. Synopses usually start or end with a clear statement about doing or not doing a specific thing with a specific patient population. The synopsis would also include the essential information from the study or systematic review that supports this conclusion. When appropriate synopses are available, a clinician can determine a course of action in a matter of a few minutes. But it is very important that the clinician have a clear understanding that the study really does match the clinical question. Also, the problem remains that the synopsis focuses on one aspect of patient management rather than on the range of decisions needed in actual care. Synopses are sometimes written in the Critically Appraised Topics format.[1] The Clinical Bottom Line feature found in *Physical Therapy* is another example of a synopsis format. Chapter 13 discusses the creation and use of synopses in more detail.

Synthesis and Synopses of Synthesis

Haynes suggests that the next level of sources of evidence is *synthesis*. Systematic reviews are the most common example of syntheses. These reviews are based on extensive literature searches designed to find as much of the research about a topic as possible, an analysis of each article found, and then an integration of the findings of the studies. The reviews have narrative assessments of each study and often rate their quality. Many systematic reviews also include meta-analyses, which are statistical analyses that allow the results of multiple studies to be merged, thereby giving more strength to the results. Many reviews also have some visual analysis of the results, such as forest plots, that allow the reader to see the ways in which the studies have both similar and varying results. The Cochrane Collective has led the way in publishing systematic reviews, but reviews are also appearing with increasing frequency in other journals. Chapter 14 discusses systematic reviews in more depth. The next level of sources is *synopses* of *syntheses*. These sources provide clinicians reviews of systematic reviews. They are also discussed in Chapter 14.

Summaries

The next level of sources of information about evidence is *summaries*. Summaries are designed to move past the basic problem of the previous three levels. They seek to integrate findings across the full management of a patient. They offer comparisons on a full range of evidence about the multiple interventions available for a given problem. Summaries about treatment options might be found in well-designed, evidence-based textbooks. In addition, clinical decision rules or clinical prediction rules also provide summary information to help clinicians compare the utility of various diagnostic tests in actually predicting the success of particular interventions. Summaries are very helpful because they much more closely approximate the actual decisions clinicians need to make, but they are, at the same time, much harder to find. Chapter 15 discusses the creation and use of summaries.

Systems

Haynes has placed *systems* at the top of his pyramid as a source of information about evidence. Systems allow full integration of evidence in the literature with the clinician's decision making at the point of care with the patient. To make the information available at the point of care, systems are often integrated into electronic medical records (EMR). As clinicians enter their patients' data in real time into the EMR, the system can provide clinicians with on-the-spot access to summaries and synopses, prompt them with the next option point, query them about their decisions if they seem to fall outside the parameters of the evidence, and provide information to the clinician. If the strength of the evidence supports it, systems can even be designed to deter the clinician from making a poor choice. They generally don't prohibit the clinician's decision, but instead prompt the clinician to reconsider by making queries and providing information. Systems are the best way for clinicians to access and use evidence in the course of everyday care, since the results are available almost instantly and the clinician does not have to stop to search for other data. However, as you might have suspected, there are very few examples of functioning systems, especially in physical therapy. Chapter 15 also talks in more depth about the creation and use of systems.

We have presented these six levels by moving *up* Haynes's pyramid, since this is often the way clinicians think of the search process and it mirrors the availability of different sources of evidence. Haynes advises, however, that clinicians search *down* the pyramid, since finding information at a higher level has so much more utility.

Return to the PICO question developed about Mr. Ketterman: In patients with Alzheimer's Disease (AD) with functional limitations related to deconditioning **(P)**, will an impairment-based exercise program for endurance **(I)** versus a planned increase in daily activities **(C)** be more effective in restoring function **(O)**? A search of the literature identified the following sources of evidence at each of the levels in the evidence pyramid.

SOURCE	EVIDENCE	INFORMATION FOR THE CLINICIAN
Systems	None found	
Summaries	Scottish Intercollegiate Guidelines Network (SIGN). Management of patients with dementia. A national clinical guideline. Edinburgh (Scotland): Scottish Intercollegiate Guidelines Network (SIGN); 2006;Feb. 53 (SIGN publication; no. 86).	A detailed guideline for the full management (medical, pharmacological, and nonpharmacological) of patients with AD
Synopses of Syntheses	Centre for Reviews and Dissemination. Physical activity and behavior in dementia: A review of the literature and implications for psychosocial intervention in primary care (structured abstract). Database of Abstracts of Reviews of Effects.1, 2011. Abstract and Commentary for: Eggermont LH, Scherder EJ. Physical activity and behavior in dementia: A review of the literature and implications for psychosocial intervention in primary care. Dementia. 2006;5(3):411–428.	A four-page summary of a longer systematic review. The practice recommendation is that exercise should include walking, should be of 30 minutes duration, and should occur several times a week.
Syntheses	Forster A, Lambley R, Hardy J, Young J, Smith J, Green J, Burns E. Rehabilitation for older people in long-term care. Cochrane Database of Systematic Reviews. 3. 2010	A detailed review of 49 articles that assessed many rehabilitation-based interventions, including exercise and activities of daily living, with the conclusion that these interventions were safe and reduced disability

SOURCE	EVIDENCE	INFORMATION FOR THE CLINICIAN
Synopses of Studies	Larson EB, Wang L, Bowen JD, McCormick WC, Teri L, Crane P, Kukull W. Exercise in people age 65 years and older is associated with lower risk for dementia. Ann Intern Med. 1/17/2006; 144(2):I20	An accurate one-page summary of the study below, written primarily for patients, with the conclusion that exercise may have the benefit of reducing he risk of dementia related to AD
Study	Larson EB, Wang L, Bowen JD, McCormick WC, Teri L, Crane P, Kukull W. Exercise is associated with reduced risk for incident dementia among persons 65 years of age and older. Ann Intern Med. 2006;144:73–81.	A description of a prospective cohort study of 1740 people over 65, designed to identify if exercise is related to rate of development of AD. Incidence rate of development of AD in people who exercise was 13 per 1000 person-years, compared to 19. 7 per 1000 person-years in people who didn't exercise.

As you can see, each source provides a clinician with different information. The individual study provides information from one group of subjects, and its synopsis does this in a more accessible format. But the systematic review provides information from 49 articles, representing over 3000 subjects, giving the clinician much more information in one place. The synopsis of a systematic review also summarizes a full review in only four pages. Finally, the clinical practice guideline provides information about all aspects of management of AD. At this time, no systems addressing this topic were found, but may well become available in the future.

CONCLUSION

This chapter started with a description of the process of writing a good clinical question, as the question drives everything else we do in seeking answers. We identified some concerns in identifying the type of literature that we need to seek. The goal should be to search for literature that has been peer reviewed, whose design matches the type of question we want to answer, and that is at the highest possible level of source of evidence. Chapter 11 will give more detail on how to go about actually finding such research. But it is essential to keep in mind that finding useful evidence for clinical decisions may still be difficult. Chapter 12 will talk about some of the ways you can determine just how good the evidence is and if it is good enough. Clinicians cannot wait for the "perfect" evidence; they need to act and act on the best evidence they can find. Section IV will discuss in greater detail how clinicians can integrate the best evidence they can find with their own sound decision making and with patients' preferences to make the best decisions possible in the real world of clinical care.

SELF-ASSESSMENT

1. Refer to Mr. Ketterman's case in the Appendix and write three background questions about things that puzzle you about his medical status.
2. Refer to Mr. Ketterman's case in the Appendix and write three PICO questions that will help you choose diagnostic, prognostic, or outcome measurements to use in planning his care.
3. Refer to Mr. Ketterman's case in the Appendix and write two more PICO questions that will help you choose interventions for his care.

CONTINUED LEARNING

- Based on one of the PICO questions you wrote about Mr. Ketterman, or any other PICO question of interest to you, identify an article in the peer-reviewed literature that addresses the question. Then, using an Internet search or other sources, find an article written by a vendor or by a consumer group.

1. What differences do you see in these two types of information?
2. How can you help patients see these differences and make wise choices about their care?

REFERENCES

1. Strauss SE, et al. *Evidence-based Medicine*, 4th ed. Elsevier Churchill Livingstone; 2011.
2. Center for Evidence Based Medicine, University of Oxford. http://www.cebm.net/index.aspx?o=1157 Accessed on March 21, 2010.
3. Daly A, Raza A. *Journal Club Handbook*, Birmingham Women's Hospital; 2008.
4. Haynes RB. Of studies, syntheses, synopses, summaries, and systems: The "5S" evolution of information services for evidence-based healthcare decisions. Evid Based Med. 2006;11:162–164.
5. DiCenso, Bayley L, Haynes RB. Accessing pre-appraised evidence: Fine-tuning the 5S model into a 6S model. Evid Based Nurs. 2009;12:99–101.

chapter 11

Finding the Evidence

Connie Schardt, MLS, AHIP, FMLA

Knowledge is of two kinds. We know a subject ourselves, or we know where we can find information upon it.

—SAMUEL JOHNSON

•

✳ Mr. Ketterman's Case

Mr. Ketterman has several common health problems. I know there is a lot of information out there to help me understand his illnesses and plan his care. But I really don't know how to find it from credible sources. And I don't have hours available to do the searching. (*See Appendix for Mr. Ketterman's health history.*)

INTRODUCTION

Finding answers to clinical questions can be a rewarding activity once you become familiar with the resources available to you and understand effective searching techniques. This chapter will focus on finding the evidence to clinical questions, where it is stored and how you can efficiently retrieve it. We will also suggest methods to manage the retrieved references and discuss how to keep current with new information.

As we discussed in Chapter 10, questions that occur during the care of patients usually fall into one of two broad categories: background questions and foreground questions. Background questions are concerned with general knowledge that helps us to understand the process of disease. According to Strauss,[1] these questions have two parts: a root question such as "what" or "how" or "why" and an aspect of the disease or condition in question. These types of questions are usually answered with textbooks that provide general descriptions, overviews, and summary information. Foreground questions, often framed as PICO questions, are concerned with the management issues of individual patients with specific problems. Evidence based practice is centered on the care of specific patients and therefore provides a framework for addressing these foreground questions. Foreground questions are usually answered by current research, either in the form of filtered resources that select, analyze, and summarize studies as systematic reviews and preappraised topics or by primary studies that are reported in journals as original research, found through unfiltered research.

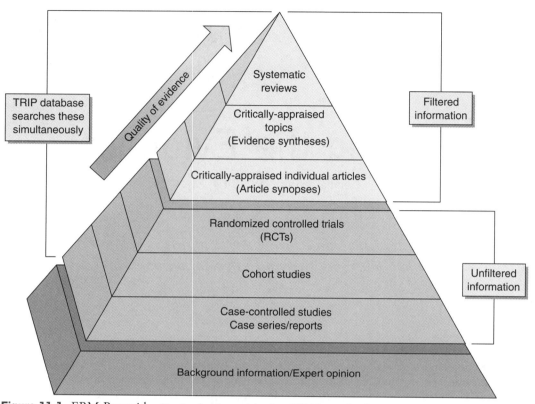

Figure 11-1 EBM Pyramid. *(Reprinted with permission from EBM Pyramid and EBM Page Generator, copyright 2006 Trustees of Dartmouth College and Yale University. Produced by: Jan Glover, David Izzo, Karen Odato and Lei Wang.)*

FILTERED RESOURCES

Filtered or preappraised resources have undergone a process of critical appraisal that systematically assesses the study for its methodology and validity, its results, and its relevance to making an informed clinical decision. Evidence-based practice requires the availability of current filtered evidence about diagnosis, treatment, and prevention of health disorders. Filtered evidence is characterized by a process of critical appraisal that evaluates the study for soundness of methodology, significance of results, and applicability to patients. The quality of the evidence is often visualized in the evidence pyramid, which shows the organization of resources based on the quality and comprehensiveness of the evidence (Fig. 11-1).

Filtered information can be quick to search and is validated for sound methodology. Examples of filtered resources relevant to physical therapy include: PEDro (Physiotherapy Evidence Database), Cochrane Database of Systematic Reviews, and the National Guideline Clearinghouse. (See Chapters 13–16 for detailed descriptions of these forms of filtered information.)

PEDro

PEDro Physiotherapy Evidence Database (www.pedro.fhs.usyd.edu.au/) is an initiative of the Centre for Evidence Based Physiotherapy (CEBP) at the University of Sydney. It was developed to give rapid access to references and abstracts of randomized controlled trials, systematic reviews, and evidence-based clinical practice guidelines in physiotherapy. Most randomized controlled trials in PEDro have been rated for quality to help discriminate between trials that are likely to be valid and interpretable and those that are not. Searching is by words in the title or abstract and by broad categories of therapy, problem, body part, or study methodology. The results are displayed by type of study: systematic review, clinical trial, and practice guideline. The clinical trials include a critical appraisal score, which is documented in the full record. The database is small, with only about 19,000 records as of April 2011; it is updated monthly and focuses exclusively on selected relevant studies in physical therapy.

Cochrane Database of Systematic Reviews

The Cochrane Collaboration is an international, not-for-profit organization providing up-to-date information about the effectiveness of health care. The Cochrane Library (www.thecochranelibrary.com/) is a collection of databases that contain high-quality, independent evidence to inform health care decision making. There are several databases within the Cochrane Library. The one most relevant to physical therapy is the Database of Systematic Reviews. Cochrane systematic reviews represent a thorough review of the literature on a single topic, with conclusions based on high-quality studies that have been evaluated for validity, significance of the results, and applicability to patient care. There are several Cochrane Review Groups, including the Back Group, Bone, Joint and Muscle Trauma Group, and Musculoskeletal Group, which have developed systematic reviews on topics that are of interest to physical therapists. The full text of the Cochrane systematic reviews is only available online through a subscription service. Searching is by words in the title or abstract or by Medical Subject Headings (MeSH). The Cochrane Collaboration provides free access to the abstracts of their systematic reviews from their Web site at www.cochrane.org/reviews/index.htm.

The National Guideline Clearinghouse

The National Guideline Clearinghouse (www.guideline.gov) is a free, comprehensive database of evidence based clinical practice guidelines. Criteria for inclusion in the database include:

1. systematically developed statements that include recommendations, strategies, or information that assists physicians and/or other health care practitioners and patients make decisions about appropriate health care;
2. production under the auspices of medical specialty associations, agency, or organization; and
3. documented systematic literature search and review of existing scientific evidence published in peer-reviewed journals; and
4. availability of the full text of a guideline that was developed and reviewed within the last 5 years.

Searching is by text words and by browsing disease categories.

UNFILTERED RESOURCES

Unfiltered information usually requires a more focused search strategy and the need to critically appraise the study before applying the results to a patient. The unfiltered resources are often much larger and more comprehensive databases, such as PubMed and CINAHL (Cumulative Index to Nursing and Allied Health Literature).

Medline/PubMed

Medline is the U.S. National Library of Medicine's (NLM) premier database; it contains over 17 million references to journal articles in the life sciences with a concentration on biomedicine. Biomedicine includes the areas of behavioral sciences, chemical sciences, and bioengineering as they relate to basic research and clinical care, public health, health policy development, and related educational activities. PubMed is NLM's search service, which provides access to MEDLINE and the other databases of the National Center for Biotechnology Information (NCBI). (There are other search services, such as Ovid, Inc and MDConsult, which also provide a search interface to the Medline database.) A distinctive feature of Medline is that each reference is read by a subject expert who then indexes or tags the article using standardized terminology called Medical Subject Headings or MeSH. MeSH helps organize and identify articles on specific topics within the database. Due to its enormous size, searching requires a well-thought-out search strategy that includes subject headings and text words that can then be limited to specific parameters. While there is a growing number of free full-text articles linked from PubMed, to obtain the full text of most articles requires personal subscription or access to a medical library.

CINAHL (Cumulative Index to Nursing and Allied Health Literature)

The CINAHL database from EBSCO indexes over 3000 journal titles in nursing, allied health (including physical therapy), biomedicine, complementary medicine, and consumer health information from 1982 to the present. It includes approximately 2,300,000 records for articles, books, pamphlets, dissertations, government publications, audiovisuals, software, and proceedings. CINAHL is an indexed database, using CINAHL Subject Headings, many of which are similar to MeSH. Unlike PubMed, CINAHL requires a subscription and is therefore usually available only through medical libraries or professional associations. It is important to note that while these databases are the primary resources for finding journal articles, they may not index all the journals in the field of physical therapy and rehabilitation medicine. Several studies have shown that PubMed is the more comprehensive database for physical therapy journals, followed by PEDro and CINAHL.[2,3] Thus a thorough literature review may require searching all of these resources and databases. See Table 11.1 for a summary of these databases.

Tutorials

Most databases will provide tutorials or additional help with understanding the search techniques related to the database. Medical libraries also develop their own tutorials and search aids. Some examples:

- PEDro: http://pedro.org.au/english/search-help/
- PubMed: http://nlm.nih.gov/bsd/disted/pubmed.html
- http://mclibrary.duke.edu/training/pubmed
- CINAHL: http://support.epnet.com/training/tutorials.php
- http://mclibrary.duke.edu/training/cinahlebsco

Table 11.1   Summary of Primary EBM Resources for Physical Therapy

Resource	Topic/Coverage
PEDro	Developed specifically by and for physical therapists; abstracts of randomized controlled trials, systematic reviews, and evidence based clinical practice guidelines in physiotherapy; 19,000 records as of 5/2011; Most trials in the database have been rated for quality to help discriminate between trials that are likely to be valid and interpretable, and those that are not. *Access:* http://pedro.org.au/ [Free]
Cochrane Database of Systematic Reviews	Systematic reviews, most using meta-analysis, from the 50 Collaborative Review Groups. Focused topic summaries. Gold standard for systematic reviews. One systematic review per topic; *Access:* http://thecochranelibrary.com/view/0/index.html [Abstracts available for free at Web site]
National Guideline Clearinghouse	A public resource for evidence based clinical practice guidelines. *Access:* http://guidelines.gov/ [Free]
PubMed	PubMed provides more comprehensive coverage of the biomedical journal literature (Medline); since 1960+; uses MeSH indexing; over 17 million citations *Access:* http://ncbi.nlm.nih.gov/pubmed/ [Free; access to full-text articles may require a fee or subscriptions]
CINAHL Cumulative Index to Nursing and Allied Health Literature	CINAHL indexes journal articles, books and book chapters, dissertations, audiovisual materials, and other formats; since 1982+; subject coverage focuses on nursing and the allied health disciplines, including physiotherapy, health education, and nutrition. Includes references to journals, books, dissertations, conference proceedings, and other publications; *Access:* http://ebscohost.com/cinahl/ [Fee-based]

THE SEARCH STRATEGY

Before you start your search for relevant information, you need to have a clear understanding of what you are looking for (the clinical question) and where you might find it (the resources). The basic steps of conducting a literature search are shown in Figure 11-2.

Focus the Question

Determine the important concepts that need to be present in the article or information you find. The PICO framework, discussed in Chapter 10, provides a model for developing a well-focused question. A well-defined clinical question can lead to a well-focused search strategy. It will also be useful in identifying the most relevant articles that address the specific question and patient.

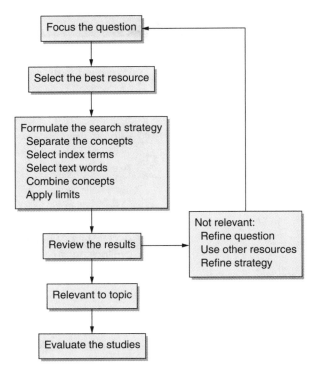

Figure 11-2 Search Process.

Select the Best Resource

The well-formed clinical question will help guide your selection of the resources most likely to provide useful results. PEDro and Cochrane are considered filtered resources because the studies included in these small, specialized databases have been critically appraised and therefore provide some assurance that the studies are valid and the results reflect sound scientific methodology. PubMed and CINAHL are much broader in scope but do not evaluate the quality of the studies. Additional work and time will be needed to determine the validity and significance of the results of studies found in these databases.

Formulate the Search Strategy

There are several steps in formulating the search strategy:

* **Separate the concepts:**
  After selecting the most appropriate resources, you need to be familiar with how each resource is constructed and therefore the best way to retrieve relevant information from it. Use the concepts of your clinical question to form your search strategy.
* **Select index terms:**
  Medline and CINAHL use standardized terminology (called MeSH and CINAHL Subject Headings) that helps the researcher find all articles on a topic regardless of the exact words used by the author. This is especially helpful when there may be several ways to describe the same concept. For example, articles that discuss using electrodes to deliver pain relief may refer to this as "TENS" or "electroanalgesia" or "Transdermal

Electrostimulation." However, the index term or subject heading in Medline and CINAHL is "Transcutaneous Electric Nerve Stimulation" and therefore all articles that discuss this concept will be indexed under this term. These index terms or subject headings are relatively easy to find. Most databases will provide a list of them (in Medline this is the MeSH Database; in CINAHL it is the CINAHL Subject Headings) or will automatically "map" (or translate) your search term to an appropriate subject heading.

- **Select text words:**

  Text words, on the other hand, are the words that the authors used in the title or abstract. Common problems with text words are that you need to include all the synonyms for a concept in a comprehensive search strategy, and while the word might appear in the abstract that does not guarantee the article is about it. (For example, "TENS" may appear in the abstract because the author stated that "the patients were not given TENS therapy. . . .") Text words are useful when the concept has no equivalent subject heading, is a unique word or phrase, or is a new concept that has not yet been assigned a subject heading. Often the most effective search strategy uses a combination of index terms and text words to retrieve as much useful information as possible.

- **Combine concepts:**

  Search terms can be combined using the Boolean logic of "OR" to broaden or "AND" to narrow the retrieval. Using the logic of AND requires that *all terms selected are in the same citation*, whereas using the logic of "OR" requires that *at least one of the selected terms is in a citation*. These combining terms or Boolean logic are a universal language for all databases and search engines and must be applied correctly to get the best results (Fig. 11-3).

- **Apply limits:**

  Depending on the question and the amount of information retrieved from your search of the topic, you may want to limit the final results to a specific age group, language, type of study, or years of publication. Each database has its own set of limits that can be applied to further refine the search. PubMed offers a unique method for limiting retrieval to the most appropriate study methodology based on the type of clinical question being asked. Once you have a set of articles that address your topic, copy your final set number with the # sign into Clinical Queries, select the type of question category (therapy, diagnosis, prognosis, etiology, or clinical prediction), and select a narrow or broad strategy. The system will automatically add a short search strategy proven to get at the most appropriate study methodology based on the type of question selected.

OR – either term in same citation

AND – both terms in same citation

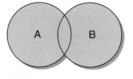

A = TENS
B = electrical stimulation therapy

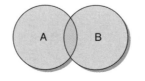

A = TENS
B = back pain

Figure 11-3 Boolean Logic.

Table 11.2 Example of Indexing Terminology for Article

Percutaneous electrical nerve stimulation for low back pain: a randomized crossover study.

PubMed–MeSH

- Adult
- Cross-Over Studies
- Electric Stimulation Therapy
  Methods
- Exercise Therapy
- Female
- Humans
- Low Back Pain therapy
- Male
- Pain Measurement
- Quality of Life
- Single-Blind Method
- Transcutaneous Electric Nerve
  Stimulation

CINAHL Subject Headings

Electric Stimulation: Low Back Pain–Therapy

Crossover Damage: Random Assignment: P-Value:
Chi Square Test: Research Instruments: T-Tests:
Funding Source: Adult: Middle Age: Male: Female

Review the Results

Review the titles and abstracts for relevance to the clinical question. If they are not relevant to your question, you may need to modify your search strategy, refocus your question, or select another resource. Searching is an iterative process that may take several attempts before reaching a satisfactory retrieval. One way to improve your search strategy is to identify a highly relevant citation and then view the complete record for the indexing terms assigned to it (Table 11.2). This may give you suggestions for additional terms to use in refining your search strategy. If the results are relevant, then they should be evaluated to determine if they can be applied to patient care. (See Chapter 12.)

Here is an example of search strategies (conducted 4/25/2011) from the resources we have just discussed for the question: In patients with back pain, does the use of TENS or electrical stimulation provide effective pain relief?

DATABASE	SEARCH STRATEGY	RESULTS
PEDro	electrical stimulation [Abstract & Title] lumbar spine, sacro-iliac joint or pelvis [Body part]	93 practice guidelines, systematic reviews, or clinical trials
Cochrane Database of Systematic Reviews	electrical stimulation [Title, Abstract, Keywords] and "back pain"[Title, Abstract, Keywords]	10 systematic reviews

DATABASE	SEARCH STRATEGY	RESULTS
PubMed	#1 back pain[MeSH Terms] #2 tens [title, abstract] #3 Transcutaneous Electric Nerve Stimulation[MeSH] #4 #1 AND (#2 OR #3) #5 #1 AND (#2 OR #3) Limits: Randomized Controlled Trial	49 citations
CINAHL	S1 (MH "Transcutaneous Electric Nerve Stimulation") S2 (MH "Back Pain+") S3 S1 AND S2 S4 S3 Limiters—Publication Type: Research	34 citations

SEARCH ENGINES

Search engines are computer programs designed to help find information on the public Web. They look for content matching specific criteria, usually words or phrases, and retrieve a list of items that contain the exact words or character strings. The items are usually displayed in a ranking that may depend on the frequency of the words and their location in the page or document rather than their relevance to the topic.[4] Google Scholar is a subset of Google that searches across disciplines and published sources, including peer-reviewed papers, theses, books, abstracts, and articles, from academic publishers, professional societies, preprint repositories, universities, and other scholarly organizations. The results are ranked according to a number of criteria such as full text, number of times cited by other authors, and the publication in which the article appears. It is important to note that although Google Scholar is a good way to limit your search in Google to the published literature, there is no way to know exactly what journals were included in the search.[5]

There are some specialized search engines that search across a well-defined subset of EBM-related Web sites, such as TRIP (Turning Research Into Practice). The purpose of the TRIP Database (www.tripdatabase.com) is to allow health professionals easy access to the highest-quality material available on the Web to support evidence based practice. TRIP, based in the UK, searches across over 90 Web sites of high-quality medical information, providing direct access to abstracts from journals (such as the BMJ, JAMA, and NEJM), practice guidelines, textbooks, (such as eMedicine and the Merck Manual), systematic reviews, and evidence based synopses (such as POEMS, Bandolier, and BestBets). In addition, TRIP provides a link to conduct the search in PubMed using the Clinical Queries feature.

Because search engines query across many different Web sites, you can only search by text words or words that appear on the Web page. This means that you may have to try several different word combinations or synonyms before you find exactly what you need. It also may result in retrieving a very large number of items, many of which may not be relevant. Search engines such as Google will include all types of Web sites, including commercial, personal, governmental, and educational, making it the responsibility of the searcher to figure out which sites provide the most authoritative, unbiased, and accurate information.

Here is an example of search strategies (conducted 4/25/2011) from the search engines we have just discussed for the question: In patients with back pain, does the use of TENS or electrical stimulation provide effective pain relief?

DATABASE	SEARCH STRATEGY	RESULTS
TRIP	electrical stimulation and back pain	151 citations (articles, guidelines, synopses, textbooks, etc.)
Google	(electrical stimulation or tens) and "back pain"	401,000 results (commercial, blogs, articles, etc.)
Google Scholar	(electrical stimulation or tens) and "back pain"	5920 results

ACCESS TO RESOURCES

One common misconception about the resources is that "everything is available for free on the Internet." Although some of the resources may be free because they are older material or provide limited access to just abstracts, getting to authoritative, full-text information often requires subscription fees and access to a medical library. The Internet is the communication platform that allows libraries and health care professionals, as well as businesses, to provide access to databases and products for their patrons, customers, or audience. The resources listed in this chapter are usually available at most medical centers or community hospitals with library services. A medical librarian can help you access these databases, provide advice on the most efficient search strategies, and help obtain copies of relevant articles.

If you do not have access to a medical library, there may be other ways to access some of these resources. The National Library of Medicine coordinates the National Network of Libraries of Medicine (NN/LM) (http://nnlm.gov), whose mission is to provide health professionals and the general public with health information resources and services. They do this through outreach programs and an extensive network of hospital and academic medical libraries. Area Health Education Centers (AHEC) are also involved in supporting education and training for health care professionals. These regional and statewide programs support health libraries and coordinate access to information services and resources. (www.nationalahec.org/)

Resources Available From the American Physical Therapy Association (APTA)

The American Physical Therapy Association (APTA) (www.apta.org) offers a members-only service that provides access to CINAHL, the Cochrane Library, and selected research journals through the association Web site. The *Open Door: APTA's Portal to Evidence-Based Practice* provides members with easy access to journals and other resources relevant to clinical practice whenever and wherever they need it. In addition, the *Open Door* maintains a list of current research articles and an e-mail alert system to keep current on new additions and searching tips for the *Open Door* project. Another service of APTA is the *Hooked on Evidence* Web site. This represents a "grassroots," member-generated effort to develop a database containing current research evidence on the effectiveness of physical therapy interventions. To be included in the database, studies must involve human subjects, examine at least one physical therapy intervention, report outcomes, and be published in an English-language, peer-reviewed journal. This service is discussed in greater detail in Chapter 14.

MANAGING THE EVIDENCE

Once you have retrieved a set of citations or references from a database or Web site, you may need a way to organize the items so that you can review and use them at a later time. This is especially true if you are conducting ongoing research, writing a paper, or require more time to review the material. Most of the large database systems offer advanced features that provide storage space, folders to save search strategies and specific citations, and e-mail alerts for new citations. In PubMed this feature is called MyNCBI. After a short registration process that requires you to create an account with an ID and password, *MyNCBI* allows you to save a search strategy that can then be rerun at a later date. Search strategies can also be rerun to display only the new citations added to the database since that last time the strategy was run. Selected individual citations from searches can be saved temporarily to the ClipBoard or permanently saved to the Collections folder in MyNCBI. Both the Clipboard and Collections eliminate duplicates and collect the citations into one set, which can then be exported to EndNote or other bibliographic management software. CINAHL has a similar feature called MyEBSCOHost, which provides folders for keeping track of search strategies and selected citations.

Reference Management Software

Reference management software allows you to download and organize references from the major databases, create bibliographies in customized formats, and easily incorporate references into working manuscripts. The references can be entered manually or imported directly from databases, such as PubMed and CINAHL. You should check with your medical library to find out which programs might be supported at your institution. In addition, there are a growing number of Web sites that provide free online reference management tools.

The most popular software programs are EndNote (endnote.com/) and RefWorks (www.refworks.com/). These programs have similar functionalities, but they can vary in level of difficulty, cost, operating system compatibility, and sharing options. (See http://hsl.unc.edu/Services/guides/citationmanager_comparison.cfm for a chart comparing these two programs.)

The most popular free online programs are Connotea (http://connotea.org/), citeulike (http://citeulike.org/), Mendeley (http://mendeley.com/), and Zotero (http://zotero.org/). Wikipedia offers a detailed comparison of these programs at: http://en.wikipedia.org/wiki/Comparison_of_reference_management_software#Reference_list_file_formats.

KEEPING CURRENT WITH NEW EVIDENCE

The amount of new information added to databases and the Web is staggering and can present a challenge to health professionals who need to keep current on specific research topics and their own professional literature. As an example, 2000 to 4000 completed references are added each working day to PubMed. Fortunately, many of the databases provide automated current awareness services that allow professionals to easily review new research.

PubMed through its MyNCBI service allows you to generate an e-mail alert whenever new citations are added to the database that match a specific search strategy. When a citation is added to the database, an e-mail message is sent with the abstract. This alert service can also be generated for table of contents of current issues of journals indexed in the database. (See http://ncbi.nlm.nih.gov/sites/myncbi/about/ for more information.) MyEBSCOHost from CINAHL offers a similar service. Many individual journals also offer an automated table of contents service; however, most require an individual subscription to activate their service.

In 2011, the American Physical Therapy Association unveiled *PTNow* (http://apta.org/PTNow/), a Web-based portal designed to give physical therapists easy access to various types of evidence. It allows users to find original, assessed, and synthesized evidence for both background and foreground questions; to search related Web sites; to ask questions of experts; to access information on diagnostic, prognostic, and outcome tools; and to download patient education materials.

Blogs, Wikis, and RSS Feeds

The Web has evolved from a static, view-only platform to an interactive and engaging tool for exchanging ideas and conversing about issues. This evolution, sometimes referred to as Web 2.0, utilizes social networking tools to encourage communication. Some of these tools, specifically blogs and wikis, are being used to share news, information, and opinions and to create a greater sense of community among people with common interests. A blog is a Web site, usually authored by an individual, that offers commentary and news on a particular subject. The content can include text, images, links to other Web pages and multimedia, and the option for readers to leave comments in an interactive format. Posts are updated frequently and presented in chronological order with links back to older material. One of the great appeals of blogs is that they use very simple editing screens that do not require any experience with HTML or Web-authoring tools. This may help explain the estimates of over 50 million blogs in existence. Most of these are authored by individuals and cover a very wide array of topics from the very personal journals to social and professional issues to important medical information. Blogs can be very useful sources of current information, but like any other resource from the Internet, you must evaluate the blog for authorship, potential bias, and authoritativeness before you accept and use the information presented.

A wiki is a collaborative Web site that allows a group of people to develop and edit content on a topic. One of the most well known wikis is Wikipedia (en.wikipedia.org), the largest, free, online encyclopedia currently available on the Internet. Like blogs, the quality and value of the content of wikis can vary dramatically, and it is important to always read the content with a critical eye. However, wikis tend to focus more on providing content and information, rather than opinions and personal accounts.

Examples of blogs and wikis related to physical therapy:

- Concepts in Orthopaedic and Sports Medicine Rehab
  (http://orthosportsrehab.blogspot.com/)
- MyPhysicalTherapyspace.com
  (http://blog.myphysicaltherapyspace.com/)
- PT Think Tank (http://ptthinktank.com/)
- Physiopedia (www.physio-pedia.com).

RSS (Really Simple Syndication) is an easy way to manage all the new content that is being published daily on the Internet. The RSS feed provides a mechanism for readers to receive current, unread content from blogs, wikis, and other Web sites at a central point or Web page, called a "feed reader." This eliminates having to go out and visit each blog, wiki, or Web site to read what has been newly published. The feed reader can organize the selected feeds by subject area and displays the newest unread postings on a single Web page. RSS is also being used by PubMed and CINAHL to allow searchers to generate an RSS feed of a specific search strategy to display the new results in a feed reader (rather than e-mail), with links back to the citations in the database. Example of RSS feed readers are Google Reader (www.google.com/reader/) and Bloglines (www.bloglines.com/).

MOBILE DEVICES

Over the last several years smart phones and tablets have become common devices for accessing information resources. Many of them are Web-based, so users can access Internet resources just as they would do from desktop computers. In response to this growing use, libraries and resource producers are reformatting their pages and products to conform to the size of a smart phone or tablet screen. A second way that these devices can access resources is through specific programs or applications (often referred to as "apps"). These applications are usually self-contained and downloaded to the device so that they can function without being connected to the Internet. There are 100s of medical applications available for a variety of operating systems, including Apple, RIM, Android, and Symbian.

Applications can be grouped around three activities: patient education, reference, and clinical tools. Check your local medical librarian, iTunes Apps Store, or Android Market for other applications. Blogs and wikis are also excellent sources for reviewing and ranking medical applications.[6]

Examples of apps for patient education include *Shoulder Decide* or *Knee Decide* by www.orcamd.com; for reference, *Muscle Anatomy* by Blaine King; and for clinical tools, *Goniometer* by Jinfra or *Stop Watch and Timers* by SkyPaw Co Ltd.

CONCLUSION

The practice of physical therapy requires finding current relevant evidence to answer clinical questions about the care and management of patients. Formulating a well-focused question and becoming familiar with the resources available to you can make finding information easier and more productive. The next step, once you have found relevant studies or information on your question, is to evaluate the evidence for validity and review the results for applicability.

SELF-ASSESSMENT

1. Using one or two of the questions you developed in Chapter 10 about Mr. Ketterman's care, use the filtered resources discussed in this chapter to find answers to your questions.

2. Now try to find answers to the same questions using unfiltered resources.
3. Compare the types of evidence that you find using both of these search approaches.
4. If you are unable to find any answers in half an hour, reach out to reference or medical librarians or colleagues to get help.

CONTINUED LEARNING

- Visit *PTNow* and some of the blogs or wikis discussed in this chapter. Prepare a presentation on the resources you find there for your colleagues.
- Use some of the tutorials identified in the chapter and then present these search options to your colleagues as ways for them to find information to support their practices.
- Visit a few of the myriad resources available for patients (Web sites, blogs, wikis, apps, etc.) and determine which ones and why you will recommend them to your patients.

REFERENCES

1. Straus SE et al. Evidence-based medicine: How to practice and teach EBM, 4th ed. Edinburgh; New York: Elsevier/Churchill Livingstone; 2011.
2. Wakiji EM. Mapping the literature of physical therapy. Bull Med Libr Assoc. 1997;85:284–288.
3. Maher CG, Moseley AM, Sherrington C, Herbert RD. Core journals of evidence-based physiotherapy practice. Physiotherapy Theory and Practice. 2001;17:143–51.
4. http://en.wikipedia.org/wiki/Search_engines#Search_engine_bias Accessed on May 10, 2011.
5. http://en.wikipedia.org/wiki/Google_Scholar Accessed on May 10, 2011.
6. http://www.webpt.com/blog/post/top-10-ipad-apps-physical-therapists Accessed on May 10, 2011.

chapter 12

Elements of Good Research Practice

Nowadays people know the price of everything and the value of nothing.

—OSCAR WILDE

•

✳ Mr. Ketterman's Case

I know I need to read the articles about Mr. Ketterman's care, but I just don't know where to start. I often read just the Abstract or the Introduction and the Conclusion because all that information in the Methods and Results just confuses me. But, I know I'm missing a lot of important information! *(See Appendix for Mr. Ketterman's health history.)*

INTRODUCTION

Having found evidence that relates most closely to a clinical question, the next step in the evidence based practice (EBP) process requires the careful reading and critiquing of the evidence. But this is perhaps the most daunting task facing clinicians who wish to practice in an evidence based manner—determining whether evidence found in the literature can be of value to their patients. As the sophistication of physical therapy research increases, the task of evaluating any research report for its accuracy and truthfulness becomes more challenging. After all, the evidence can only be of value to your patient if it is derived from a valid study. Validity, used here to mean trustworthiness, is an essential characteristic of any individual study. The more the results of a study can be trusted, the greater its validity in helping to make an informed clinical decision. An understanding of some of the methodological and analytical standards for conducting valid, high-quality clinical research experiments is a good starting point to build one's critical appraisal abilities. In this chapter we will focus on understanding the elements of good research. Chapters 13 through 16 will then apply the principles of good research practice to the various types of evidence, ranging from single studies to systems (Fig. 12-1).[1]

It is not the intention of this text to provide direction for researchers, nor to be a full source of all the details of research design and management that a clinician might find interesting. Rather, we have attempted to identify the essential elements that should be considered in

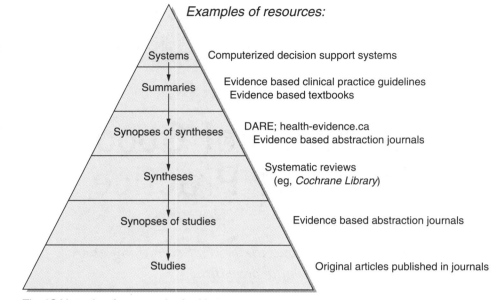

The 6S hierarchy of pre-appraised evidence

Figure 12-1 Sources of Information About Evidence. *(From DiCenso A, Bayley L, Haynes RB. Accessing pre-appraised evidence: Fine-tuning the 5S model into a 6S model. Evid Based Nurs. 2009;12:99–101.)*

assessing the literature. Because there are many such elements and you may wish to focus on them specifically when reviewing articles, we provide an overview of what will be covered in this chapter (Box 12.1).

RESEARCH DESIGN

We will compare two large categories of research designs, experimental research designs and observational research designs. The research design is selected by the investigator based on the research question of interest. As you have seen in Chapter 10, questions may relate to selecting the best examinations in order to determine a diagnosis for the patient or may relate to the risks and benefits of a particular intervention. Experimental research designs provide the strongest evidence for causal relationships between an intervention and an outcome of care. They are the designs typically used to demonstrate the efficacy of an intervention. Efficacy is a measure of the capacity of an intervention to actually produce a change. Observational research designs can also provide good evidence for intervention studies and are more frequently used to study diagnostic or prognostic questions. They are designs typically used to demonstrate the effectiveness of an intervention. Effectiveness is a measure of the ability of the intervention to bring about the expected change in the real world.

Research designs in biopsychosocial sciences stem from one of two philosophical paradigms, the quantitative paradigm or the qualitative paradigm. The difference between these two approaches as to what is knowable is described in Chapter 8, and the qualitative research paradigm and research designs are discussed there, including criteria with which you might determine the value of a study that uses a qualitative research design. The research designs described in this chapter stem from the positivist philosophy, which purports that

Box 12.1 Overview of Topics Covered in This Chapter

Research Design
- Experimental Research Designs
- Observational Research Designs

Determining Value in Studies of Clinical Interventions
- Criteria for Evaluating Internal Research Validity
- Did the Research Design Maximize the Prevention of Bias?
- Did the Selection and Treatment of Subjects Avoid the Introduction of Bias?
  - Obtaining the Best Sample of Subjects for the Study
  - Proper Assignment of Subjects to Groups
  - Tracking Subjects Through the Study
  - Controlling What Study Subjects Know
- Did the Selection and Methods of Interventions and Measurement of Outcomes Avoid the Introduction of Bias?
  - Selection of Interventions
  - Measurement of Outcomes
- Evaluating External Validity
- Evaluating Statistical Conclusion Validity
  - Descriptive Statistics and Point Estimates
    - Homogeneous and Heterogeneous Data
    - Normal Distribution
    - Visual Representations of Measures of Central Tendency and Dispersion
  - Inferential Statistics and Hypothesis Testing
    - Variables and Hypotheses
- Evaluating Outcomes: Effect Size and Number Needed to Treat
  - Power
- Summary of Statistical Conclusion Validity

Determining Value in Studies of Diagnostic/Prognostic Accuracy
- Did the Selection of Subjects Avoid the Introduction of Bias?
- Did the Selection of Measures and Procedures Avoid the Introduction of Bias?
- Were the Statistical Estimates Developed and Presented Without Bias or Error?
- Other Statistics Found in Observational Research

---

truth is independent of the investigator and knowable through direct and carefully controlled observations, interventions, and measurements of subjects. There are many rubrics that categorize research designs in medical science, with discrete definitions and methodological characteristics. In this text we will describe several of the designs most commonly found in literature useful to physical therapists and identify the questions that are useful for determining the value of findings derived from each.

Experimental Research Designs

Two categories of quantitative research designs are useful for organizing one's thoughts (Fig. 12-2). The first category is experimental research, within which we will discuss the type of experimental research that epitomizes this category, the randomized controlled trial (RCT). An experimental research design is selected when the investigator wishes to examine if a

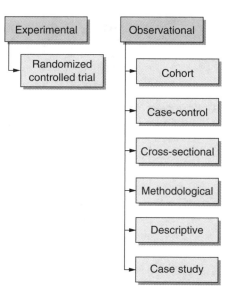

Figure 12-2 Research Designs for Studies.

cause-and-effect relationship exists between one or more interventions and the subsequent outcomes. Traditional criteria for true experimental research designs include *random selection or allocation* of research subjects to groups, the *inclusion of a control group* for comparison to a treatment group, and *purposeful manipulation* (dose, frequency, or duration) of the treatment variable. Of these three criteria, randomization of subjects is often considered the single most important element. Randomization of subjects to treatment groups helps ensure that the groups will be equivalent on important measures at the beginning of the study, thus giving the best measure of the relative effects of the two contrasted treatments. These research designs also employ tightly controlled research methods in order to provide the strongest possible statement about observed differences in groups at the end of the experiment.

In addition to true experimental research designs, some researchers may use a variety of designs that are similar to experimental research but do not quite meet all the rigorous requirements of true experimental research. In the past, these designs might have been referred to as quasi-experimental. Quasi-experimental designs share the purpose of establishing a cause-and-effect relationship between the treatment and the outcome, but fall short of the design standards of true experimental research, perhaps because it is unfeasible to randomly assign subjects or to use a control group.

Many aspects of good experimental research design are difficult to accomplish in physical therapy research, and more recently, some have used the term, practical clinical trials (PCTs) to indicate a research design that is not quite as rigorous as that found in a RCT.[2] Califf recommends such designs, commenting in an Institute of Medicine Roundtable on Evidence-based Medicine, "the sheer volume of clinical decisions made in the absence of support from randomized controlled trials requires that we understand the best alternative methods when the classical RCTs are unavailable, impractical, or inapplicable."[2] Investigators have called for clinical trials that, although perhaps somewhat less rigorous, will better meet the needs of the clinician and the patient by including a comparative or alternate therapy that is relevant to the choices of the patient.[3-5] Whether these PCTs are considered to be experimental or non-experimental research is not as important as making a clear judgment about the value of each study to you and your patient.

Observational Research Designs

The second category of research designs is termed observational designs, or nonexperimental designs. While within this category there are many, quite different designs, each of them shares one characteristic: they are conducted by making careful observations of clinical practice as it happens, or happened, rather than planning a controlled test or manipulation of treatment. Patient care goes on as planned, and close observations are made about relationships among variables, treatments, and outcomes. These designs are used when the knowledge to posit testable hypotheses for experimental research is unavailable; when the phenomenon of interest is too complex to be assessed with a clinical trial; or when the purpose of the study is not related to interventions, but to the quality of the tests or outcomes of care. Observational research designs are quite varied; some are most useful in answering questions about interventions, although lacking the strength of the RCT, and some are best suited to questions about diagnostic accuracy of tests or the natural history of an illness.

Brief definitions of the major observational research designs follow:

• Cohort: In this design, the researcher is typically interested in describing the *future health outcomes* in one cohort of subjects who have an exposure to a risk factor or will be given a certain intervention, and one cohort that is similar, but did not have either the exposure or intervention. Both groups will be followed forward in time and measured frequently to determine the occurrence of the outcome in each group.
• Case-Control: In this design, the researcher will identify two groups of subjects: the case subjects who have an outcome of interest, for example, a disease; and a group of subjects similar to them who do not have the outcome. Then the research uses medical records or interviews to *look back in time* to determine when and how each group member was exposed to the suspected causative factor.
• Cross-Sectional: With this design the researcher will identify a group of appropriate subjects and will measure their outcomes and their exposure to potential causative factors at the same time, generally just one point in time. This design is also typically used in studies of the diagnostic accuracy of tests, as the subjects are given two or more tests at one point in time.
• Methodological: These designs include repeated measures on subjects with the outcome of interest, for example, lax knee ligaments, in order to assess the reliability or validity of tests.
• Descriptive: These designs sample specific groups of subject, often using random sampling, and measure opinions or collect data about the course of an illness. These designs are useful for investigating satisfaction with health care.
• Case Study: This research design calls for careful measurement and description of typical clinical practice and is useful for documenting care given to patients with unique circumstances or responses to treatment.

DETERMINING VALUE IN STUDIES OF CLINICAL INTERVENTION

Our framework for assessing value has two components: research validity (sometimes termed experimental validity) and statistical conclusion validity. Traditional research methodologists Campbell and Stanley[5] provided one of the first frameworks for evaluating the quality of experimental research by describing the elements of research necessary to establish a causal inference. They proposed that an experiment designed to demonstrate a cause-and-effect relationship between interventions and outcomes should be judged on a set of criteria that define the *research validity*, or truthfulness, of the study. Research validity has two components, *internal* and *external*. We will focus primarily on *internal research validity*, which are those research procedures that create the greatest trust in the results of the study. For experimental studies this means having trust in the inference of the causal relationship demonstrated in the study. For observational studies, this means having trust that the phenomena being observed are accurately represented. In both designs, research validity helps to determine the extent to which bias has been controlled in the study. Bias, in a research context, refers to the tendency toward systematic errors that can arise from the design, sampling, and measurement used. Therefore, we are interested in criteria that allow us to assess how well the researchers have controlled for alternative explanations for the outcomes of the study, other than the influence of the variables of interest. These criteria are focused on the methods of the study and they will influence our confidence in its outcomes.

External research validity concerns how generalizable the findings are to patients who were not in the study. Commonly, external validity is concerned with asking how similar are the people in the study and the circumstances (time and place) of the study to our specific patients and the circumstances of the care we plan to give.

Another set of criteria developed by Campbell and Stanley[6] helps us evaluate the appropriateness of the statistical analysis of the study, or the *statistical conclusion validity*. Critiquing the internal and external *research validity* and the *statistical conclusion validity* will allow us to adequately discuss the value of the research reported in studies that appear to relate to our clinical questions (Fig. 12-3).

Criteria for Evaluating Internal Research Validity

The information needed to assess internal research validity is generally found in the methods section of a paper. This section contains very detailed descriptions of the procedures,

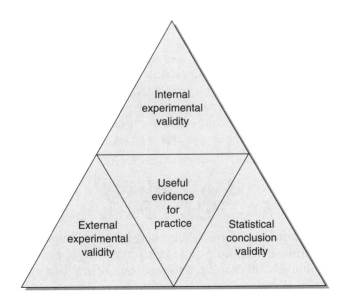

Figure 12-3 Study Elements That Identify Useful Evidence for Practice.

measures, instruments, subjects, setting, timing, and participation required of the subjects. In experimental designs, these aspects of the study design are controlled very specifically so as to have the best chance of identifying a cause-and-effect relationship between the intervention being tested, also called the independent variable, and the outcomes measured, or the dependent variables. As you read the methods section of a randomized controlled trial (RCT), you will be judging whether or not the authors exerted sufficient control to eliminate bias in the procedures, measures, sample selection, or any other important aspect of the study. Keep in mind that most authors find that the assessment of truthfulness in research is a subjective evaluation, one that places the study on a continuum from strong to weak.[7,8] We will look at three categories of good research practice:

1. selection of the correct research design,
2. selection and treatment of subjects, and
3. selection and methods of intervention and measurement of outcomes.

Did the Research Design Maximize the Prevention of Bias?

Each of these types of research designs, experimental and observational, brings strengths and weaknesses to the study of best physical therapy practice. Recent studies of the impact of research design on the evidence for practice have shown no difference in results when observational studies are compared to RCTs,[9] while others argue that this is not the case. Califf[2] provides two examples of incorrect conclusions drawn from multiple observational studies in cardiology, identified as incorrect practice only after sufficient RCTs were performed. He comments on the hope that analytical methods might enhance the causal relationships in observational studies, "... no amount of statistical analysis can substitute for randomization in ensuring internal validity when comparing alternative approaches to diagnosis or treatment."[2] The evidence to support clinical decisions in physical therapy research is comprised of both experimental and observational research designs, with some appearing less frequently than others (cohort and case-control). Table 12.1 provides a summary of examples of research designs you will find in the literature for questions about interventions, diagnosis, and prognosis in physical therapy.

Did the Selection and Treatment of Subjects Avoid the Introduction of Bias?

People who consent to participate in health care research studies may not be patients of any practitioners at the time of the study, because they do not require health care. Alternatively, they may be patients under the care of the investigator or another practitioner who has informed them about the study. In both cases, these people are referred to as *subjects* in terms of their role in a research study. This distinction is very important to the investigators conducting the study and to the clinician reading the study. The investigator must distinguish between procedures given to the patient that are tightly controlled research procedures and others that are customary care. Readers of research are interested in learning sufficient detail about the study subjects so that they can determine if the subjects in the study are sufficiently like their own patients; otherwise, the study might be of less value to their practice.

The selection and treatment of the subjects who participate in research studies can be a significant source of bias. A myriad of criteria might be used to determine if just the right study subjects were included and if all the proper procedures were used with them, including inclusion and exclusion criteria that will provide the best sample for the study, the proper

✺ **Table 12.1**	**Linking Research Designs to Research Questions for Studies**	
Type of Question	**Designs**	**Characteristic Strengths and Weaknesses for the Question**
Research questions about interventions	RCT	Randomization of subjects to treatment groups and control of both intervention and outcomes. Strongest design for these questions.
	Case Study	Detailed descriptions of interventions, but does not create generalizable knowledge from few subjects
	Cohort	Weaker than RCT, because no randomization of subjects to treatment groups, less control of intervention, but does control measurement of outcomes.
Research questions about diagnosis	Cross-Sectional (Diagnostic accuracy studies)	Subject data on two or more tests are collected at one point in time to compare the accuracy of one test against a gold standard.
	Methodological	Studies of repeated measures on subjects with the outcome of interest, addressing the reliability or validity of tests.
Research questions about prognosis	Cohort	Subjects are followed forward in time and progression of an illness may be described
	Case-control	Weaker, as subjects with the illness can only provide retrospective data on its progression. Useful if the outcome is rare.
	Descriptive	Surveys of patients with a disability to determine the course of their progress.

allocation of subjects to study groups, the importance of tracking study subjects across time, and controlling what the study subjects know during the study (Fig. 12-4).[10–12]

Obtaining the Best Sample of Subjects for the Study

One of the hallmarks of experimental research in the social sciences is the selection of a random sample of subjects, but this process is often unavailable to or cost-prohibitive for health care researchers. Instead, much of the research is conducted with samples of available subjects, called *samples of convenience*. Once a research question and an appropriate research design are selected, the next decision is, who should be in this study? The resources to study everyone to whom the research question applies, often referred to as the *population of interest*, would be unavailable in most health care research. The method of selecting a smaller group of patients to whom the research question applies is referred to as *sampling the population*, and this is

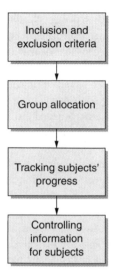

Figure 12-4 Management of Research Subjects.

undertaken with the hope of achieving a manageable group of research subjects who appropriately represent the original population. This group is called the *sample*, and good research practice requires the clear definition of who can and cannot be in the sample so as to maximize the research design's purpose to discover a causal relationship between intervention and outcome, if one exists, while not making the sample so narrowly focused that it no longer represents the population of interest. When this happens, clinicians find the research to be less useful to their own practice.

The use of criteria that a person must have to be eligible for the study, *inclusion criteria*, and those that they must not have to be eligible for the study, *exclusion criteria*, allows the researcher to recruit people to become research subjects. Some research designs may require very intricate inclusion and exclusion criteria for subsamples of the study, but we will use the structure of an RCT with an experimental and a comparison group to illustrate good sampling procedures. The first step to critique is the method used to recruit all subjects. Ask yourself if the researcher used sampling criteria that served to eliminate bias in the subjects chosen, for example, by disqualifying subjects who had multiple comorbidities to the one being studied. Having such subjects in the study could introduce competing explanations for the results. The study should provide a description of objective characteristics of the sample selected so that you might judge how similar or homogeneous a group was identified; for example, were the subjects similar in the severity of their injury or illness, the length of time since onset, and the occurrence of surgery or not? It is important that the overall sample of subjects is homogenous on important clinical, demographic, and temporal characteristics, not only to decrease sample bias but to help ensure equivalent groups once group allocation is undertaken.

Proper Assignment of Subjects to Groups

Many of the research designs described in the previous section make use of groups of subjects who receive different treatments or different levels of treatment in the study. If a comparison of X with Y is planned in the RCT, the sample will need to be assigned to one or the other group. Because the sample has generally been created using available subjects, it is crucial that the significant benefits of randomization be applied to research designs at this point. While sampling is generally not done randomly, random assignment, or allocation of subjects to groups, provides a vital element of experimental validity to the research process. Randomization helps distribute subjects with both known and unknown characteristics equally into all study groups, lending confidence that the groups were made as equivalent as possible at the beginning of the study. If the two groups are different before the study starts on some characteristic related to the intervention or the outcome, then bias has been introduced and weakened the ability to identify a cause-and-effect relationship. If one group had a very different prognosis for recovery than the other, imagine how that would influence your thinking about the outcome of the study. Again, the study should provide an objective description of the equivalency of the groups, using tables or charts, and often a statistical test, as evidence of the effectiveness of the randomization procedure.

There are several methods to accomplish random assignment of subjects to research groups, most of which depend on whether or not the whole sample is available for randomization at the start of the study, or if randomization must be done consecutively as subjects are enrolled. This is the case for most studies that use a sample of convenience. In this case, an ordered list of subject identification numbers is randomized and subjects are assigned to groups as they enter the study. Clinical trials often use another assignment technique called matching assignment, which allows the investigator to exert some control over the equivalency of the groups in addition to that provided by randomization. In matching assignment, each subject is categorized on an important and possibly confounding variable, for example sex or leg length, matched with another subject with similar characteristics, and then randomly assigned to a group, such that there are similar numbers of women in each group or equal numbers of subjects with short leg lengths in each group. In this way, the researcher does not leave it to chance (the randomization process) to equally distribute subjects with known attributes that might introduce bias into the study, should they by chance all end up assigned to one group.

We will discuss later in the chapter the importance of keeping clinicians who are involved in treating or measuring research subjects unaware, or blind, to the group assignment of the subjects. However, it is also considered important to know whether or not the person enrolling subjects into the study is aware of the group to which the next subject enrolled will be assigned. Good research practice will keep this consecutive order assignment concealed from the person enrolling subjects to avoid a bias introduced by the clinician who may not want a potential subject to be assigned to the control group. This practice is called *allocation concealment.*

Tracking Subjects Through the Study

Bias can be introduced into a study if the researcher loses track of subjects who do not complete their participation. If the study takes place over days, weeks, or months, it is likely that some study participants will become ill, reinjured, discouraged, or in some way no longer willing or eligible to participate in the study. Other participants may recover sooner than anticipated and no longer wish to participate in the study. Still others stop participating and the researcher never learns why. It is important to account for each subject at the end of the study, and particularly so if these dropouts have happened with differential frequency among the groups. At the end of the study, researchers should remain confident that the randomization performed so carefully at the beginning is not negatively affected by differential rates of attrition in the groups. Standard schematics or flow diagrams are typically provided in a study to document the progress of participants through each stage of a clinical trial (Fig. 12-5).[13,14]

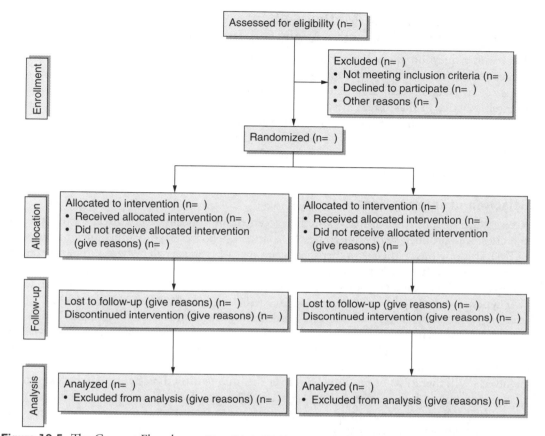

Figure 12-5 The Consort Flowchart. *(From Schulz KF, Altman DG, Moher D, for the CONSORT Group. CONSORT 2010 Statement: Updated guidelines for reporting parallel group randomized trials. BMJ. 2010;340:c332.)*

Controlling What Study Subjects Know

Controlling who knows what, when, in an experimental study is an important tool for avoiding various types of biases introduced by those involved. Here we discuss controlling what the subjects know specifically about their involvement. Good research practice requires that all potential and enrolled subjects be fully informed as to the procedures that will be used in the study so that they might make the best judgment about their involvement. In some studies, a subject will learn from the informed consent process that they have a one in three chance to be in a group that gets exercise A, exercise B, or no exercise at all. The subject is told in the informed consent document whether or not they will know to which group they have been randomly assigned and how that randomization will take place. In studies of medications, it is easier to keep subjects blind to their group assignment than it is in studies of procedures, surgeries, or physical therapy interventions. Thus the ability to include this good research practice is limited in rehabilitation research. When the subject cannot be blinded from the group assignment, then care is taken to utilize outcome measures that may be less influenced by the subject's knowledge of his or her group assignment, for example, physiological measures of body temperature, wound healing, and range of motion; however, it is not certain that these measures could be influenced by the subject themselves.

Did the Selection and Methods of Interventions and Measurement of Outcomes Avoid the Introduction of Bias?

To answer a question about which intervention may have a better effect on health outcomes, the researcher must make many choices for the conduct of the study. Methodological decisions focus on two major components: the study procedures and the study measurements. Good research practice in these areas must blend a keen focus on the research question with an eye to avoiding bias in all decisions about procedures and measures. For example, the most intricately designed study procedures could be wasted if the selected outcome measures are not the best or are performed in a biased manner. We will look first at the decisions to be made about the study procedures regarding interventions.

Selection of Interventions

A researcher wishes to investigate whether eccentric or concentric quadriceps strengthening exercises will produce better outcomes for patients who received a total knee arthroplasty (TKA). It is obvious to the researcher that either type of exercise will be better than no exercise, so there is no need (and perhaps an ethical concern) for having a control group that receives no exercise. The researcher knows one of the study variables will be type of exercise, and only two types, eccentric and concentric exercise, will be studied. What about the dose of the exercise for each type? Should subjects perform the intervention exercises daily or less frequently? How many repetitions of each exercise? Should subjects be required to visit an outpatient physical therapy clinic or perform the intervention as a home program? How many days or visits should be expected until an effect can be found? Will exercise equipment be involved? Will therapists be required to deliver the intervention directly? If so, what bias might that introduce? It is very difficult to keep the treating physical therapists in clinical trials unaware of (blind to) the group assignment of the subjects, but good research practice requires that the researcher consider whether this can occur in the study, to avoid the bias introduced by a research team member who might favor one group outcome over another.

Measurement of Outcomes

The second set of methodological decisions concerns the measurement of the outcomes of the study. In the study of choice of exercises for patients who have undergone TKA, the investigator must decide what outcomes to choose in order to determine which exercises are better for the patients. Over the years, investigators of physical therapy clinical trials have expanded the types and numbers of outcome measures considerably. Today, a clinical trial is likely to have a mix of outcome variables, often classified as primary and secondary, based on the importance to the investigators and to patients. The measures may be selected to assess physical and social well-being, as well as outcomes that address the processes of care, such as patient satisfaction. A wide range of measures can be selected that represent elements of the WHO International Classification of Functioning, Disability, and Health (ICF) model.[15,16] Applying this model, described in Chapter 1, to the selection of outcome measures could result in assessing body structures and functions with, for example, ROM or strength about the knee and a 6-minute walk test and assessing activities and participation with, for example, the Knee injury and Osteoarthritis Outcome Score (KOOS),[17] The *Guide to Physical Therapist Practice* includes a compendium of over 800 tests and measures from which to select the measures used in a study.[18]

With so many available measures, what criteria might be used to select the best ones for a specific study? Two fundamental principles of measurement are the reliability and validity of the measure.[19] These characteristics of measurement provide the clinician and researcher with confidence that they can rely on scores derived from these tests to be dependable (reliable) and accurate (valid). It is important to remember that no test or measurement process is ever perfect, and errors of one type or another are associated with every outcome measure. This is particularly true for measures that require the interaction of the therapist with the patient, as compared to tests that the patient completes independently, like a survey. Reliable measures are ones for which repeatable scores would be achieved when the test is administered more than once, over a time period in which it can be reasonably expected that the phenomenon of interest does not change, for example, two measures of isometric quadriceps force production measured on a dynamometer, taken 30 minutes apart. Valid measures are said to be accurate, and by that we mean they measure what we intend for them to measure, and not another phenomenon. If we believe that an isometric quadriceps force production test on a dynamometer is an accurate measure of the concept of quadriceps strength, then the measure can be said to be valid for the purpose of the study. When there are several tests that purport to measure the same concept, studies are performed for the purpose of comparing one test to another and thereby establishing a description of the validity of one test in comparison to another. We will expect the author of the clinical trial to report the reliability and validity of the primary outcome measures in the study as a means of assuring us that the best tests for the study were selected.

Two other important decisions should be evaluated when considering the methodological aspects of measurement in a study: the timing of the measurements and who takes them. In general, the closer in time measures are taken to the phenomenon of interest, the less error will be represented in the score. In designing the study of eccentric versus concentric quadriceps strengthening exercises over a 12-week period, the researcher must decide when to take the measurements. The two obvious time periods to be selected are before the study starts and when it ends. If the pretest measure is taken too long ahead of time, an unexpected occurrence might cause the subject to become weaker before the study starts, thus introducing error into that subject's score. Good research practice will include measures closely timed to specified points in the study for all subjects. One other aspect to consider in terms of the usability of the study to your practice is whether enough measures were taken, especially follow-up measures, ones that typically follow the conclusion of the study. Follow-up measures allow assessment of the long-term effects of interventions, so that clinicians might learn how to best time interventions over an episode of care for their patients.

The most important methodological decision related to outcome measures is whether or not the person taking the measures is blinded to the group assignment of the subjects. If the clinician giving the intervention cannot be blinded, it is very important that a different person take the measures. Even this amount of blinding of the measurer can be difficult in physical therapy studies, since interventions often change the appearance of a subject's physical body. In such studies, the timing of the measurements may need to be adjusted, or instructions given to subjects not to reveal his or her group assignment, as well as other safeguards put in place to maximize the objectivity of the clinician taking the measurements.

Evaluating External Validity

One additional aspect of good research practice that you might consider in determining the value of a study to your practice is how generalizable the results are to your practice. This is referred to as the *external validity* of the study. External validity asks, can we apply the results from a sample of patients in the controlled environment of the experiment to real life? If the controlled aspects of the setting, the subjects, and the timing of the study design are similar to your practice environment and patients, then the study findings will be generalizable to your patients. If the methods of the study bear little resemblance to how you might carry out the intervention in your practice, then you cannot be as confident that you will find the same outcomes as reported in the study. Generally, these are questions a clinician must answer based on his or her best clinical judgment. The desire to improve internal validity can sometimes result in less external validity; the reverse is also true.

Evaluating Statistical Conclusion Validity

Statistical conclusion validity refers to the degree to which the analysis performed on the data in the study allows you to make the correct decision regarding the truth or approximate truth of the hypotheses tested. This is different from the process we just reviewed, the goal of which was to determine if we could trust the causal relationship between the intervention and the outcomes of the study, based on the methods of discovery used in the study, or its experimental validity. For most clinicians, research validity is the easier conclusion to draw about a study. For some experimental studies, the procedures described have clearly introduced some type of bias, for example, failing to mask the examiners from the subjects' group assignment. It is then both easier and logical that the reader will consider research validity before reading the data analysis and results section of the paper. With practice, the reader will begin reading the results section with some expectations in mind about the outcomes of the study. For example, you might anticipate small between-group differences because the intensity of exercise given to the experimental group was, in your clinical judgment, insufficient to create a large effect. It is best to be aware of your propensity to accept the results before you begin reading them, for the statistical analysis may indicate that a treatment was beneficial to one group of subjects as compared to another. Such statistical differences cannot be considered truthful unless you are satisfied with the experimental validity of the work.

If you are satisfied with the research validity of the study, the second component to determining the usefulness of this study to your practice is to evaluate its statistical conclusion validity. Domholdt defines this simply as your assessment as to whether or not statistical tools have been used correctly to analyze the data in the study.[20] In the following section we will present an overview of basic statistical principles and terms and define their use in analyzing the data collected in experimental and observational studies. To understand statistical conclusion validity, one must master a certain amount of measurement and statistical theory.

Norman and Streiner suggest that the main purpose for understanding statistics is to be able to distinguish true differences from natural variation.[21,p2] This is what we wish to know when reading in the results of a study that, for example, a 5-point difference on a pain scale existed at the end of a comparison between a group receiving an experimental treatment and a group receiving a standard treatment. Were these two groups truly different from each other at the end of the study, or does this difference reflect natural variation in subjects' pain response to treatment? We might also say that the difference of 5 points between the groups might have happened by chance, and this is another way to describe natural variation between and within individual subjects. Without statistics to help us make sense of this statement: "there was a 5-point difference in pain scores between groups at the end of the study," we would not be able to have confidence that this was a true difference, caused by the treatment.

There are two large families of statistics that you will find in most studies: descriptive statistics and inferential statistics. *Descriptive statistics* help define the average subject, intervention, and outcomes, as well as the variability in these data. They are important analyses to present to the reader first, in order to describe the subjects, the interventions, and the outcome measures. The subjects selected for a study are referred to as the *sample*, and the numerical

Table 12.2	Categories of Data	
Category	**Definition**	**Example**
Names	Word (letters) label used to distinguish subjects in various categories	Male/female Young/Old/Very old Positive test/Negative test Inpatient/outpatient
Numerals	Numeral label used to distinguish subjects in various categories	Group 1, 2, 3 Ankle Sprain Stage 1, 2, 3
Numbers	Numbers used to quantify measures	ROM in degrees, Strength in ft. lbs. Gait speed in seconds

measures of central tendency and dispersion calculated for the sample are called *statistics*. These calculated statistics are used to project or to infer what might happen should all possible appropriate individuals be studied. The term used for all possible appropriate individuals is the *population*. Thus, we conduct studies on selected samples of subjects in order to infer what might happen could we study the entire population. The numerical measures of central tendency and the dispersion hypothesized for a population are called *parameters*. The second large family of statistics is then termed *inferential statistics*, for they allow inferences from the sample statistics collected to the population parameters, which are generally unavailable. One can think of this as trying to discover a causal relationship in a sample from one study, which can then be recommended with confidence to the entire community.

Descriptive Statistics and Point Estimates

Data are collected to describe subjects following rules of measurement that allow consistent communication of the value of what is being measured. Data can be communicated, or measured, as names, numerals, or numbers.[20,21] It is important to distinguish numerals from numbers, as numerals generally cannot be entered into mathematical formulas because they are labels and do not have quantitative value (Table 12.2). There are four classical categories, or levels, of measurement referred to in the literature: nominal, ordinal, interval, and ratio. The distinguishing elements of these categories are the mathematical operations one can perform upon them, based on the units of the measurement and the presence or absence of an absolute zero point.

Levels of Measurement

- Nominal: words or numerals assigned to distinguishable characteristics with no absolute value nor rank
- Ordinal: words or numerals or numbers assigned to distinguishable characteristics with rank, but no equal intervals between levels
- Interval: numerals or numbers assigned to distinguishable characteristics with equal intervals, but no absolute zero point representing total absence of the characteristic
- Ratio: numbers assigned to distinguishable characteristics with equal intervals, and an absolute zero indicating total absence of the characteristic

The three types of measures (name, numerals, and numbers) can also be classified into two broad categories that tell us something about the form they may take: discrete and continuous measures. Discrete measures are those that can only assume a limited set of values (generally, a known set of values). Data measured with names and numerals are generally discrete measures. Data measured with numbers can be either discrete measures (whole numbers only, for example, number of pregnancies a woman has had) or continuous measures (those that can be represented with decimals, for example, timed up-and-go score of 13.5 seconds). These distinctions about measurement of data influence later data analysis and may influence your judgment about the precision of measurement used in a study.

One of the first tables one might find in an experimental or observational study contains descriptive data about the subjects as a total group and/or divided into their assigned groups. When you look at these tables, you often find the data for several variables provided, with specific statistics for each type of data. When more than 10 subjects are in a study, it is useful to calculate statistics that tell something about the distribution of all the scores, because there is too much information to use otherwise. (For small studies of 10 or fewer subjects you might find a table that lists each subject and their individual scores). These statistics are designed to help picture the distribution of all the scores for each variable. The descriptive statistics typically found in these tables are defined in Table 12.3. An example of such a table is found in Table 12.4.

Measures of central tendency are single values that tell you something about the mid-point in a distribution of numbers. Measures of dispersion are designed to tell you something about how variable the scores are around the measure of central tendency. The age of subjects is often reported in studies as a mean and a standard deviation; for example, in Table 12.4 the mean age of the experimental group subjects was 37 years with a standard deviation of 6.5 years. Instead of the mean, the median or the mode may be used to describe the center of the distribution if the data are discrete or if the continuous data have extreme scores, such that

Table 12.3 Measures of Central Tendency and Dispersion

Measures of Central Tendency	Symbols	Definitions
Mean	X	Arithmetic average
Median		Score that divides the distribution of all scores in half
Mode		Most frequently occurring score

Measures of Dispersion	Symbols	Definitions
Standard deviation	S or SD	Square root of the average of the squared deviations from the mean
Variance	S^2	Average of the squared deviations from the mean
Range	R	The difference between the lowest and highest score. Often presented as the lowest − highest score.
Interquartile range	IQ	The scores that bound the middle 50% of the scores

▨ Table 12.4 — Sample Table with Descriptive Data

Variable	Experimental Group	Control Group
Age, y x (sd)	37 (6.5)	38 (5.7)
Sex, female %	45	47
Onset of pain, wks, Med (R)	5 (2–15)	5 (3–6)
Pain medication doses in past week, x (sd)	18 (5)	18.5 (2.5)

▨ Table 12.5 — Confidence Intervals (CI) and Standard Error of the Mean (SEM)

Sampling Statistic Methods	Definition	Calculation
Confidence intervals	A range around a statistic within which the true value of the statistic is expected to fall, with designated certainty (90%, 95%)	For the 90% confidence interval around a mean $X \pm 1.645$ (SEM)
Standard error of the mean	Standard deviation of the sampling distributions	$SEM = s/\sqrt{N}$

the mean might be misleading to the reader. In Table 12.4, the median and range are used to describe the distribution for the variable "weeks since onset of pain," since at least one person in the experimental group had an extreme score of 15 weeks. Together, the measures of central tendency and dispersion give the reader an idea of how the distribution of all the scores for subjects in that group would look. The measures of dispersion are also selected to fit the type of measure being reported, so understanding what each means can give the reader an understanding of how spread out the scores are for that measure. For example, compare the two means and standard deviations for the variable doses of pain medication taken in the past week in Table 12.4. The two groups have similar means, but the variability in the experimental group is twice that in the control group.

These measures of central tendency and dispersion are calculated from one sample, and it is quite possible that another study reported in the literature measuring the same variable may report quite different statistics. Which descriptive data are the most accurate to use in making inferences to the population of interest? If study A reports a 5-point mean decrease on a pain scale following an experimental intervention and study B conducted on the same intervention reports a 7-point mean drop in pain scores, which can you expect to happen with your patients if you use this intervention? There are additional statistics that help enhance predictions of measures of central tendency such as means as well as inferential statistical estimates, discussed later.

The standard error of the mean (SEM) is a useful statistic to understand how stable inferences about a population mean are, and this statistic is highly influenced by the sample size. Examining the calculation of the SEM (Table 12.5), one can see that large samples will have

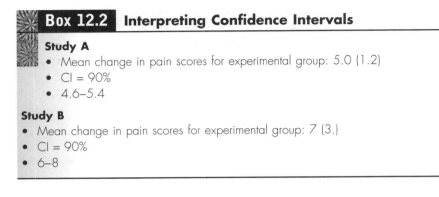

Box 12.2   **Interpreting Confidence Intervals**

Study A
- • Mean change in pain scores for experimental group: 5.0 (1.2)
  - • CI = 90%
  - • 4.6–5.4

Study B
- • Mean change in pain scores for experimental group: 7 (3.)
- • CI = 90%
- • 6–8

a smaller SEM, giving more confidence in the prediction of the population mean, while small samples will have larger errors in estimating the mean of the population. The SEM is a component of the formula for another statistic, the confidence interval (CI), which helps understand the accuracy of point estimates like the mean. This statistic is conveniently named, as it gives a range of scores within which the true value for the mean is expected to be found. The data in Box 12.2 illustrate how useful confidence intervals are to interpreting descriptive data.

Assuming that both studies enrolled 25 subjects and study B had both a higher mean and standard deviation, you can see that the range of the CIs for the two studies also differ similarly. From study A, we are 90% certain that if the true population mean is not 5, as calculated in the study, then it falls between the values 4.6 to 5.4. From study B, we are 90% certain that if the true population mean is not 7, as calculated in the study, it then falls between 6 and 8. The CI for study A is smaller than that for study B because the standard deviation around the mean found in study A is smaller. So, if you wish to know how much reduction in pain scores you might expect from this intervention, you can make use of both CIs to predict that the change to expect in your patients would be no smaller than 4.6 points and might be as high as 8 points.

Homogeneous and Heterogeneous Data

Two useful terms to understand when evaluating either a total sample of a study or the two or more groups in a sample, are *homogeneous* and *heterogeneous*. If subjects in a group have very similar scores on the measures taken, you can say the group is homogeneous in, for example, the amount of drugs they are taking during the study. If you examine the means and standard deviation/variance for a control and experimental group and find the standard deviations to be quite different, you can say the group with the larger standard deviation is more heterogeneous than the other group. Homogeneous groups are those that are composed of subjects who score similarly on the measures, and heterogeneous groups have subjects who score quite differently from each other. The statistical analysis that is performed on the measures to look for statistical differences between groups is influenced by the homogeneity of the groups in relation to each other. If the control group is quite similar in scores (for example, most subjects changed less than 5 points from pre-test to post-test) while the experimental group is extremely varied in scores (some subjects changed only 2 points and some subjects changed 15 points and everything in between), then an important assumption for the statistical analysis, homogeneity of variance, is violated and the analysis may be incorrect. Random allocation of subjects to their groups in RCTs is very important to help achieve two or more groups who have homogeneity of variance. Inspecting the descriptive statistics for each group in the study design will allow you to decide if the groups are homogeneous.

Normal Distribution

The normal curve, or bell-shaped curve, is a concept important to understanding the measures of central tendency and dispersion we have just defined. When large numbers of scores are analyzed, a typical bell-shaped distribution for that score emerges that can be defined mathematically in order to predict the probability of any one score occurring. This is very helpful to clinicians in selecting what we consider to be normal values for clinical tests, for example, defining normal systolic blood pressure. The normal distribution provides us with a mean for systolic blood pressure and also an understanding of the range of scores one could expect in patients. Particularly high or low scores, which may not be normal and could require treatment, are easier to identify.

In normally distributed data:

1. the mean, median, and mode will hold the same value, so any of these statistics can be used to describe the middle of the distribution;
2. the probability of any one score falling within the middle of the distribution, defined as the mean minus 1 standard deviation or plus 1 standard deviation, is 68%; thus the scores that cluster closely around the mean are the most frequently occurring scores;
3. the probability of any one score falling within the area of the distribution, defined as the mean ±2 standard deviations, is 95%;
4. the probability of any one score falling within the area of the distribution, defined as the mean ±3 standard deviations, is 99%; capturing almost all scores. Since only 1% of scores fall more than 3 standard deviations above or below the mean, we can understand these scores to be very rarely occurring scores.

Applying these assumptions to any presentation of a mean and standard deviation given in a table allows us to understand how widely dispersed all likely scores are. Scores that are unexpectedly high or low could represent errors of measurement or could be recognized as rare values. Many of the inferential statistical tests that are used to tell us if statistically significant relationships or differences exist between variables or groups have as an assumption that the scores are normally distributed.

Visual Representations of Measures of Central Tendency and Dispersion

A graphic figure frequently used to express the measures of central tendency and dispersion for a set of scores is called a box plot. Figure 12-6 shows the conventions used to construct a box plot. The lower and upper margins of the box are the score values occurring at the 75th percentile of the distribution (upper quartile) and the 25th percentile of the distribution (lower quartile), so the box itself illustrates what is called the interquartile range, or the middle 50% of the distribution. If the box demonstrates a wide variation in scores from the upper quartile to the lower quartile, it will be quite wide; a distribution with more closely clustered scores will be narrower. A symbol (* or +) or a line is often used within the box to indicate the median of the scores. If the median falls equally between the upper quartile and lower quartile, we understand that the scores are evenly spread in the distribution, resembling a normal distribution. If the median falls closer to the upper or lower quartile, there are more higher scores than lower scores in the distribution. In some box plots a different symbol may be found inside the box to represent the mean score.

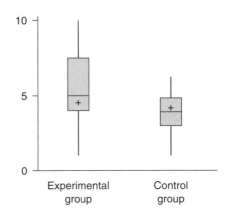

Figure 12-6 Box Plot Comparing the Measures of Central Tendency and Dispersion for Change Scores for an Experimental and Control Group.

With the use of lines extending from the box in both directions, called whiskers, the box plot also provides more data about the extreme scores on both the high and low end of the distribution. The whisker may or may not have a crosshatch line at the end of the whisker. The conventions for what the whiskers represent are less consistent than for the box portion of the plot. Traditionally, the whisker represents the score occurring closest to but not further than 1.5 times the interquartile value and is called a step, or the inner fence. (There also might be a whisker that illustrates the outer fence, or 3 times the interquartile range.) The whisker may be drawn to represent the lowest- and highest-occurring scores or the score value at 1 standard deviation above and below the mean. The whisker might also represent a confidence interval around the mean. Symbols occurring beyond the whiskers indicate outliers or extreme outliers, which indicate score values that are quite high or low. It is important to check the legend of the figure when interpreting a box plot to be certain what measures of dispersion are being plotted by the whiskers. In Figure 12-6 it is easy to quickly see that the variability in change of the scores for the experimental group was larger than the variability in the control group, thus the control group has a more normal distribution than the experimental group. The experimental group has more low scores than high scores, as indicated by the 50th percentile score occurring closer to the 25th percentile than the 75th percentile.

Inferential Statistics and Hypothesis Testing

Once you understand the distributions of the data on each measurement in the study, you can evaluate how researchers have chosen to test the hypotheses they used to design the study. To understand the hypotheses, you must be able to clearly identify the structure of the study: the variables and their roles in forming hypotheses to be tested.

Variables and Hypotheses

As you read the description of the methods of the study, you will be able to identify the variables, or measures that are important to the study design. There are two primary roles that a variable may play in the study design: the independent variable, or factor, and the dependent variable, or outcome. Independent variables are those that categorize the intervention that is being studied; for example, an independent variable might be generally termed "treatment," with one group receiving the experimental treatment and the other group receiving the control or standard treatment. The independent variables are set or manipulated by researchers to occur at the levels they desire, for example, two groups versus three groups. Most RCTs will have an independent variable that functions to study the intervention of interest; however, the number of levels of this independent variable, or number of subject groups, can vary, with a minimum of two groups. Time is another common independent variable found in studies of interventions in physical therapy. When the study design reports measuring the outcome variables before the intervention, after the intervention, and perhaps at one or more follow-up times, then we consider time to be an independent variable that the researcher chooses to manipulate. It is important to identify all the independent variables in the study, for these are the variables that the authors hypothesize may have caused the outcomes of the study.

The dependent variables are the tests and measures that the researchers choose to determine the effects of the intervention. If they study the effects of manual therapy versus traction on cervical spine pain for patients with osteoarthritis, then the changes in pain would *depend* on which type of treatment the patient received. It would be rare to find an RCT designed with only one dependent variable. It is much more likely to find many tests used, often grouped into categories, for example, impairments to bodily functions or limitations to participation and activities in daily life. Researchers may choose their outcome or dependent variables based on previous research in order to make their research comparable to other studies. Identifying the dependent variables is important to your evaluation of the statistical conclusion validity of the study because each dependent variable will be tested by a research hypothesis.

The research hypotheses are a statement of what the author believes will happen in the study to each dependent variable. For example, a research hypothesis may predict that subjects in the manual therapy group will have a greater decrease in neck pain following one treatment than will the subjects in the cervical traction group. The author will predict an outcome for each dependent variable in the study, for example, predicting that manual therapy will cause a greater decrease in pain for the experimental group as well as an increase in cervical range of motion in flexion, extension, right and left rotation, and an improvement on a functional test for the upper limbs. This goal would require six research hypotheses to be tested and the possibility for manual therapy to be favored over cervical traction on all six dependent variables or in fewer than six variables.

The study results will present the means and standard deviations measured for each group in the study on the dependent variable. Table 12.6 shows sample data. In these data, it appears that the manual therapy group showed better changes after treatment on three of the dependent variables, pain, and AROM in rotations, while the traction group had better changes in AROM in cervical flexion and extension. Some differences between groups are large and some

Table 12.6 Sample Data from a Study Comparing Manual Therapy to Traction for Patients with Cervical Spine Pain

Dependent Variables	Before Treatment (X, SD)		After Treatment (X, SD)	
	Traction	**MT**	**Traction**	**MT**
Pain	8 (2.1)	8 (2.2)	6 (2.0)	4 (1.9)
AROM Flexion	20 (6.2)	25 (5.4)	26 (5.2)	27 (4.4)
AROM Extension	10 (3.2)	14 (4.8)	24 (3.2)	20 (5.1)
AROM R Rotation	15 (2.7)	14 (2.3)	22 (3.9)	35 (11.9)
AROM L Rotation	13 (4.2)	17 (4.8)	18 (2.9)	39 (10.2)

are small. Because we can never know for certain whether these changes observed in the data between the two study groups happened by chance or were influenced by some aspect of the study design, we utilize a statistical hypothesis test to estimate how confident we are of the differences we see in Table 12.6. In other words, how likely is it that the differences between the two groups are attributable to the different treatments they received? If good research study methods, as outlined in the first part of this chapter were followed, then large differences between groups are unlikely to have happened by chance alone and are more likely to have been caused by the intervention. Therefore, each of the five variables listed in Table 12.6 will undergo a statistical hypothesis test.

There are many families of statistical tests that may be used to examine different hypotheses. Two large categories are tests of differences between means and tests of relationships between variables. Statistical hypotheses that examine differences in means between two or more groups utilize a form of hypothesis called the *null hypothesis*. The null hypothesis concerning differences in means would propose that there is no difference between the two group means, thus no true change has happened or what might be called a null event. For example, in Table 12.6, the change score for pain for the manual therapy group was 4 points and the change score for the traction group was 2. The null hypothesis to test this variable would state that although these two change scores are not the same, their difference is so small that it could have happened by chance. An appropriate statistic, in this instance a paired t-test, would be reported by the researcher to test this null hypothesis of no difference between groups. If the results of the hypothesis test are such that the null hypothesis is not likely to be true, then an alternative hypothesis is considered to be true. In this case, the difference in pain scores between the manual therapy group and the traction group are found to favor a better outcome for the manual therapy group. This would be reported as a statistically significant difference between group means. However, if the statistical test found that the size of the difference was too small to know if chance variations might have caused the difference, then the outcome of the statistical test is said to be nonsignificant.

Hypothesis testing allows us to calculate how certain we are about the comparisons we wish to make. The reported results of statistical tests often include one or more of the following statistics: the observed value of the specific statistic used, the probability statistic (p) that estimates of how likely it is that the results of the hypothesis test should be attributed to chance rather than the intervention being tested, or a confidence interval surrounding the difference score. A p value accompanying a statistical test that is lower than .05 is often considered a reasonable cutoff for attributing the outcomes of the study to the intervention, rather than to chance. A p value of .05 is interpreted as a likelihood of 5 in 100 of observing a difference between groups this large by chance alone—a rare occurrence. Here is another way to interpret a p value: if this study were repeated 100 times, with 100 different subject groups, the likelihood of finding the null hypothesis of no difference between groups is 5 times, while the likelihood of finding a true difference between groups is 95 times. A mean difference between groups may be presented with a confidence interval, for example, 2 (1.5–2.5). If the 99% CI around a mean difference score does not include the null value 0, this increases our confidence that the group differences are large enough to be attributable to the study interventions, for it is quite unlikely that the true difference score is zero.

Evaluating Outcomes: Effect Size and Number Needed to Treat

In evaluating the outcomes of the study, we can ask the question, were the groups similar at the end of the clinical trial? You will recall that several good research methods are used to ensure that the groups are similar at the beginning of the study, for example, random assignment of subjects to groups. The two groups illustrated in Table 12.6 appear to be quite similar on the dependent variables of interest to the researcher before the treatment was given. A comparison of the groups' pre-test scores is often performed, with a statistical test, to assure the reader that the randomization process worked and that the two groups are in fact similar before the intervention is given. From such comparisons of the equivalency of the groups prior to intervention, the researcher hopes to fail to reject the null hypothesis of no difference between groups. In doing so, one can conclude that the differences between groups on the dependent variables is not large enough to represent a statistical difference. When this is the case, any group differences found to be statistically significant at the end of the intervention can be more easily understood.

If the groups are statistically different at the end of the study on one or more dependent variables, our next question is, how different were they? This is a conclusion that readers can develop based on their clinical experience. Is a decrease in 4 points on an 11-point pain scale, before and after receiving manual therapy a big effect or a small effect? The statistical analysis will tell you whether or not the mean differences/change scores between groups are likely to have happened by chance or are due to the intervention. This is rather like a pass/fail decision; the hypothesis test either shows statistical significance or it does not. If it does show statistical significance, the reader can also benefit from interpreting a statistic that gives a sense of how large the differences, or effect of the treatment, were found to be.

The effect size is a statistic that nicely communicates exactly what its intent is: to tell you the relative effect of the tested intervention. The effect size statistic is calculated by dividing the difference between the two group means, or the difference between pre- and post-intervention means, by a pooled standard deviation of the two means.[20] For example, in Table 12.6 we find that the after-treatment mean pain score for the traction group was 6 and for the manual therapy group it was 4. The standard deviation for both groups was approximately 2. The ES statistic for pain scores would be calculated as 6 – 4/2 = 1. An ES of 1 tells us that the relative change caused by the intervention was approximately equal to 1 standard deviation in pain scores. Since the standard deviation tells something about the variability in the data for pain scores, evaluating the magnitude of the change score against the typical variability in the group's pain scores helps us understand how big an impact, or effect, the manual therapy treatment had. If we examine the effect of both treatments, comparing pre-tests to post-tests, we see that the effect within the traction group was 1 while the effect within the manual therapy group was twice as large, with an ES of 2.

Another statistic, the number needed to treat (NNT) can be useful in interpreting the magnitude of a comparison of treatments in a RCT.[22,23] This statistic is calculated by identifying the percentage of successful outcomes in the control group versus the experimental group, calculating the difference, and dividing that difference into 1 (this formula is described later in the chapter). The resulting number provides an estimate of the number of patients who would need to be treated, in order to have one more successful case than if you had used the control or comparison treatment. For the NNT analysis, the data must be dichotomous, for example, successful outcome versus failure. Any continuous data can be translated into this dichotomous format by selecting a cutoff point to define success and failure. A NNT of 1 would indicate that every patient treated with the experimental treatment will have a successful outcome, while a NNT of 7 would indicate that you could expect to treat 7 people before you increased your success rate by 1 person, with the new treatment compared to the old treatment. A NNT of −1 would indicate that in every case, the control treatment will produce a better outcome. The NNT statistic is helpful in comparing the relative effectiveness of competing treatments, such that the treatment with the lowest NNT should be considered preferable, given similar costs and side effects of treatment. This statistic is not yet found with regularity in the physical therapy literature, but it is thought to be a clear and intuitive statistic for clinicians to use to compare clinical practice alternatives.

Power

As you read the results section of a paper, identify each hypothesis test that is reported and find in either table or text the result of the test. Your focus should be on identifying the statistically significant findings, as those are the ones on which the author will focus. If not all dependent variables measured in the study are found to have statistically significant changes in the desired direction, the author will discuss this finding in the paper, identifying perhaps methodological issues that precluded the anticipated results. One of the most common reasons identified for failure to find statistically significant results has to do with the power of the study. The power of the study is an expression of the capability of the study to find statistically significant results of a certain desired size when in truth there is a difference.[19] Researchers can use simple calculations to determine the power of their study to find differences between treatments. The calculation requires knowledge of the typical variability in the primary dependent variable, an estimate of the desired effect size of interest to the researcher, and the sample size. By adjusting these elements the researcher can plan for sufficient subjects to assure the statistical conclusion validity of the study. If the researcher does not allow for a customary number of dropouts in the methods and the study is plagued by large attrition rate, the power of the study could be compromised. It is not uncommon for a study to be underpowered for examination of all important variables.

As we evaluate the power of a study, we use one or more criteria that indicate how small a change, or difference between groups, we wish to be able to find in the study. Two terms with unique definitions may be provided by the author: the minimum detectable change (MDC) or the minimal clinical important difference (MCID). The MDC is defined as the smallest change in score that can be statistically detected beyond random error.[24] The MCID is often identified by the researcher as a sufficiently large change score between groups that would justify a change in practice. Both of these values can be calculated from data found in previous studies of the intervention of interest (for example, the mean change score or multiplying the desired effect size by the standard deviation) using one of several formulas. For instance, if a study of manual therapy compared to cervical traction to reduce cervical spine pain found a mean change score in the experimental group of 3 points, an investigator may set 3 points as his MCID for a study of the effects of manual therapy in patients with lumbar spine pain. These statistics are useful to understand in reading studies, as they alert the clinician to the likely magnitude of changes that might be expected from the intervention, and they show that the author designed the study with sufficient power to find those differences, if, in fact, they existed.

Summary of Statistical Conclusion Validity

We have covered some of the basic concepts that will allow the reader of a randomized clinical trial to comprehend the basic statistical approach to the results section of the study. We focused on the principles of data analysis that will permit you to examine the data presented in the study, read the tables and figures, and confirm what the author provides in the text. An understanding of concepts such as variability within the data in one group or between two or more groups helps you to accept the statistical validity of the study. If you wish to master additional statistical concepts, you will find some recommended resources at the end of the chapter.

DETERMINING VALUE IN STUDIES OF DIAGNOSTIC/PROGNOSTIC ACCURACY

As clinicians we require research evidence to allow us to select the best interventions for our patients; for example, evidence that will support the choice of manual techniques, the dose of exercise, the timing of treatment, or the decision not to treat at all. But these intervention choices are only useful in the context of our clinical judgment about the patient's diagnosis and prognosis, important first steps in the patient management model. So we must also seek good research evidence to support our diagnostic and prognostic decisions. Diagnostic accuracy studies focus on evaluating clinical tests against the best available gold standard tests to determine how accurate our clinical tests are at finding patients that have and do not have a certain diagnosis.[4] Studies of patient prognoses are designed to learn the likely course of recovery for patients in similar groups, with or without certain characteristics, for example, those patients who are likely to reinjure a joint if they return to sport with or without a protective brace. In physical therapy literature, we have experienced a significant increase in diagnostic accuracy studies, but there are fewer studies that help us understand a patient's prognosis, especially the long-term outcomes of our care. The criteria for good research practice are similar for both these types of research questions, so we will focus on diagnostic accuracy studies in this discussion. As with the criteria for determining value in the previous section on intervention studies, the goal is to avoid the influence of bias in the design and analysis of these studies. We will discuss three categories of good research practice: the selection of research subjects, the selection of measures and procedures, and the statistical estimates.

Did the Selection of Subjects Avoid the Introduction of Bias?

The methods used in observational studies to assess the diagnostic accuracy of clinical tests can have a large impact on the truthfulness of the statistical estimates for the examination. The research design options for observational studies is primarily defined by the selection of subjects: cohort studies identify subjects before any exposure has happened and follow the subjects forward; case-control studies identify subjects with the disease and those without the disease and retrospectively evaluate their exposure to the variable of interest; and cross-sectional designs select subjects and perform tests at the same point in time. Our first set of quality criteria will then focus on the research design selected or how the subjects were identified.

The selection of appropriate research subjects is as important in ensuring quality in diagnostic accuracy studies as it is in clinical trials. The investigator will carefully identify the target population of patients and establish inclusion and exclusion criteria that provide a group of research subjects who are likely to need the diagnostic test under study. Subjects who have no injury at all or are so clearly impaired as to make a diagnosis obvious should be excluded from diagnostic accuracy studies.[25] If these subjects are not excluded, the results of the study will be biased, usually overestimating the accuracy of the test. If the study fails to have a heterogeneous sample of subjects with a range of severity of the suspected impairment, spectrum bias may be introduced.[26,27] Spectrum bias occurs when the sample selected for the study contains subjects at the furthest extremes of the diagnostic spectrum, while ignoring subjects in the middle of the spectrum. Spectrum bias in diagnostic accuracy studies has been linked to the selection of a case-control research design. Boyer et al[28] performed a systematic review of diagnostic studies of clinical examinations for diagnosing carpal tunnel syndrome, finding spectrum bias in 65% of the 23 highest-quality studies, all of which used a case-control research design and were determined to have overestimated the accuracy of the tests.

To judge the adequacy of the sampling and research design, the author must provide a detailed description of the sampling methods and of the subjects' participation in the study so that you know the number of dropouts in the study. A flowchart similar to what you would expect in a RCT would be helpful.

Did the Selection of Measures and Procedures Avoid the Introduction of Bias?

The research design preferred for diagnostic accuracy studies is cross-sectional, requiring one group of subjects who receive two or more tests in a closely determined time frame. Enrollment of subjects into these studies is usually sequential and prospective, but some retrospective studies of diagnostic accuracy are reported. These studies are of less value to the clinician because so many of the following procedural aspects of the study cannot be controlled. A diagnostic accuracy study will be performed to assess a new or existing test, the index test, against a reference test or gold standard. In physical therapy research, the reference test is assumed to be the most accurate test or group of tests available to diagnose an impairment in body structures or functions or in participation in desired social activity. Any differences between the index test and the reference test are assumed to be attributable to errors in the index test.[29-31] It is important that the index test not be considered a part of the reference test, for example, choosing to compare a subtest score on the SF-36 to the total score on the SF-36. (The SF-36 is a standardized measure of health-related quality of life with subsets of items that provide scores in eight separate health domains as well as the composite score.) When this is done, it is likely the results will over-estimate the accuracy of the index test.

The procedures used to administer the tests in the study are also very important to the value of the study. The first aspect to consider is whether all subjects received both the index test and the reference test. If the reference test is expensive or could cause the subject discomfort or other risks considered inappropriate for that subject, the result is that a nonrandom group of study subjects receive both tests, and this could introduce a selection bias into the findings. This is less of a concern for diagnostic accuracy studies in physical therapy, but if not all subjects can receive the reference standard, the best research practice would require a random sample of study subjects to be selected for the reference test. This practice will also control for additional selection bias if only subjects who receive a certain score on the index test are given the gold standard test.

The timing of the two tests is also a criterion on which to evaluate the study. If the measures are not taken in close proximity, there is a chance of finding disease progression bias. This can occur when the subject's status changes, for better or worse, in the intervening time between measures. This must be evaluated for each study, taking into consideration how likely it is that the subjects' status might have changed. If the measures are assessing physiological properties like heart rate or blood pressure, the index and reference measures should be taken at the same time or very close in time. Other diagnostic clinical tests use imaging results as a reference standard and may be taken days apart. The author should carefully describe the decisions for the timing of the measures in these types of studies, and you will find value when you believe that the phenomenon being measured has not changed between index and reference testing.

Diagnostic accuracy studies should contain detailed descriptions of how each measure was performed, including figures or photos if helpful. This is important both for replicating the study findings or using the tests in your clinical practice and for your assessment of the appropriateness of the test. For tests of physical performance or assessment of joint structures, knowledge of the tester's position, the subject's position, the direction and magnitude of force application, and many other aspects of the test will be crucial to your assessment of the value of the test to your practice. It is also important to evaluate who performed each test, to assure that the testers were blind to the outcomes of the reference test if they were taking the index tests, and vice versa. The tester who takes the first measure will not be at risk for knowing the second test results, but even if the order of testing is randomized, the author should state the procedures taken to ensure that each tester had no knowledge of the other test results for subjects.

Were the Statistical Estimates Developed and Presented Without Bias or Error?

The next elements to evaluate in a paper reporting the diagnostic accuracy of a test are the results and estimates provided for each test. If the previously discussed methods of procuring the test results from the correct subjects have been followed, the next step is to interpret the results of the statistical analysis used by the authors. There are a variety of statistics used to analyze the data on the index test. We will define several of the most common and discuss the interpretation of each. Descriptive data (for example, frequency counts) for the subject's scores on the two tests will provide the first level of analysis of the accuracy of the index test.

The simplest way to examine diagnostic accuracy is to dichotomize the results of each test as either positive or negative. This will occasionally require collapsing data from a test that has more than two categories of outcome, for example four grades of tendon lesions might be collapsed by denoting the highest three grades of injuries as positive tests and the lowest grade as a negative test. When the test scores are not categorical but continuous data, a cutoff point must be selected to indicate when a positive test should be recorded. Table 12.7 provides a description of a typical 2 × 2 cross tabulation table that provides this first level of analysis for the results of diagnostic accuracy studies and the basic framework that allows the construction of diagnostic accuracy estimates. Table 12.8 gives the calculations for each of the statistical estimates and a brief description of how to interpret each one.

Table 12.7 | A 2 × 2 Cross-Tabulation Table Showing Descriptive Data for a Diagnostic Accuracy Study

		Reference Test	
		Positive Test	**Negative Test**
Index Test	Positive Test	30 Tpa	5 b FP
	Negative Test	c 10 FN	d 55 TN

Index Test = new or existing test under study
Reference Test = the gold standard diagnostic test
TP = true positive; TN = true negative; FP = false positive; FN = false negative

Table 12.8 Statistical Estimates Found in Diagnostic Accuracy Statistics

Estimate	2 × 2 Table formula	Definitions	Calculations from Table 10	How This Estimate May Help You Select a Clinical Test
Sensitivity	$a/(a + c)$	The proportion of true positive results for the index test	75%	A high value, close to 100%, indicates an index test that is very sensitive to finding patients that truly have the injury. Therefore, if you find a negative result on a highly sensitive index test, you can generally assume that the subject does not have the injury.
Specificity	$d/(b + d)$	The proportion of true negative results for the index test	92%	A high value, close to 100%, indicates a test that is very specific for identifying subjects who truly do not have the injury. Therefore if you find a positive result on a highly specific index test, you can generally assume the subject has the injury.
Positive predictive value	$a/(a + b)$	The proportion of the subjects with positive index test results who actually have the injury	86%	If a person tests positive on the index test, this percentage tells you how likely it is that the person truly has the injury.
Negative predictive value	$d/(c + d)$	The proportion of the subjects with negative index test results who actually do not have the injury	85%	If a person tests negatively on the index test, this percentage tells you how likely it is that the person truly does not have the injury.
Positive likelihood ratio	Sensitivity / (1 − Specificity)	The likelihood ratio of a positive index test	9.4	If a client has a positive test, a high value for this statistic will tell you how much more likely a positive test is in a subject with the injury versus a subject without the injury.
Negative likelihood ratio	(1 − Sensitivity) / Specificity	The likelihood ratio of a negative index test	.27	If a client has a negative test, a low value for this statistic will tell you how much more likely a negative test is in a subject with the injury versus a subject without the injury.

The basic diagnostic accuracy statistics allow the clinician to select tests and measures with the best statistical conclusion validity. We would desire tests that have both high sensitivity and specificity such that incorrect classification of patients is minimized, but few tests would fall into this category. The sensitivity of a test is perhaps the easiest statistic to understand, for it means that the test items were sensitive enough to identify individuals who fall into the true positive category, a positive test, and actually have the diagnosis. It is useful to have screening tools with high sensitivity, for if a patient tests negative on a highly sensitive screening tool, you are more confident in ruling out that diagnosis. A mnemonic for this situation is SNOUT, i.e., highly Sensitive test, Negative test result, rule the diagnosis OUT. The specificity of a test describes its ability to find individuals in the true negative category, a negative test, and do not have the diagnosis. Highly specific tests are good at finding individuals who do not have the diagnosis, so a positive test result on a highly specific test tells the clinician to pay attention to that result, for it may rule in the diagnosis. The mnemonic for this situation is SPIN, i.e., highly Specific test, Positive test result, rule the diagnosis IN.[26,32]

The positive and negative predictive values (PPV and NPV) are proportions that can be calculated from the 2×2 table by working the table "horizontally" rather than "vertically," as is done to calculate sensitivity and specificity.[20] As with the sensitivity and specificity statistical estimates, we also wish for high PPV and NPV. However, these two statistical estimates are influenced by the prevalence rate of the diagnosis for all subjects in the study. The prevalence expresses the percentage of the population of interest who have the diagnosis at any given point in time.[20] If the prevalence of the diagnosis is high in the study sample, this increases the predictive value of a positive test and decreases the predictive value of a negative test, and the converse is true if the prevalence of the diagnosis is very low in the study sample.

Likelihood ratios give us a proportion of subjects (with either a positive or negative test) that contrasts those who really have the diagnosis versus those who do not. For example, a likelihood ratio of a positive index test examines just those who tested positive on the index test, making a ratio of those with the diagnosis in the numerator and those without the diagnosis in the denominator (those with diagnosis/those without diagnosis). You can also think of this as a ratio of true positive subjects (TP) to false positive subjects (FP). It is clear, then, that we wish a positive likelihood ratio statistic to be high for an index test. Likelihood ratios greater than 10 or less than 0.1 are considered to be characteristic of tests that are quite strong.

Other Statistics Found in Observational Research

We will conclude this section with a discussion of additional statistics terms which may be found in observational studies that address either diagnostic accuracy or the impact of an intervention. Some simple statistics calculated from frequency data that are helpful to understand include ratios, proportions, and rates.[20]

Ratios are created by dividing one frequency by another and are expressed using a colon (:). Proportions are calculated by dividing a subset frequency by the total frequency. Rates are calculated by expressing a proportion over a period of time. We will illustrate these statistics with hypothetical data for mechanisms of glenohumeral joint dislocation.

Your outpatient physical therapy clinic provides coverage for the sports teams at three area high schools, enrolling 800 student athletes. In the past year, you treated 40 student athletes with a diagnosis of glenohumeral joint dislocation, 38 of which were anterior in direction and 2 of which were posterior dislocations.

- The *ratio* of anterior to posterior dislocations is $38/2 = 19{:}1$. There were 19 anterior dislocations for every posterior dislocation patient.
- The *proportion* of student athletes who experienced an anterior dislocation is calculated as $38/40 = 0.95 \times 100 = 95\%$.

The *rate* of occurrence of anterior glenohumeral dislocations is calculated as $38/800 = 0.0475$; and the rate of occurrence of posterior glenohumeral dislocations is calculated as $2/800 = 0.0025$. These small decimal values are often multiplied by a constant to express the rate in easier-to-understand terms; for example, if we multiply the rate of anterior dislocations by a constant of 1000, the reported rate of anterior dislocations would be 47.5 student athletes in 1000 in the past year.

If the study examines how proportions may differ for groups of subjects, the calculation of risks and odds may be used. Suppose we chose to follow the 40 athletes in our practice who experienced shoulder dislocation because we wish to understand the influence of their rehabilitation on the occurrence of redislocation of the shoulder. Buteau et al have described a high prevalence of reoccurrence of glenohumeral dislocation in athletes in their case report on the use of a new piece of exercise equipment, the body blade, which oscillates to provide resistance in upper-limb strengthening programs.[33] Looking retrospectively at the experiences of these injured athletes, we find the data reported in Table 12.9. Surprisingly, one-half of the injured athletes were not referred for rehabilitation, but were only immobilized in a sling; and the other half were referred for physical therapy, including the use of the body blade! The frequency data in this 2×2 table can be translated into several statistical estimates: risk ratios, absolute risk reduction, number needed to treat, and odds ratios. It is not common to find a 2×2 table presented in a research report; however, these statistical estimates are often used to describe how the groups differed.

One can quickly see that the risk of reinjury to the athlete's shoulder was higher for the immobilization-only group than the experimental/body blade group. A calculation of the

Table 12.9 Risk Ratios and Odds Ratios

	Athletes Received Treatment with Immobilization Only	Athletes Received Treatment with Immobilization Followed by Body Blade Exercises	
2nd Dislocation Occurred Within 2 Years	17 (a)	8 (b)	25
No Re-dislocation Occurred Within 2 Years	3 (c)	12 (d)	15
	20	20	

Risk of 2nd dislocation for athletes receiving immobilization only (control) $a/(a + c) = .85$ (also termed the Control Event Rate—CER)
Risk of 2nd dislocation for athletes receiving body blade exercises $b/(b + d) = .40$ (also termed the Experimental Event Rate—EER)
Risk ratio (Relative Risk): EER/CER; $.40/.85 = .47$
Absolute Risk Reduction (ARR): CER − EER: $.45$
Number Needed to Treat (NNT): $1/\text{ARR}: 2.22$
Odds of subject with a 2nd dislocation being in the control group: $a/b = 2.125$
Odds of subject without a 2nd dislocation being in the control group: $c/d = .25$
Odds ratio: $(a/b)/(c/d) = 8.5$

absolute risk reduction allows the subsequent calculation of the number needed to treat; in this instance, it is quite low at 2.22, indicating that you would need to treat only two athletes with shoulder dislocation with the body blade to decrease their risk of reoccurrence of their dislocated shoulder. The odds ratio is constructed from the odds of a person in the immobilization group having or not having a second dislocation; in this case the odds of the control subjects having a second dislocation are much higher than the odds that they did not have a second dislocation. The odds ratio of 8.5 indicates that a person with a second dislocation is 8.5 times more likely to have been in the immobilization group than in the body blade group. Odds ratios are often presented with a confidence interval, so you can observe the upper and lower bound for this estimate. Odds ratios are also used to indicate the magnitude of relationship between more than two groups and an outcome variable, and in this type of analysis, one of the groups is used as the reference standard, and odds ratios are calculated for each of the other groups in reference to that group. For example, if we seek to understand the impact of age on balance, and we group our subjects into four age groups, odds ratios may be presented to express the likelihood that the groups have different balance performance.

CONCLUSION

This chapter has provided an overview of important elements that should be considered when assessing the value of experimental and observational research as it is used to help determine the accuracy of diagnostic and prognostic measures and the worth of interventions for patients. The primary focus in discussing each of these elements has been to help assure that the researchers have done what can be done to reduce the risk of bias in conducting their research and in presenting the results. It is only through such efforts that you can determine the level of confidence you should have in applying the results of the study to patient care. These elements were discussed in the context of an individual study, but they apply to all of the sources of evidence that we will discuss in subsequent chapters.

SELF-ASSESSMENT

1. Find an article that supports an intervention provided to Mr. Ketterman. Identify each of these features in the article:
   a. Design
   b. Methods intended to reduce bias in selection and management of subjects
   c. Methods designed to reduce bias related to selection of interventions and measurement of outcomes
2. Using the same article, identify the information that would determine external validity.
3. Using the same article, identify the descriptive and inferential statistics. Do they support the conclusions reached by the authors?
4. Find an article that supports a diagnostic/prognostic test used in Mr. Ketterman's care. Identify each of these features in the article:
   a. Methods intended to reduce bias in selection and management of subjects
   b. Methods intended to reduce bias in the selection of measures and procedures
5. Select a diagnostic/prognostic article that presents ratios, proportions, and rates. How can you use these data as you make decisions about Mr. Ketterman?

CONTINUED LEARNING

- There are some excellent texts that provide more detail about research design and methods in physical therapy. They include:

DiFabio R. *Essentials of Rehabilitation Research: A Statistical Guide to Clinical Practice*, Philadelphia: FA Davis; 2013.
Domholdt E. *Rehabilitation Research: Principles and Applications*, 3rd ed. St. Louis: Elsevier Saunders; 2005.
Fetters L, Tilson J. *Evidence-Based Physical Therapy*, Philadelphia: FA Davis; 2012.
Jewell DV. *Guide to Evidence-based Physical Therapist Practice*, 2nd ed. Ontario, Canada: Jones and Bartlett Learning LC; 2011.
Portney L, Watkins M, *Foundations of Clinical Research*, 3rd ed. Pearson Prentice Hall, 2009.

1. Select and become familiar with one of these texts so you can use it to explore questions you have as you read the evidence.

- Internet search sites can also be useful for learning more about specific methodological decisions and statistical tests. Select terms for articles as you are reading the evidence and explore what you can learn about them through Internet searching.

REFERENCES

1. DiCenso A, Bayley L, Haynes RB. Accessing pre-appraised evidence: Fine-tuning the 5S model into a 6S model. *Evid Based Nurs.* 2009;12:99–101.
2. Califf RM. Evolving Methods: Alternatives to Large Randomized Controlled Trials. In: The Learning Health Care System: Workshop Summary. Roundtable on Evidence Based Medicine. Institute of Medicine of the National Academies. Washington, DC: The National Academies Press; 2007:84–92.
3. Tunis S. Practical Clinical Trials. In: The Learning Health Care System: Workshop Summary. Roundtable on Evidence Based Medicine. Institute of Medicine of the National Academies. Washington, DC: The National Academies Press; 2007:57–60.
4. Olsen L, Aisner D, McGinnis JM. Roundtable on Evidence-Based Medicine. In: The Learning Healthcare System. Washington DC: The National Academies Press; 2007.
5. Campbell DT, Stanley JC. *Experimental and Quasi-Experimental Designs for Research.* Boston: Houghton Mifflin Co.; 1963.
6. Campbell DT, Stanley JC. *Experimental and Quasi-Experimental Designs for Research.* Boston: Houghton Mifflin Co.; 1966.
7. McKibbon A. et al. Finding the evidence. In: Guyatt G., Rennie D. (eds). *Users' Guides to the Medical Literature: A Manual for Evidence-Based Clinical Practice.* Chicago: JAMA and Archives; AMA Press; 2002.
8. Guyatt C, Devereaux M, Straus. *User's Guides to the Medical Literature: Essentials of Evidence-Based Clinical Practice.* 2000.
9. Concato J, Shah N, Horwitz RI. Randomized, controlled trials, observational studies, and the hierarchy of research designs. NEJM. 2000.
10. Guyatt G, Rennie, D, eds. 1B1 Therapy. JAMA and Archives. Chicago: AMA Press; 2002.
11. Heneghan C, Badenoch D. *Evidence-Based Medicine Toolkit*, 2nd ed. BMJ Books Blackwell Publishing; 2006.
12. Greenhalgh T. *How to Read a Paper: The Basics of Evidence-Based Medicine*, 3rd ed. BMJ Books, Blackwell Publishing; 2006.

13. Schulz KF, Altman DG, Moher D for the CONSORT Group. CONSORT 2010 Statement: Updated guidelines for reporting parallel group randomized trials. BMJ. 2010;340:c332.
14. Altman DG, et al: The revised Consort statement for reporting randomized trials: Explanation and elaboration. AIM. 134(April);2001:8.
15. Eden J, Wheatley B, Mc Neil B, Sax H (eds). *Knowing What Works in Health Care: A Roadmap for the National Institute of Medicine.* Washington DC: National Academies Press; 2008.
16. Steiner WA et al. Use of the ICF Model as a clinical problem-solving tool in physical therapy and rehabilitation medicine. Phys Ther. 82(11, November);2002; 1098–1107.
17. Roos EM, Lohmander LS. The Knee Injury and Osteoarthritis Outcome Score (KOOS): From joint injury to osteoarthritis. Health Qual Life Outcomes. 2003;1:64.
18. APTA. *Guide to Physical Therapist Practice,* 2nd ed. Alexandria, VA: American Physical Therapy Association; 2001.
19. Jewell DV. *Guide to Evidence-Based Physical Therapist Practice,* 2nd ed. Ontario Canada: Jones and Bartlett Learning LC; 2011.
20. Domholdt E. *Rehabilitation Research: Principles and Applications,* 3rd ed. St. Louis: Elsevier Saunders; 2005.
21. Norman GR, Streiner DL. *Biostatistics: The Bare Essentials,* 3rd ed. Shelton, CT: People's Medical Publishing House; 2008.
22. Dalton GW, Keating JL. Number needed to treat: A statistic relevant for physical therapists. Phys Ther. 2000;80:1214–1219.
23. Moore, A. What is an NNT? Bandolier. www.medicine.ox.ac.uk/bandolier Accessed April 2009.
24. Turner D. et al. The minimal detectable change cannot reliably replace the minimal important difference. J Clin Epidem. 2010;63:28–36.
25. Jaeschke R et al. Diagnostic tests. In: Guyatt G, Rennie D, eds. *Users' Guides to the Medical Literature: A Manual for Evidence-Based Clinical Practice.* Chicago: JAMA & Archives, AMA Press; 2002.
26. Cook C, Cleland J, Huijbregts P. Creation and critique of studies of diagnostic accuracy: Use of the STARD and QUADAS methodological quality assessment tools. J Man Manip Ther. 2007;15(2):93–102.
27. Lijmer JG et al. Empirical evidence of design-related bias in studies of diagnostic tests. JAMA. 1999:282:1061–1066.
28. Boyer K et al. Effects of bias on the results of diagnostic studies of carpal tunnel syndrome. J Hand Surg Am. 2009;Jul–Aug;34(6):1006–1013.
29. Whiting PF et al. Sources of variation and bias in studies of diagnostic accuracy: A systematic review. Ann Intern Med. 2004;140:189–202.
30. Whiting PF et al. The development of QUADAS: A tool for the quality assessment of studies of diagnostic accuracy included in systematic reviews. BMC Med Res Method. 2003;3:25.
31. Whiting PF et al. Evaluation of QUADAS: A tool for the quality assessment of diagnostic accuracy studies. BMC Med Res Method. 2006;6:9
32. Pewsner D, Battaglia M, Minder C, Marx A, Bucher HC, Egger M. Ruling a diagnosis in or out with "SpPIn" and "SnNOut": A note of caution. BMJ 2004;329:209–13.
33. Buteau JL, Eriksrud, MS, Hasson, SM. Rehabilitation of a glenohumeral instability utilizing the body blade. Physiother Theory and Prac. 2007;23(6):333–349.

chapter 13

The Individual Study as a Source of Evidence

It is better to read a little and ponder a lot than to read a lot and ponder a little.

—Denis Parsons Burkitt

•

✳ Mr. Ketterman's Case

I found an article contrasting aerobic endurance exercises with strength training of the upper limbs for patients with heart failure, but I'm not really sure if the study was done properly. So I don't know if I should apply this evidence to my care. *(See Appendix for Mr. Ketterman's health history.)*

INTRODUCTION

Evidence based practice is built on a process that begins with a clinician's need to know something in order provide the best care to the patient. The clinician translates the information needed into an answerable question and then efficiently finds the best type of evidence related to the question. In this chapter we will focus on determining the utility of individual studies, the base of the 6S pyramid described by DiCenso et al.[1,2] shown in Figure 13-1, in helping to make good clinical decisions. Since individual studies are the most prevalent form of evidence that clinicians use, it is important to know how to assess them. We will provide the reader with the most currently used criteria, based on the principles discussed in Chapter 12, to assess the value of evidence derived from experimental and observational research.

STUDIES

As Schardt tells us in Chapter 11, as of 2011, there are over 17,000,000 individual articles referenced in Medline, so it is clear that the individual study is the most common form of evidence available to clinicians. In addition, most of these studies are published in journals that use masked peer review. As we discussed in Chapter 10, this means that experts in the field have reviewed the authors' report of their research methods and findings and have found

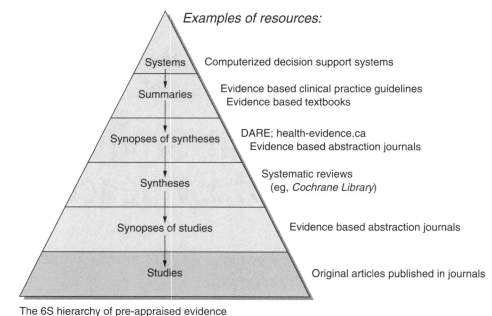

The 6S hierarchy of pre-appraised evidence

Figure 13-1 Sources of information about evidence. *(From DiCenso A, Bayley L, Haynes RB, Accessing pre-appraised evidence: Fine-tuning the 5S model into a 6S model. Evid Based Nurs. 2009;12:99–101.)*

them acceptable for publication, without knowing who the authors were. These studies can be found at all of the many sources reviewed in Chapter 11.

Studies Focused on Physical Therapy

Physical therapists can and should find articles of interest in all major health care literature. Journals with a broad focus, such as the New England Journal of Medicine (NEJM), the Journal of the American Medical Association (JAMA), the British Medical Journal (BMJ), journals with a specialty focus such as the Journal of Bone and Joint Surgery (JBJS), Neurology, Pediatrics, Journal of the American Geriatric Society, the Archives of Internal Medicine, and journals that focus on rehabilitation, such as the Archives of Physical Medicine and Rehabilitation, can all provide many articles that address the care physical therapists provide to their patients. In addition, there are now many journals published all over the world that focus specifically on physical therapy. Box 13.1 shows a list of many of these journals.

The articles in these journals cover a wide range of topics, but the ones of specific interest to physical therapists primarily fall into two groups: studies that address diagnostic or prognostic accuracy and studies that assess the efficacy and effectiveness of interventions. The standards set by peer-reviewed journals vary, and, of course, the generalizability of even the best research will vary based on the patients in question; therefore it is imperative that clinicians review studies carefully to determine their value to their clinical decision making. There are several published checklists that can be used to evaluate single studies. In addition to the CONSORT checklist[3,4] and the PEDro scale[5] used for RCTs (randomized controlled trials), the STARD checklist[6,7] and the QUADAS instrument[8,9] can be used for studies of diagnostic accuracy, and the STROBE scale can be used to evaluate observational studies in epidemiology.[10] Olivo has performed a systematic review of a range of criteria used to assess RCTs in

Box 13.1

English-Language Journals Whose Editors Belong to the International Society of Physiotherapy Journal Editors (ISPJE)

Advances in Physiotherapy
Bangladesh Physiotherapy Journal
Hong Kong Physiotherapy Journal
Indian Journal of Physiotherapy and Occupational Therapy
International Journal of Physical Therapy
International Journal of Physiotherapy and Rehabilitation
International Journal of Therapy and Rehabilitation
Journal of Geriatric Physical Therapy
Journal of Hand Therapy
Journal of Manual and Manipulative Therapy
Journal of Neurologic Physical Therapy
Journal of Orthopaedic and Sports Physical Therapy
Journal of Physical Therapy Education
Journal of Physical Therapy Science
Journal of Physiotherapy
Journal of Physiotherapy Research and Practice
Journal of Science and Medicine in Sport
Manual Therapy
New Zealand Journal of Physiotherapy
Nigerian Journal of Medical Rehabilitation
Physical Therapy
Physical Therapy in Sport
Physical Therapy Reviews
Physiotherapy
Physiotherapy Canada
Physiotherapy Ireland
Physiotherapy Research International
Physiotherapy Singapore
Physiotherapy Theory and Practice
Physiotherapy. The Journal of the Indian Association of Physiotherapists
South African Journal of Physiotherapy

medicine, finding no single scale that is recommended for physical therapy research.[11] Using the principles laid out in Chapter 12, we have developed a set of questions that you can use in reading and assessing articles.

ASSESSING STUDIES OF DIAGNOSTIC/ PROGNOSTIC ACCURACY

The first steps in patient care management are to determine an accurate and useful diagnosis and to determine the prognosis of the patient with that diagnosis. If we have not done this accurately, then we cannot begin to determine appropriate interventions, as the success of

---

Box 13.2 Determining the Value of a Study of Diagnostic Accuracy

Sample
1. Did the sample selected for the study represent an appropriate range of subjects who might require the test?
2. Did all the subjects take all the tests?

Measures
3. Is the gold standard test likely to correctly identify a subject?
4. Is the index test a part of the reference test?

Procedures
5. Did all the subjects receive both the index test and the reference test? If not, did a random sample of the subjects receive both?
6. Was the timing of the index and reference measures sufficiently close?
7. Were the tests described with sufficient detail?
8. Were the testers blind to the results of the preceding test?

Statistics
9. Were the same clinical data available in the study as would be available when the test is used in practice?
10. Are all test results reported, even if they are not clearly interpretable?

Adapted from Whiting PF, et al. The development of QUADAS: A tool for the quality assessment of studies of diagnostic accuracy included in systematic reviews. BMC Medical Research Methodology. 2003,3:25 and Whiting PF, et al. Evaluation of QUADAS, a tool for the quality assessment of diagnostic accuracy studies. BMC Medical Research Methodology, 2006;6:9.

---

interventions is linked to their application for certain diagnoses. It is useful to be reminded that physical therapists are most often making diagnoses of impairments and dysfunction. As we discuss aspects of diagnostic accuracy studies, we will use a checklist of questions designed to help you to determine whether or not good research practices have been used to eliminate bias or errors and control for variability in these investigations.[8,9] Box 13.2 summarizes the recommended questions to use to determine the value of a study of diagnostic accuracy. These questions can be used in a formal way, by completing a checklist, or more informally by having them in mind as you read the article.

As discussed in Chapter 12, studies of diagnostic or prognostic accuracy generally use observational designs. This is because these studies ask questions fundamentally different from those addressed in interventional studies. For example, in diagnostic accuracy questions, cross-sectional studies are common so that it is possible to distinguish whether the test can accurately select those subjects who really have the disease. In prognostic studies, longitudinal studies are common so that the prediction ability of the test can be determined by what actually happened to the subjects over time. Because these designs do not offer some of the protections against bias that can occur in a controlled experiment, it is imperative to look carefully at the other mechanisms the researchers used to reduce the potential for bias.

Therefore, it is important to focus on the sample of subjects used in these studies. So the first questions address the appropriate documentation of the sample.

- *Did the sample selected for the study represent an appropriate range of subjects who might require the test?*
- *Did all the subjects take all the tests?*

When the researchers do not meet these criteria, they should offer information about why they were not able to do so. This allows the reader to determine how much these issues limit the usefulness of the study.

It is also important to have clear information about the tests being assessed in the studies. In some situations there is a gold standard, a test that is known to have very good discriminative ability. Perhaps the study is designed to determine how a cheaper or more clinically practical test, referred to as an index test, compares to this gold standard. In some other cases, there is no gold standard but there is a clinical standard, a test that is widely used, and the study is designed to see if the new index test might actually be an improvement. The management of the measures used in a diagnostic accuracy study can be assessed with these questions:

- *Is the gold standard test likely to correctly identify a subject?*
- *Is the index test a part of the reference test?*

The researchers also need to use careful procedures designed to reduce the effects of the variability that can occur in conducting and interpreting the tests. The researchers should have put into place the same type of procedures used in experimental designs to blind data collectors to the status of the subjects they are evaluating.

- *Did all the subjects receive both the index test and the reference test? If not, did a random sample of the subjects receive both?*
- *Was the timing of the index and reference measures sufficiently close?*
- *Were the tests described with sufficient detail?*
- *Were the testers blind to the results of the preceding test?*

Finally, the way the researchers managed and reported the data needs to be assessed. Many clinical diagnoses are based on interpretation of test results. What clinicians already know when they look at the next data point can influence how they interpret that data point.[12] Therefore, it is important that the clinical data is managed in the study just as it would be in clinical practice. In addition, all test results, even if they are not totally clear, need to be included if accurate sensitivity and specificity are to be calculated.

- *Were the same clinical data available in the study as would be available when the test is used in practice?*
- *Are all test results reported, even if they are not clearly interpretable?*

If all of these questions can be answered with a yes, then the clinician can have confidence that the researchers have designed their studies in a way to minimize the effects of bias or variability on their results (validity) and can move on to determining if the results can be appropriately applied to individual patient care (generalizability).

ASSESSING STUDIES OF CLINICAL INTERVENTIONS

When you are looking for evidence that will help you select the best intervention for your patient, you will likely search for studies that test the effectiveness of various treatments on certain outcomes that are of importance to your patient. The randomized controlled trial (RCT) is considered a strong research design for such a question. We will use this research design to illustrate the criteria by which you will determine if a study of interventions is of

Box 13.3 Determining the Value of a Clinical Intervention Study

Research Design

1. Was the research design appropriate for the research question? Did the authors use the strongest possible design to allow a causal relationship between the intervention and the outcome?

Sample

2. Were the subjects chosen for the study the right ones?
3. Were the subjects randomly allocated/assigned to treatment and comparison groups?
4. Were the groups similar at the beginning of the study on measures that matter to you?
5. Did few subjects drop out of the study?
6. Were the subjects blinded to which group they were assigned?

Interventions

7. Were the interventions selected for each group clearly described and clearly different?
8. Did subjects receive a sufficient dose of treatment?
9. Was the clinician giving the interventions blind to the assignment of group members?

Measurement

10. Were the right tests and measures used? Ones matched to the purposes of the study, across a range of outcomes; ones that are reliable and valid?
11. Were the observers who took the measurements blind to the group assignment of the subjects?
12. Was the timing of the measures appropriate?

Statistics and Outcomes

13. Were all subjects who started the study accounted for at the end of the study?
14. Were all subject data analyzed in the groups to which they were assigned? (Intention to treat analysis)?
15. Were the groups similar at the end of the trial? How much did things change for each group and between groups?

Adapted from Schulz KF, Altman DG, Moher D. for the CONSORT Group. CONSORT 2010 Statement: Updated guidelines for reporting parallel group randomized trials. BMJ. 2010;340:c332. Altman et al: The revised Consort Statement for reporting randomized trials: Explanation and elaboration. AIM, April 2001; 134:8, and PEDro Physiotherapy Evidence Based Database. Australian Physiotherapy Association. www.pedro.org.au Accessed on June 9,2010.

value to you. The criteria are broadly useful to critique studies that use a variety of research designed to understand the efficacy and effectiveness of interventions. Box 13.3 contains a checklist to be used to evaluate the research validity of a clinical trial.

The first item in the checklist reflects our decision about the rigor of the research design selected by the investigator for the study:

- *Was the research design appropriate for the research question? Did the researchers use the strongest possible design to demonstrate a causal relationship between the intervention and the outcome?*

Chapter 12 provides information about many research designs. As we discussed there, the best design to demonstrate a causal relationship is the RCT, with its three essential features of *random selection or allocation* of research subjects to groups, the *inclusion of a control group* for comparison to a treatment group, and *purposeful manipulation* (dose, frequency, or duration) of the treatment variable. Sometimes the researchers cannot achieve each of these fully, so it is important for the clinician to recognize the limits of the study and the other actions taken by the researchers to provide useful, trustworthy data.

Descriptions of the sample and its selection are important because they contribute both to the trustworthiness or validity of a study and to the clinician's decision about the generalizability of the study to the clinician's patients.

- *Were the subjects chosen for the study the right ones?*
- *Were the subjects randomly allocated/assigned to treatment and comparison groups?*
- *Were the groups similar at the beginning of the study on measures that matter to you?*
- *Did few subjects drop out of the study?*
- *Were the subjects blinded to which group they were assigned?*

As you read the study, ask yourself how well controlled the study was in regard to the selection and treatment of subjects. Consider if the description of the subjects provides you with the information you need to decide if you can apply the findings to your patients. Because of the nature of physical therapy, subjects often cannot be blinded to the group to which they are assigned, so it is important to be sure that at least the evaluators are blinded.

The information about the specific methods used in the study is also important for trustworthiness and generalizability.

- *Were the interventions selected for each group clearly described and clearly different?*
- *Did subjects receive a sufficient dose of treatment?*
- *Was the clinician giving the interventions blind to the assignment of group members?*

As you read the study intervention procedures, you will use your clinical reasoning and expertise to evaluate each of these methodological decisions. Do they make sense to you, and can you imagine that these are the right decisions to provide the best opportunity for finding an effect for one type of exercise over the other? Or does your experience tell you that one or more of the researcher's decisions are likely to have introduced bias or errors? Recall the example used in Chapter 12 about a research study designed to investigate whether eccentric or concentric quadriceps strengthening exercise will produce better outcomes for patients who received a total knee arthroplasty. Your clinical judgment about the methods can tell you, for example, if sufficient time was allowed for the intervention to have an effect. Were the subjects in the concentric group clearly required to work less than those in the eccentric exercise group? Because of the nature of physical therapy, the physical therapist giving the exercise interventions is very likely to know to which group the subject was assigned. If so, do the methods identify ways that the evaluation function is separated from the practitioner function and that the evaluator is blind to the assignment? In addition to your clinical wisdom, you would hope to find the authors describing the evidence in the literature that informed their decisions about each step of the procedures.

Next we need to consider carefully the decisions made by the researchers about the tests and measures selected to demonstrate the differences in the results of the intervention across the groups in the study.

- *Were the right tests and measures used? Ones matched to the purposes of the study, across a range of outcomes; ones that are reliable and valid?*
- *Were the observers who took the measurements blind to the group assignment of the subjects?*
- *Was the timing of the measures appropriate?*

Often the tools are not ones that are suitable for use in the clinic, but we still need to use clinical judgment to determine if the measures address outcomes that are clinically meaningful for this patient population. Are the tools able to reliably and validly identify a clinically meaningful difference? Does the timing of the measures match what we know clinically about healing and recovery times for our patients? As we have mentioned above, it is very difficult to have subjects and providers of the intervention blinded to assignment, but it is imperative that the observers or evaluators are.

The final criteria we suggest for our checklist of determining the value in a RCT are related to the decisions made about the election and interpretation of statistics and the reporting of the outcomes.

- *Were all subjects who started the study accounted for at the end of the study?*
- *Were all subject data analyzed in the groups to which they were assigned?*
- *Were the groups similar at the end of the trial? How much did things change for each group and between groups?*

First, we examine the issue of subject attrition in the study. Previously, we included criteria to assess whether there were few subjects who dropped out of the study. We return to this concern because it can greatly affect the statistical analysis if this happened in the study. The author should account for the participation of all subjects who started the study, and those who, for example, completed one post test versus all follow-up testing sessions. The PEDro scale for assessing value in a RCT requires that data on an important outcome of the study was reported from 85% or greater of the subjects assigned to the group.[5] It is particularly important to assess whether the subject attrition happened differently within the study groups, for if one group lost 2% of subjects and the other lost 20% of subjects, the groups may no longer be as equivalent as they were at the start of the study. In clinical trials with several measurement points, it is usual to lose some subjects, so a method of analysis has been developed to address this problem, called intention to treat analysis. This analysis requires the researcher to analyze the subjects' data in the groups to which they were originally assigned, rather than analyze the data including changes in study protocol or deleting data for a subject who dropped out of the study. These occurrences can provide a biased statistical analysis by only including subjects who completed every aspect of the study, while dropping from the analysis subjects who were not responding to the intervention and chose to drop out. There are several methods of handling these problems in the data statistically, and the authors should describe for the reader exactly how they handled missing data and attempted to analyze all subject data in the originally allocated groups.

The last criterion stems from the statistical analysis of the magnitude of the effect of the intervention, when compared to a control or contrast group. As you read the study results, you will form opinions as to the importance of the differences the authors found, both within each group over time and between the groups. If this criterion is not met to your satisfaction, either because of a poor analysis or because the study was not sufficiently large to detect a minimal clinically important difference (MCID), it is not likely that the study will have any value for your patients. Thus it is appropriate that the final criterion is the most important: how big a difference did this intervention make? Is this difference large enough for you to decide to use this intervention, either for a particular patient or as a change in your typical practice for this patient population?

CONCLUSION

In this chapter we recommend criteria that will assist you to critique the various types of research that can inform your decisions with your patients. As you evaluate a study for any given clinical decision, you may find that you weight one or more criteria more heavily, and this practical approach to evaluating the value in the evidence makes good sense. We have recommended a total of 15 questions that can guide you to your decision about the value to you and your patients of any single RCT. Does a study need to meet every criterion? Few will meet every criterion as tightly as you might wish, for clinical research is a complicated process prone to many unexpected or unplanned events. As you evaluate a research report of a RCT, you may find some of the 15 criteria less important, given the intervention under study. Each decision you make about the value of a study may be adjusted as you read a new study with better design and controls in place. But it is very likely that you will learn something about your practice decisions from any study you critique, as the process of critical appraisal strengthens one's clinical reasoning capabilities.

In the next chapters you will learn about a variety of what we term filtered evidence—studies that have been critiqued for you. These are efficient sources of evidence and often provide stronger evidence than any one study can. However, when any single study is important for you to incorporate into your clinical reasoning, the principles discussed in this chapter will help you draw your own conclusion about the value of the study to you and your patient.

SELF-ASSESSMENT

1. Return to the articles that you used in Chapter 12, Self-Assessment, Questions 1–5, and use the questions we have presented in this chapter to assess their value to you.
2. What advice would you give the therapist who is caring for Mr. Ketterman based on your assessment?

CONTINUED LEARNING

- One of the best ways to develop better skill in an area is to teach about it. Develop a presentation to share with your colleagues that is based on the questions here. Then lead them in a regular analysis of literature that reports on care for groups of patients that you treat frequently.

REFERENCES

1. DiCenso A, Bayley L, Haynes RB. Accessing pre-appraised evidence: Fine-tuning the 5S model into a 6S model. Evid Based Nurs. 2009;12:99–101.
2. Haynes RB. Of studies, syntheses, synopses, summaries, and systems: The "5S" evolution of information services for evidence-based healthcare decisions. Evid Based Med. 2006;11:162–164.
3. Schulz KF, Altman DG, Moher D, for the CONSORT Group. CONSORT 2010 Statement: Updated guidelines for reporting parallel group randomized trials. BMJ. 2010;340:c332.
4. Altman DG et al. The revised Consort Statement for reporting randomized trials: Explanation and elaboration. AIM. April 2001;134:8.

5. PEDro Physiotherapy Evidence Based Database. Australian Physiotherapy Association. www.pedro.org.au. Accessed on June 9, 2010.
6. Cook C, Cleland J, Huijbregts P. Creation and Critique of Studies of Diagnostic Accuracy: Use of the STARD and QUADAS Methodological Quality Assessment Tools. J Man ManipTher. 2007;15(2):93–102.
7. STARD statement. http://www.stard-statement.org/. Accessed on May 3, 2011.
8. Whiting PF, et al. The development of QUADAS: A tool for the quality assessment of studies of diagnostic accuracy included in systematic reviews. BMC Medical Research Methodology. 2003;3:25.
9. Whiting PF, et al. Evaluation of QUADAS, a tool for the quality assessment of diagnostic accuracy studies. BMC Medical Research Methodology. 2006;6:9.
10. vonElm E, Altman DG, Egger M, Pocock SJ, Gotzsche PC, Vandenbroucke JP. STROBE initiative. Lancet. 2007;October 20:1453–1457.
11. Olivo SA, Macedo LG, Gadotti IC, Fuentes J, Stanton T, Magee DJ. Scales to assess the quality of randomized controlled trials: A systematic review. Phys Ther. 2008:88(2):156–175.
12. Chang PJ. The rationale selection and interpretation of diagnostic tests. In: Erkonen WE, ed., *Radiology 101*. Lippincott Williams & Wilkins, 1998.

chapter 14

Synopses of Studies

Kathleen Parker

The massive explosion of information has made us all a little batty.

•

✳ Mr. Ketterman's Case

I know that there is a lot of information that could help me with Mr. Ketterman's care, but it's really hard for me to read and analyze each article, one at a time. Isn't there something that can help me understand if and how I should apply an article to my patients? (See *Appendix for Mr. Ketterman's health history.*)

INTRODUCTION

There are several sources of information that we can use to help us find and organize evidence for use in daily practice. In Chapter 12 we discussed how to differentiate among individual studies and in Chapter13 how to assess *individual studies*. But looking at one study at a time can be time-consuming. The amount of information that is now available is staggering. One analysis of the quantity of material available electronically shows that in 2010 there were over 988 exabytes (1 exabyte equals 1 quintillion bytes) of information available on the Internet. This is equivalent to over 18 million times the number of books ever printed.[1] There are now many examples of abstractions of individual studies that help bring some meaning out of this amazing mass of information for clinical practice. In this chapter we will discuss *synopses of individual studies* (Fig. 14-1).[2] As DiCenso et al tell us, "The advantages of a synopsis of a single study over a single study are 3-fold: first, the assurance that the study is of sufficiently high quality and clinical relevance to merit abstraction; second, the brevity of the summary; and third, the added value of the commentary."[3]

SYNOPSES OF STUDIES

Synopses are designed to provide clinicians with direct, quick advice about specific clinical action by providing a brief, focused abstract of a study. A synopsis can be as brief as a single sentence, such as the title of many of the review articles in some evidence based journals. A review of the titles in Box 14.1 shows that while single sentences might provide some general guidance, they usually do not give clinicians sufficient information about the specificity of an intervention to be useful in treatment planning. However, the single sentence can tell clinicians if reading the review, and perhaps the article, would be worthwhile.

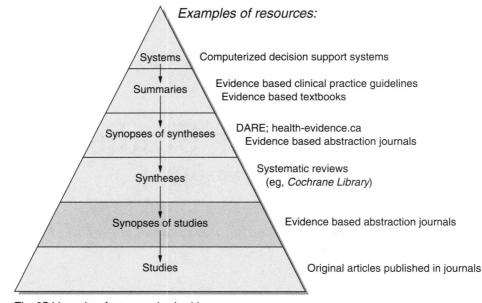

The 6S hierarchy of pre-appraised evidence

Figure 14-1 Sources of Information About Evidence. *(From DiCenso A, Bayley L, Haynes RB. Accessing pre-appraised evidence: Fine-tuning the 5S model into a 6S model. Evid Based Nurs. 2009;12:99–101.)*

Box 14.1 Examples of Single-Sentence Synopses

A. Review: Oral vitamin D prevents nonvertebral and hip fractures in a dose dependent manner in patients >65years of age (Denman M. EBM. October 2009;14(5):148–149)

B. Review: Back exercise interventions prevent self-reported episodes of back problems in adults but ergonomic education does not (Margo K. EBM. August 2009;14(4):116–117)

C. An exercise and telephone follow-up programme reduced emergency readmissions and improved quality of life in older people (Finlayson K. EBM. August 2009;14(4):120)

D. Review: Exercise may moderately improve depressive symptoms (Mead G. EBMH. August 2009;12(3):77)

The next option in a synopsis is a brief extraction of the study to support a specific conclusion. These brief extractions are usually kept to one page or less to facilitate the clinician's being able to see *quickly* the recommendation for action and to understand the supporting data for this recommendation. The full text of the review articles listed by title only in Box 14.1b. can be found at http://ebm.bmj.com. Although the full text does not provide the detail needed to replicate the intervention, it does demonstrate the value of the intervention as compared with many other interventions, and it does so in less than one page.

As this example demonstrates, the synopsis includes the essential information from the study that supports a specific conclusion. Synopses usually start or end with a clear statement or recommendation about a specific clinical action with a specific patient population. When appropriate synopses are available, a clinician can determine a course of action in a matter of a few minutes. As with all evidence the utility of a synopsis depends on how well it matches

Box 14.2	**Some Journals and Web Sites That Provide Abstracts or Synopses**

Evidence-Based Decision Making Journal Club (icu-10.med.usyd.edu.au/ebdm/)
Evidence-Based Dentistry
Evidence-Based Medicine
Evidence-Based Mental Health
Evidence-Based Nursing
Evidence-Based Spine-Care Journal
International Journal of Evidence-Based Healthcare
Journal of Evidence-Based Dental Practice
Journal of Evidence-Based Social Work

the clinician's question. The synopsis also still has the problem that it typically focuses on one aspect of patient management, rather than the range of decisions needed in actual care.

Published Synopses That Apply to Physical Therapist Practice

There are several sources of synopses available for physical therapists. One primary source can be the synopses created for other health care practitioners that address issues related to the physical therapist's management of patients. As we have mentioned above, there are now many journals that are designed specifically to provide synopses of the original literature published elsewhere. Box 14.2 lists a compilation of journals across the health care continuum with a primary focus on assessment of evidence in a synopsis format to help clinicians find information easily and review it quickly. In addition to journals that have this as a primary focus, many clinically oriented journals that report original research also have sections that are devoted to reviews of their own or other articles written specifically to guide clinicians. For example, "ACP Journal Club" is a monthly feature of *Annals of Internal Medicine;* "Current Best Evidence" is a regular feature in *The Journal of Pediatrics,* and "Practice Oriented Evidence that Matters (POEMS)" can be found in the *Journal of the American Academy of Physician Assistants.*

There has also been a growth in the number of entirely Web-based sources that focus on providing synopses of research selected from many journals and organized by specialty or patient problem. These include *Essential Evidence Plus,* which has grown from the original POEMS project by the *Journal of Family Practice* into a site where readers can find synopses of original research and of systematic reviews, as well as assistance with determining probability levels and coding patient care for accurate documentation. Another example of a Web-only resource is *Journal Watch,* from the publishers of *The New England Journal of Medicine,* that includes reviews of articles from over 300 journals and that organizes these reviews in 13 specialties and for 20 patient topics. Both sites will also provide the subscriber with a daily digest of new material as it is added to the site. (Links to active sites for these resources, and the ones described below, can be found at the F.A. Davis Web site associated with this text.)

All of these sites require a fee for the license or subscription, but there are also sites that provide synopses without charge. A very good example of these is *Evidence Updates,* which is a collaboration between the *British Medical Journal* and McMaster University. Over 120 journals are scanned for relevant articles, prerated for quality by research staff, and then rated for clinical interest and relevance by practitioners. Each subscriber then receives regular e-mails with a list of the articles with links to the article abstract.

There are several examples of synopses that exist specifically for rehabilitation or physical therapy. Each uses a different format and may have a different primary focus, but they all provide clinicians with ready access to short descriptions of studies with some assessment of their value or statement of their clinical implication.

Rehab+, part of McMaster University's evidence based practice initiative and a subset of *Evidence Updates*, provides selected abstracts from 130 clinical journals. The articles are pre-rated for quality by a research staff and then reviewed by a panel of practicing clinicians for relevance to practice and for newsworthiness. Each registrant to *Rehab+* receives e-mail alerts with links to the article abstract (as published with the original article) along with the article's relevance and newsworthiness ratings. Figure 14-3 shows an example of the notification that each registrant receives. As of this writing, registration is free.

Rehab+ for: 3/27/2010

☆ rehabplus@mcmasterhkr.com to me   show details Mar 27 (5 days ago) ↩ Reply ▼

Dear Dr. Hack:

New articles: colleagues in your specialty have identified the following article(s) as being of interest:

Article Title	Specialty	Relevance	Newsworthiness
Surgical versus non-surgical treatment for acute anterior shoulder dislocation. Cochrane Database Syst Rev	Hand Therapy	6	4
Therapeutic ultrasound for osteoarthritis of the knee or hip. Cochrane Database Syst Rev	Mobility	5	4
A systematic review of nursing rehabilitation of stroke patients with aphasia. J Clin Nurs	Neurological	6	5
Physical performance and subsequent disability and survival in older adults with malignancy: results from the health, aging and body composition study. J Am Geriatr Soc	Mobility	4	4
Evidence for predictive validity of remission on long-term outcome in rheumatoid arthritis: A systematic review. Arthritis Care Res (Hoboken)	Musculoskeletal	5	5
Measures of activity limitation on admission to rehabilitation after stroke predict walking speed at discharge: an observational study. Aust J Physiother	Mobility	5	5
Physical conditioning programs for improving work outcomes in workers with back pain. Cochrane Database Syst Rev	Work and Work Injury	7	6
Efficacy of community-based physiotherapy networks for patients with Parkinson's disease: a cluster-randomised trial. Lancet Neurol	Neurological	7	6
Manipulation or mobilisation for neck pain. Cochrane Database Syst Rev	Manual Therapy	7	5
	Work and Work Injury	6	5
	Chronic Pain	6	5
	Neurological	5	4
Dose response and efficacy of spinal manipulation for chronic cervicogenic headache: a pilot randomized controlled trial. Spine J	Chronic Pain	7	5
Surgery for cervical radiculopathy or myelopathy. Cochrane Database Syst Rev	Chronic Pain	6	5

Figure 14-2 Example of Notification from Rehab+.

Another interesting offering designed specifically for physical therapists is the Evidence Express program available from Evidence in Motion. Although the material provided by Evidence Express is not synopsized in any way, it is filtered based on the subscriber's preferences and then provided in a regular e-mail. The subscriber identifies the general area of interest (e.g., orthopedic, neurological, women's health) and then can view and alter a list of selected authors, journals, and newsfeeds. The e-mail then contains all items that fit this filter with links to the abstracts of the articles. The premise of this service is that this provides relevant material in one e-mail.

New sites will continue to develop. From time to time we will post information about them at the FA Davis Web site.

"The Bottom Line" is a feature of *Physical Therapy* that provides a translation of study findings into clinical practice for selected clinical research articles published in that journal. Each "Bottom Line" asks and answers questions about the research, such as:

- What problems did the researchers set out to study, and why?
- Who participated in the study?
- What new information does this study offer?
- What new information does this study offer for patients?
- How did the researchers go about the study?
- If you are a patient, what might these findings mean to you?
- What are the limitations of the study, and what further research is needed?

This feature is published as a companion to the article of interest in both paper and electronic format.

Collections of Synopses Relevant to Physical Therapy

There are two more advanced and organized resources available that are frequently used to conduct searches for synopses of relevant material in physical therapy. These are *Hooked on Evidence* and *PEDro* (Physiotherapy Evidence Database).

Hooked on Evidence

Hooked on Evidence is a service of the American Physical Therapy Association (APTA). It is a database of article extractions built by contributions from members of the APTA. At this writing, it includes only articles related to interventions, not to diagnosis or prognosis. Articles are selected by the reviewers or suggested by the managers of the database and specific data are extracted in an organized format. Extraction is done by choosing from among preset options in drop-down menus. The data presented for each article include:

- Design type
- Study population characteristics including number, dropout rate, and inclusion and exclusion criteria
- Blinding status

- Narrative description of the interventions received by all treatment and control groups
- List of all outcome measures
- Absolute and standardized mean differences with confidence intervals for each continuous outcome measure
- Odds ratio, risk ratio, and number needed to treat for each dichotomous outcome measure

There is also a link to the article abstract at PubMed. The articles can be found by searching keywords, which produces a list of all relevant articles, or by choosing clinical scenarios that represent typical patient populations in physical therapy. If the user chooses a scenario, the related articles are organized by design type (see Fig. 14-4a). Beginning in 2013, *Hooked* is available in read-only format to all users. APTA membership or an annual subscription fee.

PEDro

PEDro is an acronym for *Physiotherapy Evidence Database*, which is produced by the Centre for Evidence-Based Physiotherapy at the University of Sydney. *PEDro* also focuses on interventional questions and provides information about randomized controlled trials (RCTs), systematic reviews, and evidence based clinical practice guidelines. The contents can be searched based on therapy type, patient problem or impairment, body part, specialty practice, and by type of article (RCT, systematic review, guideline). See Figure 14-4a and b for an example of search results. All RCTs are rated by trained volunteers to identify those trials that are more likely to be valid and to contain sufficient information to guide clinical practice. The PEDro scale for this rating includes 10 items: random allocation, concealed allocation, similarity at baseline, subject blinding, therapist blinding, assessor blinding, greater than 85% follow-up for at least one key outcome, intention-to-treat analysis, between-group statistical comparison for at least one key outcome, and point and variability measures for at least one key outcome. Items are scored as either present (1) or absent (0) and summed for a total score for the study.[4–6] Each citation includes the score, with a breakdown of each item, an abstract, and a link to full text, when available. At the time of this writing, *PEDro* is free to all users through support from several physical therapy member organizations, insurers, and licensing authorities.

CREATING SYNOPSES

The intent of a synopsis, as we have said, is to make information readily available to clinicians about the clinical implications of any particular study. But, even with the many published sources of synopses there remains a vast amount of research that is of interest to clinicians that has not been synopsized. Several techniques have been developed that can be used by clinicians to produce their own synopses to fill this gap.

Appraisal Worksheets

Many evidence based practice authors and groups have developed worksheets for individual practitioners to use in developing their own synopses of individual studies. These worksheets are usually organized around the purpose of the study. For example, Jewell identifies different appraisal issues for studies about diagnostic tests, prognoses, and interventions as studied by both experimental and observational designs (see Chapter 12).[7] These categories are very similar to the worksheets developed by the Center for Evidence Based Medicine.[8] The Critical

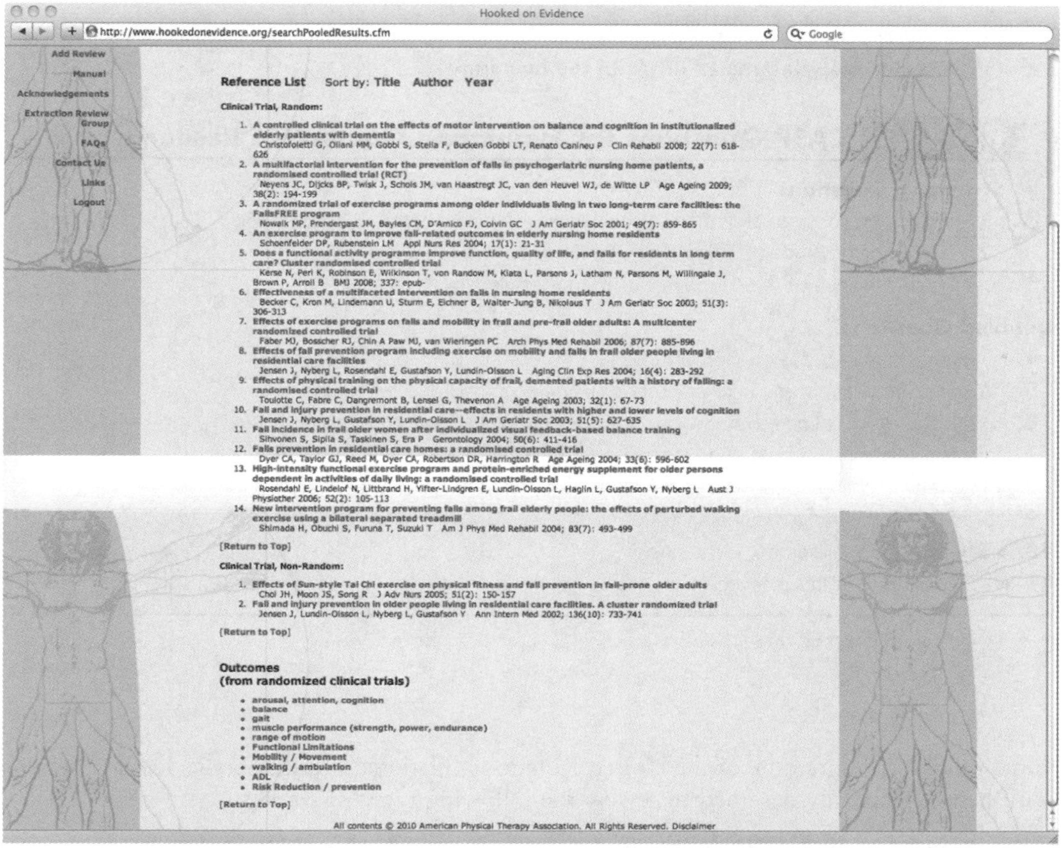

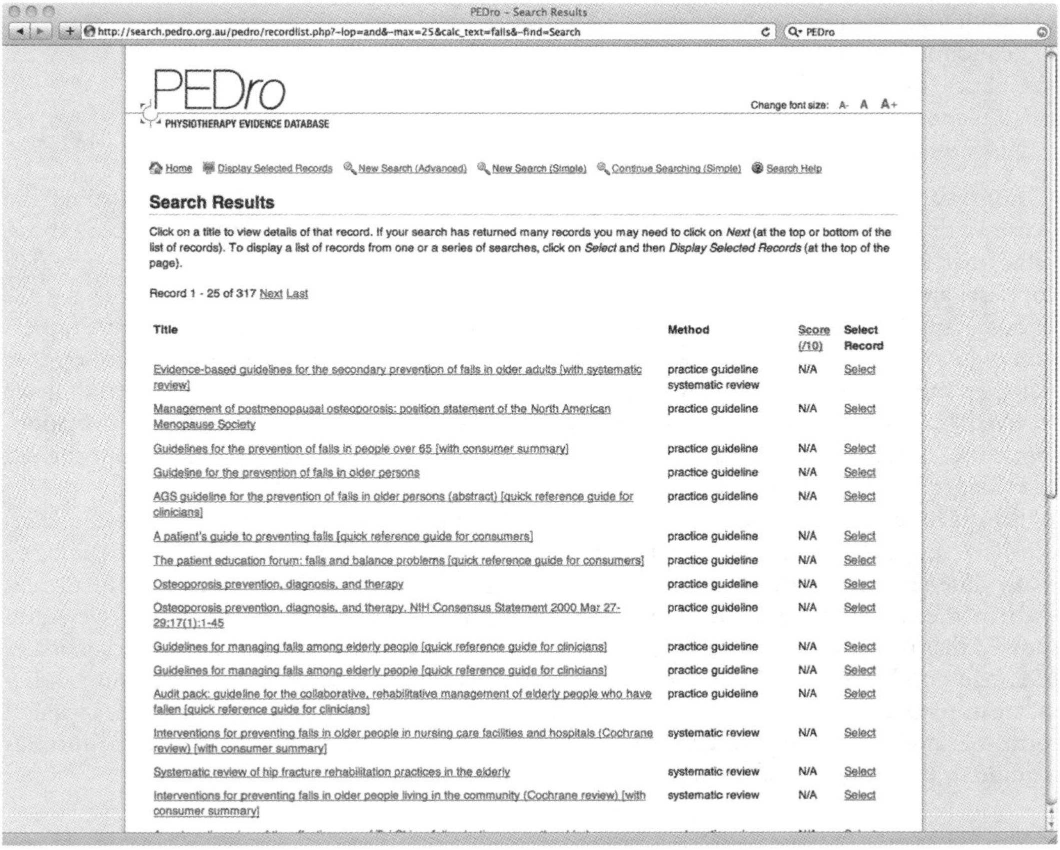

Figure 14-3a, b Examples of the Results When Searching on the Word "falls" in (a) *Hooked on Evidence* and (b) *PEDro*.

Box 14.3 **CASP Questions for Evaluating Qualitative Research***

Screening Questions
1. Was there a clear statement of the aims of the research?
2. Is a qualitative methodology appropriate?
3. Is it worth continuing? If so, move on to the detailed questions

Detailed Questions
4. Was the research design appropriate to address the aims of the research?
5. Was the recruitment strategy appropriate to the aims of the research?
6. Were the data collected in a way that addressed the research issue?
7. Has the relationship between researcher and participants been adequately considered?
8. Have ethical issues been taken into consideration?
9. Was the data analysis sufficiently rigorous?
10. Is there a clear statement of findings?
11. How valuable is the research?

---

*www.sph.nhs.uk/sph-files/casp-appraisal-tools/Qualitative%20Appraisal%20Tool.pdf/view

Appraisal Skills Programme of the United Kingdom's National Health Service has a variety of worksheets specifically designed to review the following types of studies:

- Randomized controlled trials (RCTs)
- Qualitative research
- Economic evaluation studies
- Cohort studies
- Case-control studies
- Diagnostic test studies[9]

Appraisal forms generally have similar structures. They are designed to demonstrate the worth of the study in helping clinicians make decisions, highlighting many of the issues about value that are covered in Chapter 12. The questions from the CASP qualitative research appraisal are shown in Box 14.3.

Some appraisal forms are designed to resemble scales, with assigned points for each question, which can then be summed to give an overall score. However, this single number does not give other readers much information about the reasons that an article may not have received full points, thereby causing clinicians to lose what may be valuable information. Therefore, it may be best to simply review the full scoring sheet when deciding about the use of evidence from a reviewed article.

Efforts have been made to bring more standardization to these worksheets, so that clinicians can have more confidence in their use to help guide care. This is especially needed, since so many different scales are available. One analysis showed that there are at least 21 distinct scales used in the literature to appraise work of relevance to physical therapy.[10] This review also showed that up to that time, while many of the scales appear to measure the appropriate issues (i.e., had good face validity), none of these scales had been tested for reliability and validity as measurement tools. The best advice at this time is for a clinician to choose an appraisal form that highlights the major concerns for the particular type of study and use the form as a guide to thinking and as a record of the analysis.

In a related effort, evidence based researchers have developed statements to guide authors of study reports about the elements that should be included in reports of particular kinds of studies. These include CONSORT for randomized controlled trials,[11] STARD for diagnostic studies,[12] STROBE for observational studies,[13] and QUALRES for qualitative research studies.[14] In turn, these statements are also used by researchers in designing their studies and by journal editors in reviewing reports for publication. But the authors of the statements caution that they are not designed, nor validated, to be used by readers in assessing quality of evidence.[12]

Critically Appraised Topics

When there is no worksheet suitable for appraisal, clinicians can create a more narrative synopsis. Perhaps the most familiar form of narrative synopsis is the Critically Appraised Topic (CAT), as described in *Evidence-Based Medicine* by Straus et al.[15-16] A CAT is a one- or two-page summary of all of the steps involved in an evidenced-based approach to the literature. CATs are generally created by clinicians for their own use, either personally or in groups. They are written because clinicians want to document their review of a specific article for future reference themselves or to share with their colleagues. Typically, a CAT is written about an interventional trial with an emphasis on RCTs; however, they can be written about groups of articles and about diagnostic or prognostic questions. The clinical question is defined, the search strategy and results are described, selected articles are cited, and details of the study are summarized, and an appraisal is done. Finally, a conclusion is given about recommended clinical behavior that reflects the strength of the methods and evidence at hand. There are several different formats for writing CATs (references). Box 14.4a shows the typical elements of a CAT. Box 14-4b shows a completed CAT written using this format.

CATs are written in response to a question that arises directly from clinical practice. As has been said, very seldom can we find a single article that exactly matches a full clinical question. Much more often the article is answering a specific part of the question. By collecting a series of CATs on the overall general topic, we can begin to bring together pieces of evidence that will eventually give us a clearer direction. Another important consideration is the nature of the clinical bottom line that serves as a conclusion derived from the study and as advice to the clinician. The bottom line is *not* a summary of the research findings. Instead, it is a recommendation to the clinician about action or clinical behavior. Clinicians need to take action. They can choose to adopt the new technique or assessment or they can choose to stay with the current option. They do not have the luxury of waiting for better research before treating the patient, as much as they might like to. The bottom line therefore needs to reflect the best judgment that can be made based on the evidence available in the study.

While it may seem that the growth of synopses means that clinicians do not need to develop their own, CATs continue to have many uses. They can help individual clinicians organize their thoughts about a specific article and build those thoughts for a body of literature by accumulating knowledge in a focused way. By writing down the findings, clinicians also greatly improve the ability to retrieve the work as they encounter similar patients in the future. They can also have a great impact if a group of clinicians collects CATs on topics related to the patient populations they see frequently. If a clinic with 10 staff members agreed that everyone would do one CAT a month, by the end of a year there would be 120 articles reviewed, with the information available to everyone in a very accessible manner. Finally, CATs are a great way to hone EBM skills, thereby also increasing our expertise in reviewing the materials prepared for us by others.[15]

Box 14.4a   The Essential Elements of a CAT

Title
The title of a CAT is the clinical question, often in PICO format (see Chapter 10) that was the reason the clinician sought out the article being reviewed. Using the clinical question means that similar articles can also be identified this way to build a series of articles about the question. Sometimes a clinical scenario, a short description of the patient case that led to the clinical question, is added.

Reviewer
This is the person who wrote the CAT. If the CAT is written as part of a personal library, the name is not necessary, but often CATs are written as part of a practice library.

Search
This section details the search strategy used by the reviewer (see Chapter 11). It includes the resources selected for the search (Medline, Cochrane, CINAHL, etc.) and the specific search strategy used, including MESH terms, specification of publication type(s), years searched, and any other details that will allow the clinician to repeat the search at a later date.

Date
Date of the search and the proposed date for reevaluation of the topic. The date of a renewed search is based on an estimate of how fast knowledge in this area is changing.

Citation(s)
The specific and full reference of the article (s) being discussed should be reported in a standardized format, such as that used by common journals or by Medline. This allows the author and readers to retrieve the article in the future.

Clinical Bottom Line
The reviewer should make a clear statement about the action recommended by the evidence in the study. This decision about what to recommend is determined after the full analysis of the article. But by placing it here, near the top of the CAT, readers can immediately see the conclusion to be drawn from the study.

Description of Study
This section should summarize in one or two paragraphs what actually happened in the study (see Chapter 12) using this format:
Design–Is the design experimental (causality) or observational (relationships)?

- *Population:* What patients were included and excluded? Was there a control group? How was assignment made to the groups?
- *Methods/Interventions:* What were the therapeutic interventions, diagnostic interventions, exposures, length of time for the activity as well as for follow-up?
- *Outcome tools/measures:* What was measured and/or counted to answer the researchers' questions?
- *What happened:* How were subjects tracked through the study; how many patients presented, were excluded, dropped out, completed protocol, etc.?

Box 14.4a The Essential Elements of a CAT—cont'd

Results

This section summarizes the results that are the actual evidence being sought. Using existing tables that are part of the study report can sometimes best summarize these data. If not provided in the study and if adequate data are provided, the reviewer should calculate important parameters such as odds ratios, relative risk reduction, and number needed to treat.

Comments

This section is the opportunity to identify the issues that could cause concern about applying the research. These concerns can be related to the actual study design and implementation (internal validity). Other concerns relate to the external validity or the generalizability of the work (see Chapter12).

Box 14.4b A Completed CAT

- *Title:*

In women who have recently become mothers does exercise and education versus education alone better increase well-being.

- *Reviewer:*

Laurie. Hack

- *Search:*

PubMed Advanced Search was used to search Medline by using the terms exercise AND education AND mothers. No limiters were used.

- *Date:*

March 31, 2010. Review search on April 1, 2011

- *Citation(s):*

Norman E, Sherburn M, Osborne RH, Galea MP. An exercise and education program improves wellbeing of new mothers: A randomized controlled trial. Phys Ther. 2010;90:348–355.

- *Clinical bottom line:*

The results of this study support the use of a program combining exercise and education in new mothers to decrease the risk of postpartum depression.

- *Description of study:*

Design—This was a randomized controlled trial.

- *Population:* Primiparous and multiparous women six–eight weeks postpartum after delivery at an Australian hospital were randomly assigned to an intervention (N = 80) and a control group (N = 81). Women medicated with a psychiatric disorder or who remained hospitalized were excluded.

Box 14.4b   A Completed CAT—cont'd

- *Methods/Interventions:* The intervention group (N = 62) received an eight-week program of one-hour group physical therapist-led exercises with their babies and a 30-minute education program. The control group (N = 73) received a written education program. (Missing participants were unable to begin the protocol because of personal reasons.)
- *Outcome tools/Measures:* The outcome tools were the Positive Affect Balance Scale (PABS) , the Edinburgh Postnatal Depression Scale (EPNDS), and questions about physical activity level.
- *What happened:* Outcomes were measured at baseline, end of intervention, and four weeks post-intervention. Two subjects were lost to follow-up in the intervention group, and three in the control group. No adverse events were reported.
- *Results:*

There was a significant between-groups difference in PABS scores over time. At baseline, risk for depression in the intervention group was 22%; in the control group 16%. At end of intervention the risk in the intervention group was 11%; control group remained unchanged. There were no differences at baseline or at end of intervention in physical activity.

- *Comments:*

The women in this article were in a rural area of Australia and were considered at risk of social isolation. Their results may not be found in all populations of postpartum women. Since activity level was the same in both groups, the differences found in outcomes are difficult to explain based on physiological effects of exercise. The socialization that was part of the intervention may also play a part; although the authors cite other research that shows social interaction alone does not produce similar changes in risk for depression.

CONCLUSION

Synopses are an excellent way for clinicians to find or create for themselves succinct assessment of research that focuses on the clinical implications of the work. They are increasingly available electronically, with options for "push" technology, to bring the information directly to the clinician. The majority of synopses remain focused on single studies that assess one aspect of care, generally a specific intervention.

SELF-ASSESSMENT

1. Based on the questions you developed for Mr. Ketterman, review recent issues of the journals listed in Box 14.2 to see if you can find examples of synopses that can help you in your practice decisions.
2. With a partner, identify two articles that can help you make decisions about Mr. Ketterman's care. Each of you should use the questions in Box 14.3 to create a synopsis of one article. Then share the synopsis. What are the strengths and weaknesses of using this approach to share information?
3. One way to see if you are on target in writing your own synopses would be to write a CAT for an article in *Physical Therapy* that also has a "Clinical Bottom Line" available online. Write the CAT before reading the "Bottom Line" and then compare your assessment with that of the expert.

CONTINUED LEARNING

- There is no better way to learn about synopses than to prepare some yourself. Ask a colleague to join you in assessing articles of joint interest and then share the synopses. This can grow to include several therapists in a practice to build a library of relevant synopses.
- Read synopses written outside of physical therapy (many of which are available in full text through public search engines) to identify the range of articles that are available to provide guidance about physical therapist practice.
- Contribute to *Hooked on Evidence* by performing an article abstraction.

REFERENCES

1. Nordenson B. Overload! Columbia Journalism Review. Nov/Dec 2008;47(4):30–42.
2. Haynes RB. Of studies, syntheses, synopses, summaries, and systems: The "5S" evolution of information services for evidence-based healthcare decisions. Evid Based Med. 2006;11:162–164.
3. DiCenso A, Bayley L, Haynes RB. Accessing pre-appraised evidence: Fine-tuning the 5S model into a 6S model. Evid Based Nurs. 2009;12:99–101.
4. Maher CG, Sherrington C, Herbert RD, Moseley AM, Elkins M. Reliability of the PEDro scale for rating quality of randomized controlled trials. Phys Ther. 2003;83:713–721.
5. de Morton NA. The PEDro scale is a valid measure of the methodological quality of clinical trials: A demographic study. Austr J Physiother. 2009;55:129–133.
6. Macedo LG, Elkins MR, Maher CG, Moseley A, Herbert RD, Sherrington C. There was evidence of convergent and construct validity of Physiotherapy Evidence Database quality scale for physiotherapy trials. J Clin Epidem. 2010:8:920–925.
7. Jewell D. *Guide to Evidence-Based Physical Therapy Practice*. Jones and Bartlett; Sudbury, MA, 2008.
8. Center for Evidence Based Medicine, University of Oxford. http://cebm.net/index. aspx?o = 1157 Accessed on March 21, 2010.
9. Critical Appraisal Skills Programme, National Health Service, United Kingdom. http:// phru.nhs.uk/pages/PHD/CASP.htm Accessed on March 21, 2010.
10. Armijo Olivo S, Macedo LG, Gadotti IC, et al. Scales to assess the quality of randomized controlled trials: A systematic review. PhysTher. 2008;88:156–175.
11. Schulz K, Altman DG, Moher D. CONSORT 2010 Statement: Updated guidelines for reporting parallel group randomized. BMJ. 2010;340:c332.
12. Bossuyt PM, Reitsma JB, Bruns DE, Gatsonis CA, Glasziou PP, Irwig LM, Lijmer JG, Moher D, Rennie D, de Vet HCW. Towards complete and accurate reporting of studies of diagnostic accuracy: The STARD Initiative. Ann Intern Med. 2003;138:40–44.
13. von Elm E, Altman DG, Egger M, Pocock SJ, Gøtzsche PC, Vandenbroucke JP. Strengthening the reporting of observational studies in epidemiology(STROBE) statement: Guidelines for reporting observational studies. BMJ. 2007;335:806–808.
14. Cohen D, Crabtree B. Qualitative Research Guidelines Project, July 2006. http://www. qualres.org/HomeGuid-3868.html
15. Strauss SE, Richardson WS, Glasziou PP, Haynes RB, *Evidence-based Medicine*, 4th ed. Elsevier Churchill Livingstone, London, 2011.
16. Fetters L, Figueiredo, E, Keane-Miller D, McSweeney DJ, Tsao, C-C. Critically appraised topics. Pediatr Phys Ther. 2004;16:19–21.

chapter 15

Synthesis of Studies Through Systematic Reviews and Meta-Analyses

Alison Bailey Hallam, PT, MS

*Organizing is what you do before you do something,
so that when you do it, it is not all mixed up.*

—AA Milne

•

✳ Mr. Ketterman's Case

I've read several articles now about exercise in patients with congestive heart failure. Some of them have very few subjects and they seem to have different results. How can I organize these results to help me make a decision about his care? *(See Appendix for Mr. Ketterman's health history.)*

INTRODUCTION

Chapters 12, 13, and 14 have been concerned with the collection of data and its analysis from individual studies and their syntheses. These are forms of primary analysis. When trying to answer a clinical question with a limited amount of time and resources, it is common to focus on finding a few, or even only one, primary resource and therefore end up with an incomplete answer.

Most clinicians would feel more confident in applying research evidence if they could find complete and valid answers, and find them more efficiently. This is where what Haynes calls a synthesis of the relevant primary data is useful (Fig. 15-1).[1,2] A synthesis, or secondary analysis, takes the form of a systematic review, where all the data on a topic is aggregated, with or without further statistical analysis, to gain a broader picture of the issue. This solves the clinician's problem of limited time and resources. It also addresses an issue frequently found in much of health care, where it is difficult to find large cohorts of subjects, and the resultant studies have a small number of participants (*ns*). Such studies individually do not

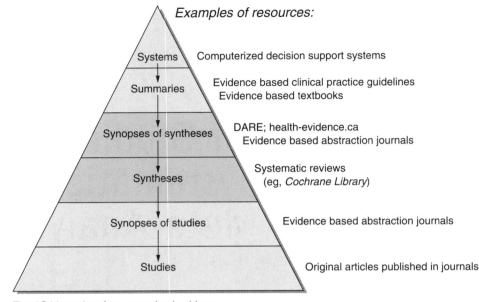

Examples of resources:

Systems — Computerized decision support systems

Summaries — Evidence based clinical practice guidelines / Evidence based textbooks

Synopses of syntheses — DARE; health-evidence.ca / Evidence based abstraction journals

Syntheses — Systematic reviews (eg, *Cochrane Library*)

Synopses of studies — Evidence based abstraction journals

Studies — Original articles published in journals

The 6S hierarchy of pre-appraised evidence

Figure 15-1 Sources of Information About Evidence. *(Redrawn with permission from DiCenso A, Bayley L, Haynes RB. Accessing pre-appraised evidence: Fine-tuning the 5S model into a 6S model. Evid Based Nurs. 2009;12:99–101.)*

provide sufficient information to guide practice. A synthesis has the advantage of collectively analyzing the results from these studies with a small number of subjects and identifying possible significant results that cannot be seen looking at one study at a time.

This chapter will consider the systematic review, with and without a meta-analysis, as a way to quickly find answers to clinical questions. It will show you how to be a discerning reader of reviews and introduce you to methods commonly used to present the results. In addition, we will also discuss synopses of syntheses, Haynes's next level up the pyramid.

SYSTEMATIC REVIEWS AND META-ANALYSES

There is a long history of reviews in every discipline; these reviews are often based on the author's resources or preferences in selection of the articles to be reviewed. Often the review is designed from its inception to support a particular point of view. However, such reviews are not the best way to apply evidence from the literature to clinical decisions. In the context of evidence based practice, we want reviews that are comprehensive and free from author bias. This has resulted in the development of a particular form of review, termed *systematic review.* "Systematic reviews are concise summaries of the best available evidence that address sharply defined clinical questions."[3] Like a good clinical study, a systematic review is prepared following a careful plan. Prestated methods for including and excluding relevant studies are used and primary studies that meet these criteria are used as "subjects" in the review. These criteria help to minimize bias and random errors.

The way in which the results are presented is called the *evidence synthesis.* The form that the evidence synthesis takes is based on the type of data reviewed. If the data are qualitative, then a *meta-synthesis* is carried out. If the data are quantitative and homogenous, then a *meta-analysis* is employed. If the quantitative data are not homogenous, then a *narrative summary* is used.[4] As Egger et al summarize, "Well conducted meta-analyses allow a more objective appraisal of the evidence than traditional narrative reviews, provide a more precise estimate of a treatment effect, and may explain heterogeneity between the results of individual studies."[5]

Finding Systematic Reviews and Meta-Analyses

Systematic reviews can be found in journals. They can also be specified as a methodology when searching in databases such as PEDro, CINAHL, and PubMed (see Chapter 11). However, systematic reviews are most easily found as a *Cochrane Review* in the Cochrane Library, which can be accessed directly, through PubMed, or through gateways, such as APTA's Open Door. A Cochrane Review is a systematic review of primary research. It is considered the gold standard of systematic reviews as it must be carried out according to a standardized and rigorous methodology. Jadad et al[6] found that Cochrane reviews are of comparable or better quality and are updated more often than reviews published in print journals. Therefore, they are a good starting point when looking for the answer to your clinical question.

There are several places to investigate within the Cochrane Library. As well as the Cochrane Database of Systematic Reviews (CDSR), the Cochrane Library includes the Cochrane Central Register of Controlled Trials (CENTRAL), with references to completed and ongoing randomized controlled trials; the Cochrane Methodology Register, with references to methodologic papers; and three other databases of systematic reviews (Database of Abstracts of Reviews of Effects—DARE), health technology assessment reports (HTA), and economic evaluations (HEED).[7]

Assessing the Quality of Reviews

The definition of systematic reviews, including meta-analyses, as provided by Chalmers and Altman[8] is, "a review that has been prepared using a systematic approach to *minimizing biases and random errors* which is documented in a materials and methods section." [Emphasis added] This seems a straightforward definition when, in fact, there are myriad sources of error and bias. Since these syntheses are so useful to clinicians seeking answers for their clinical questions, several appraisal tools have been developed to help clinicians recognize errors and biases, assess the value of the synthesis, and summarize the results from the synthesis, so that they can make good decisions about applying the results of other views. As we saw in discussing synopses of studies (see Chapter 14), evidence based researchers have developed statements to guide authors of systematic reviews and meta-analyses about the elements that should be included in these types of syntheses. The most well known of these statements is PRISMA (http://prisma-statement.org/statement.htm). In turn, these statements are also used by researchers in designing their studies and by journal editors in reviewing reports for publication. But, we will use the appraisal tool developed by the Critical Appraisal Skills Programme (CASP), which is a program within the Learning & Development Unit of the Public Health Resource Unit of the United Kingdom's National Health Service, as it is specifically designed for the reader of systematic reviews.

Ten Questions to Help You Make Sense of Reviews

The tool, 10 questions to help you make sense of reviews, is a popular and easy-to-use appraisal tool that provides a reader with an efficient and effective screen for determining the quality of a systematic review. (The tool is available for your personal use by downloading it from <http://sph.nhs.uk/sph-files/casp-appraisal-tools/S.Reviews%20Appraisal%20Tool.pdf/

view>.) This chapter will take each CASP question and present the pertinent issues. You may need to refer to previous chapters to cover methodological and statistical issues in greater detail. Each question can be answered by one of three options: Yes, Can't Tell, or No.

Screening Questions

The first two questions are designed for the clinician to determine if detailed reading of the review will be useful in answering the clinician's question.

1. Did the review ask a clearly focused question?

Consider if the question is "focused" in terms of:

- The population studied
- The intervention given or exposure
- The outcomes considered

2. Did the review include the right type of study?

Consider if the included studies:

- Address the review's question
- Have an appropriate design

In Chapter 10 we discussed the need for the research we seek to be focused on the four parts of the clinical question: Problem or Population, Intervention, Contrast intervention, and Outcome. We also discussed the importance of having the right Design type to match the question of interest (PICO + D). These two screening questions (1 and 2 above) can help clinicians determine that the review includes the right set of literature using the right designs.

One of the main issues to be considered before applying the results from a systematic review is whether or not the results are likely to be valid.[9] This issue will be revisited throughout this checklist. But, the first consideration of validity is the review's *face validity*; that is, does the topic appear to include the elements that make it relevant to the clinician, for the particular question?

Clearly Focused Question

Population: In the description of subjects, one must check that all the relevant details of the patients are provided, such as age, sex, diagnosis, and time since onset of problem. Also, these factors must be sufficiently narrow that the results are meaningful. For example, a review that looks at fracture healing rates should not combine results from teenagers through the elderly, unless they are divided into subgroups, given the inherent differences between the age groups. Physical therapists often find that a question is both clearly focused and well constructed but not *entirely relevant* to their patient. In this case, it is worth checking the review to see if a subgroup analysis has been carried out, which might be more closely related to a specific patient.

Intervention: A poor description of the intervention is frequently the downfall of a potentially good study. In many areas of physical therapy, treatment *philosophies* are compared without adequate description of the actual intervention. There is therefore no way of ensuring that treatments were equal, and they are certainly not reproducible. You may be surprised to find how few studies are included in a review of an area in which there has been much published. The application of rigorous standards for inclusion often results in a large cull of *inadequate* papers.

Contrast Intervention: Because of the nature of systematic reviews, they will not include contrast interventions, although they will discuss the interventions provided to any control groups.

Outcome: Because the decision to apply results has to be based on the changes in outcomes that the intervention produced, having a clear statement of outcomes is essential. It is also the only way that results can be compared across multiple studies.

Right Type of Studies

Applicability to Question: It can be frustrating at times to find a review of a related topic but one that does not answer your specific question. This is often the case as, through necessity, the question narrows the population, outcome, and intervention under consideration. For example, intervention studies in stroke often exclude so many comorbidities that the clinician has very few patients who match the sample.

An explanation of the importance of the information covered and how it fits into the context of previous work is a good sign. This should be followed by an explicit statement of the criteria used to choose the studies to be included in the review to protect against selection bias.

Design: Defining "appropriate" with regard to the study design is left to the clinician. Many consider the gold standard to be a randomized controlled trial (RCT), but this level of rigor has often not yet been carried out in physical therapy. And so the reviewers may have decided to accept studies that fall further down the Hierarchy of Evidence scale, such as an experimental study without randomization. In Chapter 12 we discussed several reasons, with their advantages and disadvantages, for choosing other research designs besides RCT (see Chapter 12). Of equal importance, and sometimes overlooked, is the fact that an RCT may not be the best design for a particular question. This may occur when the research question cannot be answered by a comparison at the time, for example, when there is no gold standard of treatment against which to compare. In this instance, a case series would be useful (see Chapter12). Finally, designs other than RCTs may have been considered because an RCT is unethical. This is often the case in physical therapy, where the optimal design would be to compare one intervention to no treatment.

Insisting upon carrying out reviews using only RCTs limits improvements to therapy practice. A compromise sometimes employed is the analysis of subgroups of information based on their design type. This helps to present the full spectrum of information available at the time. A good review also sets out the literature limitations in its introduction and explains its reasons for the choice of study designs included, thereby further educating the reader.

If the answers to the questions above are "Can't Tell" or "No," then the CASP authors suggest serious thought be given to whether it is worth continuing to read the review.

Detailed Questions: The Process of Review

The remaining questions focus on the quality of the review and also help the clinician determine if and how to apply the results of the review to their patients.

3. Did the reviewers try to identify all relevant studies?

Consider:

- Which bibliographic databases were used
- If there was follow-up from reference lists
- If there was personal contact with experts

- If the reviewers searched for unpublished studies
- If the reviewers searched for non-English-language studies

Identification of Studies: Including only some data available on a topic introduces systematic errors and threatens the validity of the results. A number of data sources are difficult and time-consuming to find, and yet, the effort needs to be made. Egger and Davey-Smith[10] found that among published studies, those with significant results are more likely to get published in English, more likely to be cited, and more likely to be published repeatedly, leading to English-language bias, citation bias, and multiple-publication bias. This likelihood that studies with significant results (the results show that the intervention had a significant positive, or sometimes negative, effect) are more likely to be submitted and accepted for publication than those that show no results is termed *publication bias.* Systematic reviews that do not consider difficult-to-access information may be prone to these biases. It is therefore important to note how a review has explicitly considered each of the following issues.

Databases: A sign of a high-quality review is a thorough search of the information available to answer the research question. This process should be sufficiently described to allow replication. The process begins with complete coverage of the databases used to find articles. The databases used depend on the topic, but a standard procedure within physical therapy would be to include a search of the databases in Box 15.1, all of which are discussed in greater detail in Chapter 11.

Use of Reference Lists: Researchers should explicitly state the measures they have taken to ensure thorough hand searching. At the very least, the Cochrane Collaboration should have been checked. Examples of good practice include searching through the reference lists from identified studies, systematic use of the "Related Articles" function within the databases searched, and a check of key journals over the past year (as it may take this long for them to appear in a database).

Unpublished and Gray Literature: A thorough review will take extra steps and search sources such as conference presentations, abstracts, posters, technical reports, theses, and unpublished data. These informally published pieces of work are known as gray literature. By including gray literature, a systematic review is better able to overcome publication bias.

Box 15.1	**Minimal Set of Databases to Be Included in a Thorough Systematic Review of a Physical Therapy–Related Topic**

Review Databases:
- Cochrane Database of Systematic Reviews
- Database of Abstracts of Reviews of Effects (DARE)
- American College of Physicians (ACP) Journal Club
- The Cochrane Central Register of Controlled Trials (CCTR)

Article Databases:
- Medline
- PubMed
- Cumulative Index of Nursing and Allied Health Literature (CINAHL)
- EMBASE
- Allied and Alternative Medicine Database (AMED)
- PEDro

Hopewell et al[11] investigated the impact of gray literature in meta-analyses of RCTs of health care intervention. Of five studies that compared the effect of the inclusion and exclusion of gray literature, all showed that published studies demonstrated a greater treatment effect than did the gray trials—as much as 9% when the data of three of these studies were combined. Burdett et al[12] looked at the combined effects of gray literature and non-English journals and found that they were less favorable, therefore moving the estimated treatment effect toward a null result.

A step beyond searching the gray literature is contacting researchers for unpublished data or ongoing work through discussion groups and contacting experts in the field. Davey-Smith and Egger[13] remind us of the danger in treating unpublished and published material in the same way. They suggest that unpublished data be heavily scrutinized, as it has not undergone peer review, and consideration be given to the possibility that its source may have a vested interest, for example, a manufacturer. Mosteller and Colditz[14] go so far as to recommend that data from unpublished work should be considered separately from peer-reviewed data. Therefore, a *discriminating* reader should:

- Look to see that a systematic review has searched the gray literature and included it where appropriate.
- Consider the amount and quality of the unpublished and gray literature presented. An overreliance on it would raise questions about the quality of the review.

Inclusion of Foreign-Language Information: To make the review comprehensive and accurate, evidence suggests that all articles in all languages should be included for consideration, to avoid publication bias secondary to the selective availability of data. Egger and Davey-Smith[14] suggest that "positive" findings may be more likely to be published in an international journal in English, whereas "negative" findings may be more likely to appear in a national journal in the original language. Other researchers have found that the exclusion of trials published in languages other than English did not affect the meta-analyses and therefore did not bias estimates of intervention effectiveness (Juni et al[15] and Moher et al[16]). The conclusion seems to be that the inclusion of *trials published in languages other than English* is a sign of a better quality review because the researchers have been thorough. However, evidence is insufficient at this stage to count a lack of inclusion against them. Reviews should be explicit about whether or not they used English-only publications.

4. Did the reviewers assess the quality of all relevant studies?

Consider:

- If a clear, predetermined strategy was used to determine which studies were included. Look for a scoring system and more than one assessor.

Quality of the Relevant Studies: It is essential that the reviewers choose only studies that meet certain standards of quality. The inclusion of poor-quality studies is likely to distort the results of a meta-analysis and the conclusions of the review and therefore inject bias into the review because of bias in the individual studies. As was discussed in Chapter 12, there are several types of bias that can affect internal validity, among them selection, performance, detection, and attrition bias. The quality of research is related to the means the researchers used to reduce each of these biases.

A Scoring System: A number of scales have been developed in an attempt to help the reader to assess the quality of systematic reviews and meta-analyses. Despite the large number of available scales, no single one has emerged as a clear favorite. We chose this CASP checklist because it considers the factors that are absolutely necessary to prevent types of bias and provides the best combination of effectiveness and efficiency.

Use of More Than One Assessor: Because of the subjective nature involved in choosing to include or exclude a study from a review, it is good practice for at least two assessors to have been involved in the decision making. Check to see that this has been stated, as well as a procedure for resolution of disagreements.

5. If the results of the studies have been combined, was it reasonable to do so?

Consider whether:

- The results of each study are clearly displayed
- The results were similar from study to study (look for tests of heterogeneity)
- The reasons for any variations in results are discussed

6. How are the results presented and what is the main result?

Consider:

- How the results are expressed (e.g., odds ratio, relative risk, etc.)
- How large the result is and how meaningful it is
- How you would sum up the bottom-line results of the review in one sentence

7. How precise are these results?

Consider:

- If a confidence interval were reported, would your decision about whether or not to use this intervention be the same at the upper confidence limit as at the lower confidence limit?
- If a *p*-value is reported where confidence intervals are unavailable

Integration of the Results of Multiple Studies

As we have said, often the research found on a given topic may be so disparate that the results of each study cannot be combined in any way and the reviewers must instead provide narrative summaries to help guide the clinician. But, sometimes, the research does have enough similarities in design, subjects, methods, and outcome measures that the results can be combined. This is especially helpful when the studies either have differing results or when the similar studies may have been too small to be able to glean useful effects. Finding that the research can be combined means that clinicians will have access to more powerful data to help in their decision making. Questions 5 through 7 all deal with this issue by asking if reviewers made the right decision in combining and if they combined appropriately. This combination is done through a series of statistical procedures known collectively as a *meta-analysis*. Meta-analyses are often, but not always, presented as part of a narrative review of the research studies. This means that clinicians can see the quantitative summary of the results as well as find synopses of each study. These three questions all deal with the quality of the methods used by the reviewers in combing results and will be discussed together.

Reasonableness of Combination: Clearly, the initial question a clinician must ask in reading the review is whether it was reasonable to combine the studies. There are many aspects to considering this question, as this is really an example of the old phrase "garbage in, garbage out" being true. First look at the actual articles. Does it make sense clinically to you that these articles are grouped together? Do these look like "good" articles to you based on the principles in Chapter 12?

Funnel Plots for Meta-Analysis: Earlier we discussed the problem of *publication bias*, that is, the possibility that the studies available for review overrepresent work that showed positive, large effect sizes, and underrepresent work that had non-statistically-significant results. Many authors of reviews use a *funnel plot* as the first part of their quantitative analysis to help screen for this problem. A typical funnel plot will have studies arranged by size on the vertical axis and by variance from the pooled estimate of effect size (often such measures as relative risk or odds ratio) of all the studies on the horizontal axis.[17–18] Studies with small samples tend to have greater variation in treatment effect due simply to chance, whereas the opposite is true for larger studies. Therefore when the available studies represent a range of results around the pooled estimate of effect, the cluster diagram will resemble an inverted funnel. An asymmetric funnel indicates a relationship between treatment effect and study size. If the reviewers find an asymmetrical result in the funnel plot, they have several options. One is to not proceed with further quantity analysis, but to do qualitative analysis, with a warning to the reader about the potential bias; another is to seek the gray literature discussed above and recalculate the funnel plot, since that may well result in greater symmetry; and a third is to determine reasonable causes of the asymmetry other than bias and proceed with the analysis. The important thing for the clinician is that the reviewer address the issue in a reasonable way that makes clinical sense.

Heterogeneity: While this type of assessment is a good start, using statistical analyses that take into account the variations in similar studies can provide more definitive data and removes any personal biases we may have about the studies. It is important to determine if the studies are similar enough to be grouped together. This question deals with the issue of *homogeneity* versus *heterogeneity*. We mentioned these concepts in Chapter 12 in reference to the variability in the subjects in a study. Here, we are asking how different were the populations, interventions, and outcomes studied? Are their results comparable? When you see a variety of effects of the intervention upon an outcome, it is important to be able to determine if the results are actually related to the intervention itself, and not the result of either *clinical heterogeneity*, that is, differences in populations, interventions, and outcomes themselves, or *methodological heterogeneity*, where there are differences in study design or quality.

Heterogeneity is measured statistically as part of the meta-analysis, as we discuss below. But the reviewers need to do several steps initially to make sure that it even makes sense to do the statistical analyses. The reviewer should identify issues that had good potential for causing heterogeneity at the beginning of the studies. A good review will show or state that a table of studies was developed to explore whether or not there are any unsuspected relationships that might have affected the size of the effect. If possible relationships are found, then subgroups should be established prior to even beginning the statistical analyses.

The results of each study should be displayed clearly and in a manner that allows easy comparison across studies. The format used by the Cochrane group is a good example. Here is an example taken from the systematic review, "Supportive devices for preventing and treating subluxation of the shoulder after stroke."[19] One can easily see in the summaries (Fig. 15-2) comparing Ancliffe[20] and Griffin[21] that the interventions and the outcomes are identical. However, as is often the case, there are some variations. The methods vary slightly (Griffin's study includes a placebo group), and the participants are also different (Ancliffe's subjects have more acute stroke, while Griffin's had a higher male-to-female ratio, a larger number of subjects, and a greater proportion of subjects with right hemiplegia).

Ancliffe 1992

Methods	Parallel group, single centre trial Exp: routine management (details not specified) + strapping C: routine management
Participants	Inclusion criteria: no history of shoulder pain, upper arm paralysis Age (mean): Exp/C = 69/74 years Time after stroke: Exp/C = <2/2 days Number of participants: Exp/C = 4/4 Male/Female = 4/4 Right/Left hemiplegia = 1/7 Dropouts: Exp/C = 0/0
Interventions	Strapping: one protecting pad and two strapping tapes were used. First the protecting pad was positioned on the medial surface of the upper arm to protect the axilla and allow for application of the tape. The first strapping tape began at the middle of the clavicle, continued across the deltoid muscle in a diagonal direction, along the pad under the arm. Then, a slight stretch was applied in the direction of the posterior fibres of the deltoid with the tape terminating one quarter of the way along the spine of the scapula. The second strapping tape was applied in the same direction as the first, but 2 cms below. Strapping was left on day and night and changed every three or four days.
Outcomes	Pain: number of pain-free days (<1 Ritchie Articular Index: 0 = patient has no tenderness, 1 = patient complains of pain, 2 = patient complains of pain and winces, 3 = patient complains of pain, winces, and withdraws, Bohannon 1986) after admission to study
Notes	

Risk of bias

Item	Authors' judgement	Description
Allocation concealment?	Unclear	D = not used

Figure 15-2 Examples of Qualitative Critique of Studies That Cannot Be Combined in a Meta-Analysis. *(Ancliffe A., 1992[20] and Griffin B., 2003[21].)*

If you find in a systematic review that there are apparent differences between the populations, interventions, or outcomes which you feel are sufficient to skew the results, this may be a sign of a poorer-quality review, particularly if the reviewer does not recognize the variability and discuss the implications, including the potential for future research.

Most first-time review readers, especially if they are reading in an area outside their expertise, will not feel capable of distinguishing between acceptable and unacceptable degrees of heterogeneity. In the example above, it is difficult to tell from just visual inspection whether or not the population variations prevent the groups from being comparable. In addition, because many studies are relatively small, it may be difficult to assess their results simply by examining the numerical results of individual studies (see Chapter 12). The use of a meta-analysis, combining the data from individual studies, allows the clinician to get a clearer picture of the intervention effects than does examining studies one at a time.

Presentation of Results in Forest Plots: A forest plot is part of a meta-analysis and is a way to visually present the results of the studies in the review. It provides information about the magnitude, direction, and precision of the individual effects of all the studies in one place.

Griffin 2003

Methods	Parallel group, single centre trial Exp: strapping + routine management (could include task-specific re-education for function, maintenance of ROM, provision of supportive devices for the arm) Placebo: placebo strapping + routine management C: routine management
Participants	Inclusion criteria: within 4 weeks of stroke, no history of shoulder pain, score on Item 6 of the Motor Assessment scale of less then 4, score on Ritchie Articular Index of less than 2. Age (mean): Exp/P/C = 65/62/59 years Time after stroke (mean): Exp/P/C = 10/10/12 days
	Number of participants: Exp/P/C = 9/10/12 Male/Female = 22/10 Right/Left hemiplegia = 20/12 Dropouts: Exp/P/C = 1/0/0
Interventions	Strapping: one protecting pad and two strapping tapes were used. First the protecting pad was positioned on the medial surface of the upper arm to protect the axilla and allow for application of the tape. The first strapping tape began at the middle of the clavicle, continued across the deltoid muscle in a diagonal direction, along the pad under the arm. Then, a slight stretch was applied in the direction of the posterior fibres of the deltoid with the tape terminating one quarter of the way along the spine of the scapula. The second strapping tape was applied in the same direction as the first, but 2 cms below. Strapping was left on day and night and changed every three or four days.
Outcomes	Pain: number of pain-free days (<2 Ritchie Articular Index: 0 = patient has no tenderness, 1 = patient complains of pain, 2 = patient complains of pain and winces, 3 = patient complains of pain, winces, and withdraws, Bohannon 1986) after admission to study
Notes	
Risk of bias	

Item	Authors' judgement	Description
Allocation concealment?	Yes	A - Adequate

Figure 15-2, cont'd

Forest plots can provide an amazing array of information to clinicians, once all parts of it become clear. See Figure 15-3 for an analysis of a forest plot from a review of progressive resistance training.[22]

As can be seen from the figure, the forest plot can provide all of this information in its visual display:

- The independent and dependent variable being analyzed in the plot (A)
- The number of total studies in the review being summarized in the forest plot (B)
- The authors and year of publication for each article (B)
- The results from each study (mean, standard deviation, and number of subjects in each group, (C))
- The relative weight of each study in the analysis based on its sample size (D)
- A numerical reporting of the confidence intervals for these studies (E)

Figure 1. Forest plot of comparison: 1 PRT versus control, outcome: 1.1 Main function measure (higher score = better function).

Study or Subgroup	PRT Mean	SD	Total	Control Mean	SD	Total	Weight	Std. Mean Difference IV, Fixed, 95% CI	Std. Mean Difference IV, Fixed, 95% CI
Baker 2001	63.4	29	19	60.8	30	19	1.8%	0.09 [-0.55, 0.72]	
Bean 2004	10.4	1.3	11	9.5	1.5	9	0.9%	0.62 [-0.29, 1.53]	
Boshuizen 2005	-27.5	9.6	16	-28.2	7.9	17	1.5%	0.08 [-0.61, 0.76]	
Brochu 2002	65	21	19	76	17	14	1.4%	-0.55 [-1.26, 0.15]	
Buchner 1997	69	39	22	74	28	29	2.3%	-0.15 [-0.70, 0.41]	
Chandler 1998	44.2	20.4	44	42.5	25.8	43	4.1%	0.07 [-0.35, 0.49]	
Chin A Paw 2006	39.5	8	40	40.8	9.1	32	3.3%	-0.15 [-0.62, 0.31]	
Damush 1999	81.8	18.8	33	80.7	24.2	29	2.9%	0.05 [-0.45, 0.55]	
de Vreede 2007	50.1	9.2	28	49.6	9	26	2.5%	0.05 [-0.48, 0.59]	
Donald 2000	12.7	4.7	25	11.4	4.9	20	2.1%	0.27 [-0.32, 0.86]	
Ettinger 1997	-1.74	0.4	120	-1.9	0.3	127	11.3%	0.45 [0.20, 0.71]	
Foley 2003	61.17	14.11	26	53.49	22.37	32	2.6%	0.40 [-0.13, 0.92]	
Hiatt 1994	45	22	9	53	13	8	0.8%	-0.41 [-1.38, 0.55]	
Jette 1999	-7.5	9.9	92	-9.8	12.1	104	9.1%	0.21 [-0.08, 0.49]	
Katznelson 2006	85	12	15	75	21	16	1.4%	0.56 [-0.16, 1.28]	
Latham 2003	35.6	25.9	113	38.7	28.4	117	10.7%	-0.11 [-0.37, 0.15]	
Liu-Ambrose 2005	-14.9	13.3	32	-19.8	14.4	32	2.9%	0.35 [-0.14, 0.84]	
Mangione 2005	57.7	21.1	11	48	18.9	10	0.9%	0.46 [-0.41, 1.33]	
Mikesky 2006	-30.09	13.11	57	-30.03	11.14	75	6.1%	-0.00 [-0.35, 0.34]	
Miller 2006	35.3	11.1	25	32.1	9.8	26	2.4%	0.30 [-0.25, 0.85]	
Miszko 2003	57.7	10	13	57	18	15	1.3%	0.05 [-0.70, 0.79]	
Moreland 2001	63.9	16.9	68	65.5	17.3	65	6.2%	-0.09 [-0.43, 0.25]	
Ouellette 2004	47.8	9.39	20	47.8	9.62	21	1.9%	0.00 [-0.61, 0.61]	
Schilke 1996	-7.6	3.5	10	-9.5	4	10	0.9%	0.48 [-0.41, 1.38]	
Segal 2003	120.2	15.9	82	117.6	14.9	73	7.2%	0.17 [-0.15, 0.48]	
Seynnes 2004	-0.52	0.59	8	-1	0.93	8	0.7%	0.58 [-0.42, 1.59]	
Sims 2006	12.45	2	14	12.25	1.4	16	1.4%	0.11 [-0.60, 0.83]	
Singh 1997	82.6	18.4	17	70.3	27.8	15	1.4%	0.52 [-0.19, 1.22]	
Singh 2005	71	24	18	72.8	22.6	19	1.7%	-0.08 [-0.72, 0.57]	
Topp 2002	-35.3	10.82	35	-39.7	10.82	35	3.2%	0.40 [-0.07, 0.88]	
Tracy 2004	-27.6	5.51	11	-27.4	5.04	9	0.9%	-0.04 [-0.92, 0.84]	
Tsutsumi 1997	91.9	7.5	13	75.7	26.4	14	1.2%	0.80 [0.01, 1.59]	
Westhoff 2000	-28.4	7.5	10	-23.1	6.6	11	0.9%	-0.72 [-1.61, 0.17]	
Total (95% CI)			**1076**			**1096**	**100.0%**	**0.14 [0.05, 0.22]**	

Heterogeneity: Chi² = 35.93, df = 32 (P = 0.29); I² = 11%
Test for overall effect: Z = 3.13 (P = 0.002)

Favours control Favours PRT

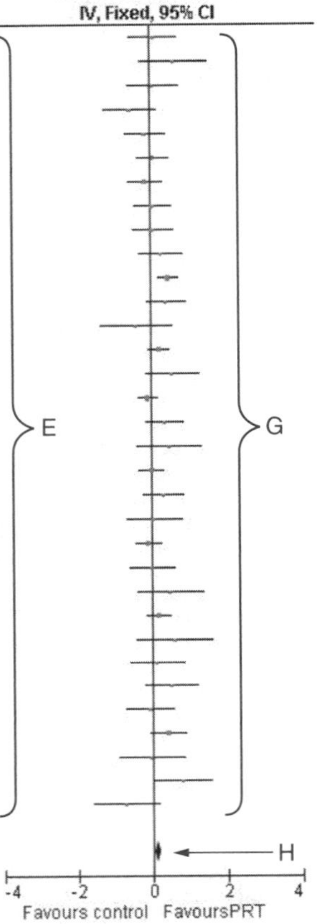

Forest plot of comparison: 1 PRT versus control, outcome: 1.1 Main function measure (higher score = better function).

Figure 15-3 Example of a Forest Plot.

- A uniform scale (e.g., standardized mean difference) to allow comparisons across the studies when a common outcome scale has not been used (E)
- Statistics (chi-square being the most common) to help determine if the level of heterogeneity is satisfactory (F)
- A plot of the relative outcomes of each study that shows:
  - By length of line, the full confidence interval
  - By size of symbol, the relative sample size, and
  - By location on each side of the centerline (no differences between groups), the direction and strength of the results (G)
- A summary line that shows the results from the integration of the studies in the review (H)

By scanning the forest plot, a clinician can immediately see the depth of literature available, the sample size and results of each study, and the individual and collective weighted results. For example, in this systematic review of progressive resistive exercise, the reviewers identified 33 studies that measured change in function (using a variety of tools) with a total of 2172 subjects. Twenty-six of these studies had results favoring progressive resistive exercise, and the weighted standardized mean difference for all the studies also favors the intervention. Because the outcome measured varied, necessitating the use of a uniform scale, we cannot identify the degree of clinical change that this represents.

Managing Heterogeneity: As we have mentioned, reviewers may decide that there are subgroups of studies based on differences in either the designs (methodological or statistical heterogeneity) or in the subjects, interventions, or outcome measures (clinical heterogeneity). Subgroup analyses can offer a solution to both of these types of heterogeneity. For example, a reviewer might divide studies into randomized controlled trials (RCTs) and nonrandomized controlled trials. In this way, analysis of the results from the RCTs will not be confounded by the potentially less reliable results from the nonrandomized studies. (See Chapter 12 for a discussion of why the results may be less reliable.) Or the reviewers may develop separate forest plots (as in our example systematic review) for studies that used different outcome measures or different subjects.

Precision of the Results: Whether or not a forest plot is provided, summary statistics are used to give readers the results of the review. Using the wrong statistics or misinterpreting the results of the statistics can result in two types of errors. It is possible to miss a clinically important result, and it is also possible to produce results that appear clinically important, but actually are not.

The most common statistics used are the odds ratio and the relative risk (sometimes expressed as a risk ratio). They are appropriately used for assessing dichotomous data, where the outcome for each participant is one of two possibilities, for example, harmed or benefited. Both of these statistics compare the likelihood of an event between two groups. The odds ratio provides the *strongest mathematical result*, but the risk ratio provides the *more easily interpreted result*.

It is important to understand when their use is appropriate and why a researcher or reviewer might choose to use one over the other. Although in everyday language we use the terms *risk* and *odds* synonymously, this is not the case in statistics. They may be used to describe the same data, but they are expressed very differently. Relative risk is often preferred because it more closely matches how we think. When the risk is 0.25, or 25%, we know that 25 people out of 100 will be affected. However, some designs prevent its use, particularly the case-control design, which selects research subjects on the basis of the outcome rather than on the exposure.

When reading a systematic review, it is important that you know which of these statistics is used. As both are graphed on a scale where the center value is 1, it is not immediately obvious which statistic is being displayed. A common mistake is the misinterpretation of odds ratios as risk ratios, causing an overestimation of the benefits and harms of an intervention. Deeks and Altman[23] suggest that use of both statistics provides the most useful information— the odds ratio could be used for mathematical *strength* while the risk ratio could then be presented for *ease* of interpretation. This is not a necessary requirement for a high-quality review, but it is a mark of deeper consideration by the review authors if it is provided.

It is also important to recognize the differences between the two for clinical relevance. This sounds obvious, but whereas a risk of 0.5 (50% chance of an event) is equivalent to odds of 1 (for every 2 people, 1 will experience an event) is easy to see, a risk of 0.95 being equivalent to odds of 19 is not.[24] Interestingly, McGettigan et al[25] found that the choice of the statistic used to present a result affected doctors' opinions or intended practices. In a systematic review of 12 RCTs, 8 compared the framing of a result as a relative risk reduction, absolute risk reduction, or number needed to treat. The authors found that the risk ratio (relative risk reduction) was viewed most positively.

Result Size and Its Meaning: Statistical significance tells us nothing about the size of the effect or its clinical relevance. For effect size, one must go back to the forest plots of relative risk and odds ratios and the summary effects of each. Be sure to review the presentation of these values, paying special attention to the midline of "no effect." The further the point estimate of effect is from the line of no effect, the greater the magnitude of the effect. But how do you determine the absolute magnitude of the effects and how much should this influence clinical practice? Are the results relevant to all your patients within the same population parameters, or only to a subset? These are questions you must answer from a clinical perspective.

Another important aspect of interpreting the results of a meta-analysis is consideration of the summary effect produced by the statistical model used. There are two: the fixed effect model and the random effects model. One of these two statistical methods will be used to analyze the pooled data. Note that our example uses a fixed effect. Because of the nature of these two analyses, a random effects model may overemphasize the importance of smaller studies with poorer quality. A fixed effect model gives preferential weighting to larger studies, thereby producing a more narrow summary effect. This may incorrectly give the impression of greater precision of the effect. Although the type of model used will not help you to determine a good-quality review from a poor one, bearing in mind the caveats of each will make you a more discerning reader, better able to interpret and apply the results appropriately.

Meta-analyses must be done carefully and appropriately to be useful to clinicians. A perceptive reader will look for the issues of bias and clinical and methodological heterogeneity, as previously discussed, as well as carefully consider the clinical meaning of the numerical values that represent the study results.

Detailed Questions: The Bottom-Line Results of the Review

Ultimately, the bottom line presented by the reviewers should explicitly answer the initial research question. This does not mean that the answer definitively shows harm or benefit, but that it provides an accurate portrayal of the data and their meaning. The bottom line in physical therapy is too often that the effectiveness of a treatment cannot be determined with the data available at the present time. Particularly in areas where research has been investigating the effectiveness of a practice that has been key to physical therapy, this may come as a surprise. Cautious interpretation may lead to suggestions for clinical practice in this case, but the reviewer should not make claims beyond the results of the current research. Updates of the review may find stronger relationships or effects in the future, but then again, perhaps not!

8. Can the results be applied to the local population?

Consider whether:

- The population sample covered by the review could be different from your population in ways that would produce different results
- Your local setting differs much from that of the review
- You can provide the same intervention in your setting

Applicability to Your Patient: The first step is to go back to the initial research question and be sure that it is answered. Sometimes the literature is not sufficiently robust at the time to provide a definitive answer, or the availability of literature is so limited that answers of significant power do not apply to *your* patient. The second step is to determine if the results are statistically significant, and if so, are they clinically important/relevant? And finally, you must determine if the results are pertinent to your specific patient(s). Sometimes a "bottom-line" that considers clinical effectiveness, as well as feasibility and meaningfulness of the intervention, will be included in the review. This is handy but still requires your judgment for applicability to your patients. Points to consider in making that judgment include:

• Are the subjects and the intervention sufficiently described to allow comparison to your patients?
• Was the intervention effective in all patient subgroups?
• Were the outcomes used in the studies relevant to your patients?

These would appear to be obvious points, but there may be subtle but important differences between your patient population and those considered in the review. For example, many studies consider the effect of muscle strength training upon the "elderly" but do not subdivide age groups. If you are treating patients primarily over 80, then a review that defines the subjects as "over 65 years" is not likely to be adequately specific, and therefore applicable, to your patients. Particularly if you are unable to find a review whose patients match your own, it is imperative that you know enough about the features that do not match to be able to gauge their relative importance. So in the previous example, you would need to investigate whether the age difference might be an important factor, and in this case the evidence would suggest that it is.

Often the issue is that your patient is not "ideal," that is, he or she would not have met the inclusion criteria for the studies due to comorbidities. In the example above, the recommendation is not clear-cut. An understanding of the pathophysiology of the disease and the proposed mechanism of action of the treatment is necessary to make a decision whether or not to apply the results to your patient.

Systematic reviews are not just carried out to ascertain treatment effectiveness. Feasibility of treatment is also an important question, so the type of study design is a consideration. Unfortunately, many of these kinds of practical clinical questions will not have been addressed in the literature, especially if they do not lend themselves to an RCT format. An example would be the decision making for cost-effectiveness.

Number Needed to Treat: If your question involves cost or time, going back to the number needed to treat (NNT, the inverse of the absolute risk reduction) may give guidance. Knowing how many people must be treated before you see benefit may help you to decide if the intervention is warranted. It is up to the clinician to decide the level of the NNT before it is worth changing practice. Some authors suggest an NNT of three or less indicates adopting the treatment.[26] However, that depends on the value of the outcome. If the outcome is the prevention of serious pain, then a much larger NNT would still be considered worthwhile. If the value of the outcome is not so clear, then a consideration of the number needed to harm (NNH) may help in the decision making (see Chapter 12 for further detail). As the NNT increases, then patient and clinic resources become more of a consideration, as more patients must receive the treatment before one new patient improves. In fact, a treatment with little resource requirements might seem preferable over one with a better NNT, if this improves overall service provision.

9. Were all important outcomes considered?

Consider outcomes from the point of view of the:

- Individual
- Policy makers and professionals
- Family/careers
- Wider community

The first aspect to consider is whether or not the outcome measures used in the studies are the same as, or relevant to, those you use in the clinic. In many areas of physical therapy, this is a big issue, as often outcome measures of activity are used when clinicians are most interested in the effects of treatment upon functional and structural integrity. For example, you are working with a stroke patient in an acute rehabilitation setting and you are interested in increasing the movement available in the affected leg to improve his safety in walking. You come across a systematic review of an intervention that uses the Functional Independence Measure (FIM) as the outcome measure, and it shows that there is a significant decrease in need for assistance while walking. But this does not tell you what aspect of movement improved to allow greater independence—was it flexibility, strength, balance? In an ideal world, the research and clinical measures would be the same; when they are not, you will need to carry out your own cost/benefit analysis and use your clinical judgment.

Another consideration will be whether the outcomes are meaningful to the experiences, values, and beliefs of your patients, as well as whether there are aspects of the intervention that are likely to upset a patient and negatively affect the outcome. To use the stroke patient example—he may feel too easily fatigued to agree to an intensive treadmill training regimen, which has been shown to be effective in similar patients but is upsetting to him.

10. Should policy or practice change as a result of the evidence contained in this review?

Consider:

- Whether any benefit reported outweighs any harm and/or cost. If this information is not reported, can it be filled in from elsewhere?

In addition to considering the positive value added by implementing such policy change, as we've discussed in preceding questions, it is essential to balance this with the potential harm from implementing the change. Recent research often includes information on mortality, morbidity, quality of life, cost-effectiveness, and patient satisfaction.[27] "Harm" is rarely measured as such; more often, data is collected on causes of dropout or side effects. This makes a benefit/harm analysis lopsided. Therefore, the best you might do is to consider benefit and cost, which were covered with NNT analysis in Question 8.

Synthesis Conclusion

Systematic reviews can provide a quick answer to your clinical questions. Despite the best attempts to make data quantifiable and systematic reviews objective, there are many opportunities throughout the process to introduce subjectivity. Regardless of the number of people involved (and sometimes because of the number of people involved), each time a decision is made about methodological quality or the presence of unacceptable heterogeneity, bias may be introduced. Ultimately, the clinicians will impose their judgment upon the quality of a review by using the guidelines above. It is hoped that by using the CASP guidelines these decision will be better informed.

SYNOPSES OF SYNTHESES

Systematic reviews are very valuable because they synthesize so much information in one place. But this very comprehensiveness means that they there are often quite long and somewhat daunting for a clinician to use. Cochrane reviews now include a "plain language" summary of the full review, but even these summaries can reach over 50 pages in length. In response to this, synopses of systematic reviews are being created, just as they have been created for individual studies.

The largest source of synopses of systematic reviews is the Database of Abstracts of Reviews of Effects (DARE). DARE was created and is maintained by the Centre for Reviews and Dissemination of the University of York (United Kingdom). Potential reviews of interventions are identified by searching leading journals, bibliographic databases, gray literature, and selected Web sites. The reviews are then assessed by two researchers who determine inclusion by assessing the reviews against these five criteria:

1. Were inclusion/exclusion criteria reported?
2. Was the search adequate?
3. Were the included studies synthesized?
4. Was the validity of the included studies assessed?
5. Are sufficient details about the individual included studies presented?

To be included, the review must meet at least four of these criteria, including 1 to 3, which are required. Each abstract includes review methods, results, and conclusions and provides a critical assessment of the systematic review. Each abstract is shared with the systematic review authors for correction of factual errors before publication. (See Fig. 15-4.) DARE can be found at many databases, such as Ovid or APTA's Open Door.

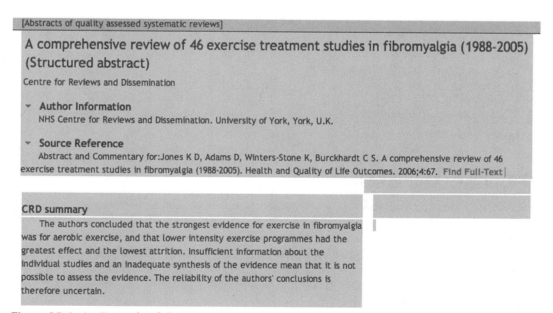

[Abstracts of quality assessed systematic reviews]

A comprehensive review of 46 exercise treatment studies in fibromyalgia (1988-2005) (Structured abstract)

Centre for Reviews and Dissemination

▾ **Author Information**
NHS Centre for Reviews and Dissemination. University of York, York, U.K.

▾ **Source Reference**
Abstract and Commentary for:Jones K D, Adams D, Winters-Stone K, Burckhardt C S. A comprehensive review of 46 exercise treatment studies in fibromyalgia (1988-2005). Health and Quality of Life Outcomes. 2006;4:67. Find Full-Text

CRD summary
The authors concluded that the strongest evidence for exercise in fibromyalgia was for aerobic exercise, and that lower intensity exercise programmes had the greatest effect and the lowest attrition. Insufficient information about the individual studies and an inadequate synthesis of the evidence mean that it is not possible to assess the evidence. The reliability of the authors' conclusions is therefore uncertain.

Figure 15-4 An Example of the Narrative Results From a DARE Abstract.

Synopses of syntheses can be found from many other sources as well; for example, they are published in evidence based journals, such as a synopsis of a systematic review of exercise to improve depressive symptoms that was published in *Mental Health*.[28] *Physical Therapy* has begun publication of a series known as Linking Evidence and Practice (LEAP). LEAP articles are based on actual patient scenarios and provide useful clinical information from systematic reviews available from the Cochrane Collaborative and other reliable sources. Their goal is to improve the application of information from systematic review to daily physical therapy practice.[29,30]

Just as the number of synopses of individual studies has increased, there will be an increase in the number of synopses of syntheses. These synopses can provide information to clinicians in a way that is clinically useful. They can also be created by clinicians as a useful way to share the literature among themselves at events such as journal clubs and as part of professional development programs.[31] There will also be an increase in articles that bring together the results of several systematic reviews.[32]

CONCLUSION

Syntheses and their synopses can serve the clinician by gathering the results of many individual studies in one source. As with all sources of evidence, the clinician must assess the quality of systematic reviews before implementing their recommendations. This assessment includes an examination of the technical components of the review but also involves a clinical judgment about the applicability of the findings to specific patient questions.

SELF-ASSESSMENT

1. Find a systematic review related to the value of aerobic exercise for improvement of cardiovascular status in patients with cardiovascular disease. Using the CASP questions, determine the quality of the systematic review.
2. Does the systematic review give you enough information to determine if the results apply to patients like Mr. Ketterman? Does it give you enough information to design a specific intervention?
3. Identify three or four systematic reviews on topics of interest to you that contain forest plots. Examine each of the elements of the forest plots and then write a few paragraphs that translate these points into a narrative. Do you prefer the graphic presentation of the forest plot or the narrative form?

CONTINUED LEARNING

- Arrange a journal club session in your practice where each participant presents systematic reviews.
- Writing a systematic review is a challenging activity but one that can help clinicians bring together a body of literature to answer important clinical questions. Writing a review is also an excellent way to gain mastery of search and assessment skills. The best guide to writing a systematic review is the Cochrane Collaboration's Handbook, which can be found at www.cochrane.org/training/cochrane-handbook.

REFERENCES

1. Haynes RB. Of studies, syntheses, synopses, summaries, and systems: The "5S" evolution of information services for evidence-based healthcare decisions. Evid Based Med. 2006;11:162–164.
2. DiCenso A, Bayley L, Haynes RB. Accessing pre-appraised evidence: Fine-tuning the 5S model into a 6S model. Evid Based Nurs. 2009;12:99–101.
3. Mulrow CD, Cook DJ, Davidoff F. Systematic reviews: Critical links in the great chain of evidence. Ann Intern Med 1997;126(5):389–391.
4. Hemingway P, Brereton N (April 2009). What is a systematic review? http://www.whatisseries.co.uk/whatis/pdfs/What_is_syst_rev.pdf Accessed on July 21, 2010.
5. Egger M, Davey-Smith G, Phillips AN. Meta-analysis: Principles and procedures. BMJ. 1997;315:1533–1537.
6. Jadad AR, Cook DJ, Jones A, Klassen TP, Tugwell P, Moher M, et al. Methodology and reports of systematic reviews and meta-analyses: A comparison of Cochrane reviews with articles published in paper-based journals. JAMA. 1998;280:278–280.
7. Grimshaw J. So what has the Cochrane Collaboration ever done for us? A report card on the first 10 years. CMAJ. 2004;171(7):747–749.
8. Altman D, Chalmers I, eds. *Systematic Reviews*. London: BMJ Publishing Group; 1999.
9. Oxman AD. Systematic reviews: Checklists for review articles. BMJ. 1994;309:648–651.
10. Egger M, Davey-Smith G. Meta-analysis bias in location and selection of studies. BMJ. 1998;316:61–66.
11. Hopewell S, McDonald S, Clarke M, Egger M. Grey literature in meta-analyses of randomized trials of health care interventions. Cochrane Database Systematic Reviews. 1,200.9
12. Burdett S, Stewart L, Tierney J. Publication bias and meta-analyses: A practical example. Int J Tech. Assessment in Health Care. 2003;19(1):129–134.
13. Davey-Smith G, Egger M. Meta-analysis: Unresolved issues and future developments. BMJ. 1998;316:221–225.
14. Mosteller F, Colditz GA. Understanding research synthesis (meta-analysis). Ann Rev Pub Health. 1996;17:1–23.
15. Jüni P, Witschi A, Bloch R, Egger M. The hazards of scoring the quality of clinical trials for meta-analysis. JAMA.1999;282:1054–1060.
16. Moher D, Pham Ba', Klassen TP, Schulz KF, Berline JA, Jadad AR, Liberati A. What contributions do languages other than English make on the results of meta-analyses? J Clin Epidemiol. 2000;53:964–972.
17. Sterne JAC, Egger M, Davey-Smith G. Investigating and dealing with publication and other bias. In: Egger M, Davey-Smith G, Altman DG, eds. *Systematic Reviews in Health Care: Meta-Analysis in Context*, 2nd ed. London: BMJ Books; 2001.
18. Egger M, Davey-Smith G, Schneider M, Minder C. Bias in meta-analysis detected by a simple graphical test. BMJ. 1997;315:629–624.
19. Ada L, Foongchomcheay A, Canning CG. Supportive devices for preventing and treating subluxation of the shoulder after stroke. Cochrane Database of Systematic Reviews. 1, 2005.
20. Ancliffe J. Strapping the shoulder in patients following a cerebrovascular accident (CVA): A pilot study. Austral J Physiother. 1992;38:37–34.
21. Griffin AL, Bernhardt J. Strapping of the hemiplegic shoulder prevents development of shoulder pain during rehabilitation. 1st Neurological Physiotherapy Conference of the National Neurology Group of the Australian Physiotherapy Association. 27–29 November 2003:Sydney, Australia.
22. Liu Chiung-ju, Latham NK. Progressive resistance strength training for improving physical function in older adults. Cochrane Database of Systematic Reviews 2009, Issue 3. Art. No.: CD002759. DOI: 10.1002/14651858.CD002759.pub2.
23. Deeks JJ, Altman DG, Bradburn MJ. Statistical methods for examining heterogeneity and combining results from several studies in meta-analysis. In: Egger M, Davey-Smith G, Altman DG. *Systematic Reviews in Health Care: Meta-Analysis in Context*, 2nd ed. London: BMJ Books; 2001.

24. Cochrane Handbook for Systematic Reviews of Interventions. www.cochrane.org/ training/cochrane-handbook. Accessed on July 31, 2009.
25. McGettigan P, Sly K, O'connell D, Hill S, Henry D. The effects of information framing on the practices of physicians. J Gen Intern Med. 1999;14(10):633–642.
26. McQuay HJ, Moore RA. Using numerical results from systematic reviews in clinical practice. Ann Intern Med. 1997;126:712–720.
27. Ciliska D, Cullum N, Marks S. Evaluation of systematic reviews of treatment or prevention interventions. Evid Based Nurs. 2007;4:100–104.
28. Review: Exercise may moderately improve depressive symptoms. Evid. Based Ment. Health. 2009;12;77–78.
29. Jette DU, Buchbinder R. PTJ helps clinicians link evidence to patient care. Phys Ther. 2010;90:6–7.
30. Lin C-W C, Taylor D, Bierma-Zeinstra SMA, Maher CG. Exercise for osteoarthritis of the knee. Phys Ther. 2010;90:839–842.
31. Oermann MH, Floyd JA, Galvin EA, Roop JC. Brief reports for disseminating systematic reviews to nurses. Clin Nurse Spec. 2006;20:233–238.
32. Taylor NF, Dodd KJ, Damiano DL. Progressive resistance exercise in physical therapy: A summary of systematic reviews. Phys Ther. 2005;85:1208–1223.

chapter 16

Summaries and Systems

Computers are useless. They can only tell you answers.

—Pablo Picasso

•

✳ Mr. Ketterman's Case

While I have found lots of literature about individual aspects of Mr. Ketterman's care, I really need help thinking about his whole plan of care. Can't I find some information that will help me through the whole process from diagnosis and prognosis to selection of intervention and choice of outcome measurements? *(See Appendix for Mrs. Ketterman's health history.)*

INTRODUCTION

As we have seen, studies (Chapters 12 and 13), synopses of studies (Chapter 14), and syntheses and synopses of syntheses (Chapter 15) all offer clinicians evidence that can help guide clinical decision making in patient-centered physical therapy care. But we also have seen that in almost all cases, this evidence is focused on one specific aspect of that care, be it diagnostic and prognostic tests or interventions. As clinicians, we want to understand the evidence about the full range of care we provide to patients. The efficiency of having the entire pattern of care reviewed becomes even more obvious when we are focusing on a patient population that represents a large part of our practice. *Summaries* and *systems*, the final two elements of Haynes's 6S pyramid (Fig. 16-1) offer us just such information.[1,2] They integrate a range of evidence across available studies and syntheses to provide guidance about management of a particular health problem.[1]

SUMMARIES

Practice Guidelines

Perhaps the most common form of summary is an evidence-based clinical practice guideline.[1–2] Because the term *guideline* is used in so many different contexts, we will take a step back to come to a common definition before proceeding with resources and examples. Eddy[3] has described in detail the different kinds of policy statements available to guide care, as is shown in Figure 16-2. Along the width (*x*-axis) of the cube is the intended use of any policy, ranging

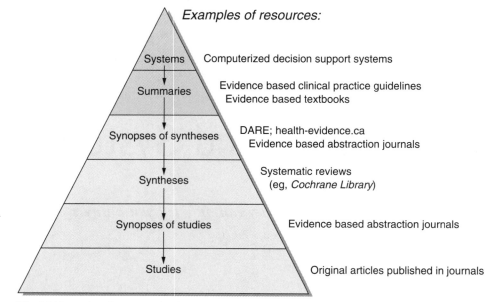

Figure 16-1 Sources of Information About Evidence. *(From DiCenso A, Bayley L, Haynes RB. Accessing pre-appraised evidence: Fine-tuning the 5S model into a 6S model. Evid Based Nurs. 2009;12:99–101.)*

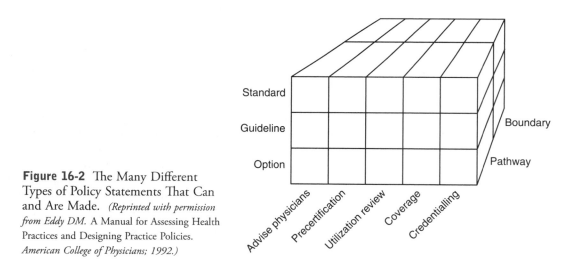

Figure 16-2 The Many Different Types of Policy Statements That Can and Are Made. *(Reprinted with permission from Eddy DM.* A Manual for Assessing Health Practices and Designing Practice Policies. *American College of Physicians; 1992.)*

from providing advice, through approvals for payment, to approvals for allowing practice, such as credentialing by facilities and insurance companies. Most of us have experienced policies governing each of these functions. In this chapter we are primarily interested in the use of policies based on evidence to provide advice, although it is certainly possible that payers and employers may develop policies based on evidence.

Along the depth (z-axis) of the cube is the type of guidance intended. Will the policy dictate a particular path to which the practitioner adheres, or will it set limits within which the practitioner chooses among various options? Again, we are familiar with these two options.

Many facilities have developed clinical paths to help provide optimal care to groups of patients.[4] The *Guide to Physical Therapist Practice* is a leading example of a boundary-type policy document. The *Guide* includes over 30 practice patterns that outline acceptable options for examination, intervention, and outcome measurement for specific patient populations.[5] It is up to the clinician to choose from among these options as appropriate for the individual patient.

Along the height (*y*-axis) of the cube is the intended flexibility range of the policy statement. The most rigorous type of practice policy is the standard. When we are able to reach a high level of certainty about what *ought* to happen, then the policy can be called a standard and the practitioner can be held accountable for meeting the standard. Penalties for lack of conformance to the standard can include loss of licensure, malpractice litigation, denial of payment, or loss of employment. Obviously, such high-stake penalties mean that the standard must be supported by a very high level of evidence that it is, indeed, the correct standard. Eddy[3] states that development and adoption of standards should be based not only the scientific evidence but also on the nearly unanimous clinical wisdom of practitioners and nearly unanimous agreement among patients about the desirability (or undesirability) of the outcome of the care adopted in the standard. At this writing, there are no published standards that are specific to physical therapy. Of course, there are standards of care that cross disciplines, such as those related to infection control, which are applicable to physical therapists. But the total number of things in health care about which relatively unanimous agreement can be reached is very small.

At the next level on this axis are guidelines. When we have enough information to make decisions about the appropriate use of a test or an intervention, and a majority of clinicians and patients would agree about the desirability (or undesirability) of the outcome of the care, then they can be considered guidelines. Guidelines serve as recommendations about what is *preferred* in practice. Clinicians may well choose to do something different, but that choice should be based on factors such as a patient's health variability and preferences. We'll discuss later the growing body of policy statements that are offered specifically to physical therapists as clinical guidelines, as well as the many guidelines that are cross-disciplinary in nature. Despite the growing number of guidelines, they still cover only a small fraction of practice.

At the third level on this axis is the category of option. A policy statement should be considered an option if there is some uncertainty about outcomes of the particular test or intervention, or if clinicians' and patients' preferences about the outcomes are unknown, unclear, or equivocal. The practice patterns in the *Guide to Physical Therapist Practice*[5] represent a good example of policy documents that offer clinicians options for selecting examination tools and interventions for identified patient groups.

The *Guide to Physical Therapist Practice* has three sections. The introduction and "Part One: A Description of Patient/Client Management" provide a framework for care (see Chapter 1). This section also includes a comprehensive listing of the various tests and measures used by physical therapists in examining patients and measuring their outcomes, as well as the interventions they provide. The second section is a compilation of several practice patterns that we will discuss later. The third section is made up of several appendices that include important resources for practicing clinicians, including many of the American Physical

Therapy Association's clinical policies, documentation templates, and a sample patient satisfaction survey.

The practice patterns are descriptions of the care that have been determined by experts to be preferred for certain categories of patients. They are not limited to randomized controlled clinical trials, and they are not systematic reviews, but rather they are summaries of the best advice from a number of experts. As such, they are *not* guidelines as we are discussing them in this chapter, but they are examples of policy documents that provide options, by setting boundaries for care for a variety of purposes, including providing advice to practitioners and recommendations for coverage and payment decisions. Because of the important roles they play in clinical practice, it is useful for all clinicians to understand them.

Patterns are developed for the four systems that represent the majority of physical therapy care: musculoskeletal, neuromuscular, cardiovascular/pulmonary, and integumentary. Each pattern contains the same elements:

- A diagnostic label based on impairments that describes the patient group from the perspective of the care that physical therapists provide. It is useful here to recognize that a diagnosis is a label that categorizes patients to improve the probability of identifying the correct prognosis and choosing appropriate interventions. As such, diagnoses are not just about pathology. In physical therapy, diagnostic groupings that can guide our care are much more often based on the patient's impairments or function. Examples from each system are:
    - Musculoskeletal: Impaired Joint Mobility, Motor Function, Muscle Performance, and Range of Motion Associated with Localized Inflammation.
    - Neuromuscular: Impaired Motor Function and Sensory Integrity Associated with Progressive Disorders of the Central Nervous System.
    - Cardiopulmonary/Vascular: Impaired Aerobic Capacity/Endurance Associated with Deconditioning.
    - Integumentary: Impaired Integumentary Integrity Associated with Partial-Thickness Skin Involvement and Scar Formation.
- The International Classification of Diseases codes that represent the pathologies typically associated with these impairments.
- A comprehensive list of the elements of examination that would typically be used to determine if the patient falls in this diagnostic category. The list, covering history, systems review, and specific tests and measures, is inclusive and represents many more tests than would actually be performed for any given patient.
- A description of the prognosis and plan of care that would typically be expected for patients in this diagnostic category.
- A comprehensive list of interventions with their anticipated outcomes that may be used for patients in this category. Again, the list represents many more items than would actually be performed for any given patient.
- Indication for reexamination, global outcomes expected in almost all cases, and criteria for discharge.

Returning now to Haynes's model, the clinical guidelines that we will be discussing in this chapter are most closely aligned with those policy recommendations that are termed guidelines by Eddy. They may be either boundary or pathway documents, and they serve a variety of purposes, ranging from advice to practitioners to coverage and payment decisions by insurers. These types of guidelines are produced by many sources. They can come from professional or health care delivery organizations and governmental agencies. What they have in common is that they are based on evidence from the literature, as assessed by a group of experts, and offer recommended patterns of care incorporating several, if not all aspects of care for a particular group of patients.

Sources for Guidelines

Many resources are available for identifying clinical guidelines. The source with the largest number of guidelines is the National Guideline Clearinghouse (NGC),[6] which is a service of the Agency for Healthcare Research and Quality (AHRQ)[7] of the U.S. Department of Health and Human Services. The NGC may be accessed by anyone at www.guideline.gov. It contains much useful information about guidelines, including:

- Structured abstracts (summaries) about the guideline and its development.
- Links to full-text guidelines, where available, and/or ordering information for print copies.
- A Guideline Comparison utility that gives users the ability to generate side-by-side comparisons for any combination of two or more guidelines.
- Unique guideline comparisons, called Guideline Syntheses, that compare guidelines covering similar topics, highlighting areas of similarity and difference. These syntheses often compare guidelines developed in different countries, providing insight into international health practices.
- An Annotated Bibliography database where users can search for publications about guideline development and implementation.
- An Expert Commentary feature written or reviewed by members of the NGC Editorial Board.

In order for a guideline to be accepted for publication at NGC it must meet all of these inclusion criteria:

- The clinical practice guideline contains systematically developed statements with recommendations, strategies, or information that assist health care practitioners and patients to make decisions about appropriate health care for specific clinical circumstances.
- The clinical practice guideline was produced under the auspices of medical specialty associations; relevant professional societies, public or private organizations, or government agencies at the federal, state, or local level; or health care organizations or plans.
- Corroborating documentation can be produced and verified that a systematic literature search and review of existing scientific evidence published in peer-reviewed journals was performed during the guideline development.
- The full-text guideline is available upon request in print or electronic format (for free or for a fee), in the English language.
- Documented evidence can be produced or verified that the guideline was developed, reviewed, or revised within the last 5 years.

It is easy to find guidelines at NGC simply by entering free text into the search box. For example, a search on knee pain produced 59 different guidelines; on stroke, 350 guidelines; on aerobic exercise, 71 guidelines.

Guidelines in Physical Therapy

Another source of guidelines, one which is much more specific to physical therapy, is the *Physiotherapy Evidence Database (PEDro)*[8] (see Chapter 14). It is also relatively easy to identify guidelines in *PEDro* simply by specifying practice guideline in the search strategy and then selecting the topics from drop-down menu choices. For example, a search for practice guidelines on the same topics as the NGC search meant selecting "lower leg or knee" from a drop-down menu, which identified 28 guidelines, selecting "neurofacilitation" and "motor coordination," which identified 5 guidelines, and selecting "reduced exercise tolerance" and "cardiothoracics," which indentified 160 guidelines.

Several professional organizations have begun development of clinical guidelines as well. The Orthopedic Section of the American Physical Therapy Association has started a project to develop evidence-based guidelines that use the International Classification of Functioning, Disability, and Health (ICF) to describe categories of patients with various musculoskeletal conditions.[9,10] These guidelines are designed to provide recommendation on all aspects of care for each condition, including examination, diagnostic classification, prognosis, intervention, and assessment of outcomes. The strength of the recommendation is based on the assessment by the authors of existing peer-reviewed literature. Figure 16-3a, b, and c shows a summary of the recommendations for the condition of heel pain–plantar fasciitis.

The American Physical Therapy Association has a major project to develop clinical guidelines for the practice of physical therapy. Its first steps are to identify all currently available relevant documents and to define the processes to be used to develop new clinical practice guidelines. Further information on the progress of this activity will be available at www.apta.org and at the FA Davis Web site for this text, as it becomes available.

Other Sources of Guidelines

In addition to these sources, many other organizations have produced guidelines. Some are for the purpose of guiding payment policy, such as those issued by insurance companies. Others are promulgated by delivery organizations, such as large corporate practices or multi-hospital systems to provide consistency in practice. Sometimes these guidelines are then made available for sale to the public.

Assessing the Quality of Guidelines

With this many sources, it is important for clinicians to assess the quality and applicability of the evidence before implementing guidelines in their own practices. When assessing guidelines, not only is the quality of the evidence important but it is also necessary to understand the level of (un)certainty of the recommendation being made. The strength of the recommendation is based on several factors in addition to the strength of evidence, including recognition of costs, potential dangers, etc. A system for assessing guidelines that takes into account both of these features has been developed and is in wide use in the EBP community, including the World Health Organization and the Cochrane Collaborative. This system is called GRADE (Grading of Recommendations Assessment, Development and Evaluation).[11–16] The GRADE system first rates the quality of evidence used to support the guideline using the following rating scheme:

Heel Pain—Plantar Fasciitis: Clinical Practice Guidelines

CLINICAL GUIDELINES

Summary of Recommendations

 PATHOANATOMICAL FEATURES

Clinicians should assess for impairments in muscles, tendons, and nerves, as well as the plantar fascia, when a patient presents with heel pain.

B **RISK FACTORS**

Clinicians should consider limited ankle dorsiflexion range of motion and a high body mass index in nonathletic populations as factors predisposing patients to the development of heel pain/plantar fasciitis.

B **DIAGNOSIS/CLASSIFICATION**

Functional limitations associated with pain in the plantar medial heel region, most noticeable with initial steps after a period of inactivity but also worse following prolonged weight bearing, and often precipitated by a recent increase in weight-bearing activity, are useful in classifying a patient into the ICD category of plantar fasciitis and the associated ICF impairment-based category of heel pain (b28015 Pain in lower limb; b2804 Radiating pain in a segment or region).

The following physical examination measures may be useful in classifying a patient with heel pain into the ICD category of plantar fasciitis and the associated ICF impairment-based category of heel pain (b28015 Pain in lower limb; b2804 Radiating pain in a segment or region):
• Symptom reproduction with palpatory provocation of the proximal plantar fascia insertion
• Active and passive talocrural joint dorsiflexion range of motion
• The tarsal tunnel syndrome test
• The windless test
• The longitudinal arch angle

 DIFFERENTIAL DIAGNOSIS

Clinicians should consider diagnostic classifications other than heel pain/plantar fasciitis when the patient's reported functional limitations or physical impairments are not consistent with those presented in the diagnosis/classification section of this guideline, or, the patient's symptoms are not resolving with interventions aimed at normalization of the patient's physical impairments.

A **EXAMINATION: OUTCOME MEASURES**

Clinicians should use validated self-report questionnaires, such as the Foot Function Index (FFI), Foot Health Status Questionnaire (FHSQ), or the Foot and Ankle Ability Measure (FAAM), before and after interventions intended to alleviate the physical impairments, functional limitations, and activity restrictions associated with heel pain/plantar fasciitis. Physical therapists should consider measuring change over time using the FAAM as it has been validated in a physical therapy practice setting.

 EXAMINATION: FUNCTIONAL LIMITATION MEASURES

Clinicians should utilize easily reproducible functional limitations and activity restrictions measures associated with the patient's heel pain/plantar fasciitis to assess the changes in the patient's level of function over the episode of care.

B **INTERVENTIONS: MODALITIES**

Dexamethasone 0.4% or acetic acid 5% delivered via iontophoresis can be used to provide short-term (2 to 4 weeks) pain relief and improved function.

 INTERVENTIONS: MANUAL THERAPY

There is minimal evidence to support the use of manual therapy and nerve mobilization procedures short-term (1 to 3 months) for pain and function improvement. Suggested manual therapy procedures include: talocrural joint posterior glide, subtalar joint lateral glide, anterior and posterior glides of the first tarsometatarsal joint, subtalar joint distraction manipulation, soft tissue mobilization near potential nerve entrapment sites, and passive neural mobilization procedures.

B **INTERVENTIONS: STRETCHING**

Calf muscle and/or plantar fascia-specific stretching can be used to provide short-term (2 to 4 months) pain relief and improvement in calf muscle flexibility. The dosage for calf stretching can be either 3 times a day or 2 times a day utilizing either a sustained (3 minutes) or intermittent (20 seconds) stretching time, as neither dosage produced a better effect.

 INTERVENTIONS: TAPING

Calcaneal or low-Dye taping can be used to provide short-term (7 to 10 days) pain relief. Studies indicate that taping does cause improvements in function.

A **INTERVENTIONS: ORTHOTIC DEVICES**

Prefabricated or custom foot orthoses can be used to provide short-term (3 months) reduction in pain and improvement in function. There appear to be no differences in the amount of pain reduction or improvement in function created by custom foot orthoses in comparison to prefabricated orthoses. There is currently no evidence to support the use of prefabricated or custom foot orthoses for long-term (1 year) pain management or function improvement.

 INTERVENTIONS—NIGHT SPLINTS

Night splints should be considered as an intervention for patients with symptoms greater than 6 months in duration. The desired length of time for wearing the night splint is 1 to 3 months. The type of night splint used (ie, posterior, anterior, sock-type) does not appear to affect the outcome.

A16 | APRIL 2008 | NUMBER 4 | VOLUME 38 | JOURNAL OF ORTHOPAEDIC & SPORTS PHYSICAL THERAPY

Figure 16-3 (a) An Example of the Summary of the Recommendations for Musculoskeletal Conditions as Presented in Guidelines from the Orthopedics Section of the APTA, with the Explanation of the Grading System Used.

(Continued on page 280)

I	Evidence obtained from high-quality randomized controlled trials, prospective studies, or diagnostic studies
II	Evidence obtained from lesser-quality randomized controlled trials, prospective studies, or diagnostic studies (eg, improper randomization, no blinding, < 80% follow-up)
III	Case controlled studies or retrospective studies
IV	Case series
V	Expert opinion

GRADES OF RECOMMENDATION		STRENGTH OF EVIDENCE
A	Strong evidence	A preponderance of level I and/or level II studies support the recommendation. This must include at least 1 level I study
B	Moderate evidence	A single high-quality randomized controlled trial or a preponderance of level II studies support the recommendation
C	Weak evidence	A single level II study or a preponderance of level III and IV studies including statements of consensus by content experts support the recommendation
D	Conflicting evidence	Higher-quality studies conducted on this topic disagree with respect to their conclusions. The recommendation is based on these conflicting studies
E	Theoretical/ foundational evidence	A preponderance of evidence from animal or cadaver studies, from conceptual models/principles, or from basic sciences/bench research support this conclusion
F	Expert opinion	Best practice based on the clinical experience of the guidelines development team

Figure 16-3, cont'd (b) Levels of Evidence and (c) Grades of Evidence.

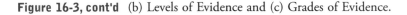

- High quality—Further research is very unlikely to change our confidence in the estimate of effect.
- Moderate quality—Further research is likely to have an important impact on our confidence in the estimate of effect and may change the estimate.
- Low quality—Further research is very likely to have an important impact on our confidence in the estimate of effect and is likely to change the estimate.
- Very low quality—Any estimate of effect is very uncertain.

The system then looks at these four factors in determining if the strength of the recommendation was appropriate:

- Quality of evidence
- Uncertainty about the balance between desirable and undesirable effects
- Uncertainty or variability in values and preferences
- Uncertainty about whether the intervention represents a wise use of resources

The system is intended to be used by developers of guidelines to alert the potential users to their quality. So one way to help clinicians be more confident about guideline use is to determine if the guideline developers have used the GRADE system. Guideline developers also use other, similar systems, such as the one illustrated in the Orthopedics Section Guidelines (see Fig. 16-3). If they do not report any such system, clinicians could still attempt to use these suggested factors in determining for themselves if the guidelines should be implemented in their setting.

The Institute of Medicine has also produced standards for the creation of clinical practice guidelines.[17] It states:

To be *trustworthy*, guidelines should

- Be based on a systematic review of the existing evidence;
- Be developed by a knowledgeable, multidisciplinary panel of experts and representatives from key affected groups;
- Consider important patient subgroups and patient preferences, as appropriate;
- Be based on an explicit and transparent process that minimizes distortions, biases, and conflicts of interest;
- Provide a clear explanation of the logical relationships between alternative care options and health outcomes, and provide ratings of both the quality of evidence and the strength of the recommendations; and
- Be reconsidered and revised as appropriate when important new evidence warrants modifications of recommendations.[17,p.3]

Clinical Decision/Prediction Rules

Another form of summary is known as the *clinical decision rule* or *clinical prediction rule*. Both of these terms are used in the literature to describe tools for clinicians that identify factors that have a high likelihood of leading to a more accurate diagnosis or more successful intervention. In general, they can be considered a specific type of clinical guideline. Most of the rules written in medicine are termed clinical decision rules and relate to the need for further diagnostic tests. This type of rule is useful to help allocate resources and reduce costs as well as ensure that the patient receives necessary testing to guide further care. In physical therapy, the rules are more likely to be termed clinical prediction rules and increasingly are developed to help identify the patient subgroup most likely to benefit from a particular intervention.

There are currently no central repositories for clinical decision/prediction rules; rather, they can be found in the typical ways that clinicians find evidence, through the use of various search engines (see Chapter11). Most clinical decision/prediction rules will be found by using clinical guidelines as a search parameter, along with appropriate search terms for the specific topic.

Physical therapists can find and apply clinical decision/prediction rules for a broad range of medical topics. For example, the decision rule on when to ambulate a patient with deep vein thrombosis (DVT) of the lower extremities was originally written to guide physicians in their decision making but has much to offer to physical therapists treating this patient population.[18,19] This is a good example of the premise of a decision rule (see Table 16.1). By applying

Table 16.1 Clinical Decision Rule for Identifying the Probability of Lower Extremity Deep Vein Thrombosis

Signs/Symptoms	Score	Explanation
Active cancer (within 6 months of diagnosis or palliative care)	1	
Paralysis, paresis, or recent plaster immobilization of lower extremity	1	
Recently bedridden >3 days or major surgery within 4 weeks of application of clinical decision rule	1	
Localized tenderness along distribution of the deep venous system	1	Tenderness along the deep venous system is assessed by firm palpation in the center of the posterior calf, the popliteal space, and along the area of the femoral vein in the anterior thigh and groin.
Entire lower-extremity swelling	1	
Calf swelling by >3 cm compared with asymptomatic lower extremity	1	Measured 10 cm below tibial tuberosity.
Pitting edema (greater in the symptomatic lower extremity)	1	
Collateral superficial veins (nonvaricose)	1	
Alternative diagnosis as likely or greater than that of deep vein thrombosis	−2	Most common alternative diagnoses are cellulitis, calf strain, and postoperative swelling

Score interpretation:
0–probability of proximal lower-extremity deep vein thrombosis (PDVT) of 3% (95% confidence interval [CI]: 1.7%–5.9%)
1 or 2–probability of PDVT of 17% (95% CI: 12%–23%)
3–probability of PDVT of 75% (95% CI: 63%–84%)
Data from Wells (Lancet) and Riddle.

this rule, the clinician can assess various clinical signs and symptoms and determine the likelihood of there being a DVT. Knowing the likelihood can guide next steps, including referral to other practitioners and the use of more extensive diagnostic tests, such as ultrasound. It can also insight into the level of urgency needed in seeking further information. For example, Riddle et al recommend, since DVT can be a life-threatening event, that any patient who scores a 3 be followed up on the same day.

Recently, there has been rapid growth in the publication of clinical prediction rules specific to interventions provided by physical therapists, particularly in the management of patients with musculoskeletal problems. Studies have presented rules in the area of management of low back, neck, knee and foot pain, and ankle sprain.[20–31]

Assessing the Quality of Clinical Decision/Prediction Rules

The premise of a well-developed clinical decision/prediction rule is that clinicians can rely on it to simplify their decision making processes and to reduce unwarranted variability in the selection of diagnostic tests and interventions. In order to warrant this trust, the rule must be developed carefully. It is recommended that there should be evidence in the literature on three critical issues before a rule be adopted. First, the rule should be *derived* by identifying potential predictors of the outcome of interest and then determining which of these predictors were present in a group of patients known to have the diagnosis or known to have successful outcomes. Then, appropriate statistical analyses, such as regression analysis, are used to determine which of the factors is more powerful in successfully predicting the outcome. The second step is to *validate* the rule by testing it in a variety of patient populations, with a variety of clinicians using the rule. This helps to assess that the first findings were not due to chance or to bias and to show that various clinicians are able to apply the rule. The third step is to conduct an *impact analysis*. Such analysis demonstrates whether clinicians are willing to use the rule and that use of the rule results in improved outcomes for patients, thereby justifying any costs associated with the rule.[32] It is common that each of these steps may be published in separate studies, often with different authors. Analyses of the clinical rules written to guide physical therapist care do not, to date, meet all of these criteria.[33,34] These critics point out that most clinical rules in physical therapy measure primarily short-term outcomes in relatively small populations, have not had sufficient validation studies, and have not undergone impact analyses.

It is therefore important for clinicians to review rules carefully before relying too heavily on them in their clinical practice. Review of the rule can help a clinician think more carefully about relevant evidence, thereby improving decision making. It can also be an opportunity to determine patient preferences in choosing tests and interventions. In addition, clinicians can begin to collect their own data about the results of the use of the rules. In some cases, this data collection can lead to additional validation studies that can support or refute the rule in particular populations and settings.

The Future of Summaries

Haynes[1] identifies a limited set of journals that are designed to provide summaries of comprehensive information in medicine: *Clinical Evidence*, which is part of the British Medical Journal Group activities (available primarily by direct subscription), and *Physician's Information and Education Resources* (*PIER*), which is published by the American College of Physicians (available only to members of the American College of Physicians).

Most physical therapists will not have access to these resources. However, there are a limited number of commissioned papers from the editors of *Clinical Evidence* that demonstrate the types of reviews they do. Box 16.1 shows the table of contents for *Putting Evidence into Practice: Palliative Care*.[35] Each section contains an explicit review of the evidence. For example, the section on prognostic accuracy presents information from a meta-analysis about physicians' consistent tendency to predict longer life expectancy than actually occurred. It also presents the evidence on prognostic scales to help improve this accuracy. The sections on intervention each start with information on valid and reliable outcome measures and provide the results from the best available evidence about the effectiveness of the various interventions. Such an evidence-based comprehensive review is surely a valuable resource for any clinician working with this patient population.

To maintain its value such a summary needs to be frequently updated. This is why these resources are typically electronic documents rather than published in paper format. Perhaps

---

Box 16.1 | **Table of Contents for *Putting Evidence into Practice: Palliative Care***

Part 1. Background
Introduction

- Demographics and disease burden
- Definitions
- Illness trajectories
- Prognostic accuracy
- Patients' care needs and preferences during advanced illness
- Patient-caregiver relationship
- Barriers to delivering effective palliative care
- Communication
- Coordination and delivery of care

Part 2. Evidence Review: Symptom Assessment and Management

- Symptom assessment
- Pain
- Dyspnea
- Fatigue
- Distress, depression, and mental health
- Delirium
- Anorexia and cachexia
- Dehydration
- Nausea and vomiting
- Constipation

---

they represent the format of the textbook of the future, particularly as their use spreads to more health professions. Certainly they represent a goal for the future, since it is clear that pre-assessed, integrated sources of evidence of great value to clinicians in everyday practice.[36]

SYSTEMS

As we have discussed, one of the features of using a pyramid (see Fig. 16-1) to represent sources of evidence is that we can see both the utility and the frequency of the sources. The source of evidence at the bottom of the pyramid, the individual study, is the most commonly available but has less immediate clinical utility. As we move up the pyramid, the sources become scarcer but more useful to the clinician in everyday practice. At the very top we find the *system*. A *system* is described as a computerized decision support system that links actual patient data with known evidence and established algorithms to provide suggestions to the clinician for management of the specific patient. This source of evidence appears to have great utility, as it occurs at the point of care and is applied in the context of the individual patient, truly representing the integration of all three aspects of evidence-based practice: clinical judgment, respecting patient choices, and using published evidence. However, such types of evidence are not widespread in health care. No examples specific to physical therapy were identified; however, this type of evidence is not widespread in health care generally. (As and if these become available in physical therapy, information will be posted at the FA Davis Network.)

Quality of Decision Support Systems

Several systematic reviews have been done to determine the effectiveness of the computerized decision support systems that have been developed. The reviews conclude that where they are available, they most often deal with specific and fairly narrow aspects of care and particular aspects of decision making and that there is some success reported in these focused areas, such as medication choices and prevention reminders.[37-41]The evidence demonstrates that there are four factors that contribute to the likelihood of the activity being successful[42]:

- the decision support is provided automatically as part of clinician's daily work;
- the decision support is delivered at the time and location of decision making;
- specific actionable recommendations are provided as part of the support; and
- the support is computer-based.

It is also important to note that success is generally measured from the perspective of the clinician, with little evidence available about changes in patient outcomes. In general, the research on more dynamic and complex systems remains inconclusive as to their actual impact on care. There are no published scoring schemes for clinicians to use to evaluate the quality of these systems, so clinicians will need to judge them based on their own sense of the utility of the support system and the information that authors make available about them.

Many writers continue to believe that computerized decision support systems have great promise to provide support for clinicians in their decision making.[42-43] Much of this confidence is based on the promise of constantly improving computer systems, coupled with growth in the use of electronic health records (Chapter 19) and the body of evidence.

CONCLUSION

Summaries and systems offer clinicians a distinct advantage over other sources of evidence, as they provide advice across the continuum of care. Currently, there are fewer sources of these types of evidences than those lower on the 6S pyramid. There are also fewer standards available to help clinicians assess the quality of these sources of evidence. However, there has been a rapid growth in the number of guidelines, particularly clinical decision/prediction rules available to help improve physical therapist practice. While there are far fewer options related to computer-based decision support systems, there continues to be promise and investment in expanding these options for clinical decision making. These are two areas that bear close attention as we move into the future.

SELF-ASSESSMENT

1. Review the material describing Mr. Ketterman's case (Appendix). Do you believe Mr. Ketterman is at risk for DVT? Review the clinical prediction rule for DVTs. Would you recommend that Mr. Ketterman's therapist change her behavior based on this rule?
2. Review the patterns in the *Guide to Physical Therapist Practice*. Which ones apply to Mr. Ketterman's care? How do their recommendations match the care that Mr. Ketterman received?

CONTINUED LEARNING

- Identify a recent clinical prediction rule that has been published for management of patient care in physical therapy. Using the guidelines identified in the McGinn[30] article, determine whether this rule meets these guidelines.
- Perform a search to determine if you can identify any new developments in clinical decision support systems for physical therapy practice.

REFERENCES

1. Haynes RB. Of studies, syntheses, synopses, summaries, and systems: The "5S" evolution of information services for evidence-based healthcare decisions. Evid BasedMed. 2006;11:162–164.
2. DiCenso A, Bayley L, Haynes RB. Accessing pre-appraised evidence: Fine-tuning the 5S model into a 6S model. Evid Based Nurs. 2009;12:99–101.
3. Eddy DM. *A Manual for Assessing Health practices and Designing Practice Policies.* American College of Physicians; 1992.
4. Sinnott, MC. The reengineering of American hospitals: Critical pathways to success. PT Magazine. 1994;2(12):55–61.
5. APTA, *Guide to Physical Therapist Practice*, 2nd ed. Alexandria, VA: American Physical Therapy Association; 2001.
6. National Guideline Clearinghouse, http://www.guideline.gov/ Accessed on June 29, 2010.
7. Agency for Health Care Research and Quality. http://www.ahrq.gov/ Accessed on June 29, 2010.
8. Physiotherapy Evidence Database. http://www.pedro.org.au/ Accessed on June 29, 2010.
9. Godges JJ, Irrgang JJ. ICF-based practice guidelines for common musculoskeletal conditions. J Orthop Sports PhysTher. 2008;38(4):167–168.
10. McPoil TG, Martin RL, Cornwall MW, Wukich DK, Irrgang JJ, Godges, JJ. Heel pain–plantar fasciitis: Clinical practice guidelines linked to the international classification of function, disability, and health from the Orthopaedic Section of the American Physical Therapy Association. J Orthop Sports PhysTher. 2008;38(4)A1–A18.
11. Guyatt GH, Oxman AD, Vist GE, Kunz R, Falck-Ytter Y, Alonso-Coello P, Schünemann HJ for the GRADE Working Group. GRADE: An emerging consensus on rating quality of evidence and strength of recommendations. BMJ. Apr 2008;336:924–926.
12. Guyatt GH, Oxman AD, Kunz R, Vist GE, Falck-Ytter Y, Schünemann HJ for the GRADE Working Group. What is "quality of evidence" and why is it important to clinicians? BMJ. May 2008;336:995–998.
13. Guyatt GH, Oxman AD, Kunz R, Falck-Ytter Y, Vist GE, Liberati A, Schünemann HJ for the GRADE Working Group. Going from evidence to recommendations. BMJ. May 2008; 336:1049–1051.
14. Schünemann HJ, Oxman AD, Brozek J, Glasziou P, Jaeschke R, Vist GE, Williams JW, Kunz R, Craig J, Montori VM, Bossuyt P, Guyatt GH for the GRADE Working Group. Grading quality of evidence and strength of recommendations for diagnostic tests and strategies. BMJ. May 2008;336:1106–1110.
15. Guyatt GH, Oxman AD, Kunz R, Jaeschke R, Helfand M, Al Liberati A, Vist GE, Schünemann HJ for the GRADE working group. Incorporating considerations of resources use into grading recommendations. BMJ. May 2008;336:1170–117.
16. Kavanagh BP. The GRADE system for rating clinical guidelines. PLoS Med. 2009;6(9): e1000094.
17. Graham R, Mancher M, Wolman DM, Greenfield S, Steinberg E, eds. *Clinical Practice Guidelines We Can Trust.* Committee on Standards for Developing Trustworthy Clinical Practice Guidelines, Institute of Medicine; 2011.

18. Wells PS, Hirsh J, Anderson DR, Guy F, Mitchell M, Gray L, Clement C, Robinson KS, Lewandowski B. A simple clinical model for the diagnosis of deep-vein thrombosis combined with impedance plethysmography: Potential for an improvement in the diagnostic process. J Intern Med. 1998;243:15–23.
19. Riddle DL, Hoppener MR, Kraaijenhagen RA, Anderson J, Wells PS. Preliminary validation of clinical assessment for deep vein thrombosis in orthopaedic outpatients, clinical orthopaedics and related research. Clin Orthop Rel Res. 2005; 432:252–257.
20. Cai C, Pua YH, Lim KC. A clinical prediction rule for classifying patients with low back pain who demonstrate short-term improvement with mechanical lumbar traction. Eur Spine J. 2009;18:554–561.
21. Childs J, Fritz J, Flynn T, et al. A clinical prediction rule to identify patients with low back pain most likely to benefit from spinal manipulation: A validation study. Ann Intern Med. 2004;141:920–928.
22. Cleland JA, Childs JD, Fritz JM, et al. Development of a clinical prediction rule for guiding treatment of a subgroup of patients with neck pain: Use of thoracic spine manipulation, exercise, and patient education. PhysTher. 2007;87:9–23.
23. Cleland JA, Fritz JM, Whitman JM, et al. The use of a lumbar spine manipulation technique by physical therapists in patients who satisfy a clinical prediction rule: A case series. J Orthop Sports PhysTher. 2006;36:209–214.
24. Currier L, Froehlich P, Carow S, et al. Development of a clinical prediction rule to identify patients with knee pain and clinical evidence of knee osteoarthritis who demonstrate a favorable short-term response to hip mobilization. Phys Ther. 2007;87: 1106–1119.
25. Flynn T, Fritz J, Whitman J, et al. A clinical prediction rule for classifying patients with low back pain who demonstrate short-term improvement with spinal manipulation. Spine (Philadelphia, PA, 1976). 2002;27:2835–2843.
26. Fritz JM, Childs JD, Flynn TW. Pragmatic application of a clinical prediction rule in primary care to identify patients with low back pain with a good prognosis following a brief spinal manipulation intervention. BMC Fam Pract. 2005;6:29.
27. Hancock MJ, Maher CG, Latimer J, et al. Independent evaluation of a clinical prediction rule for spinal manipulative therapy: A randomised controlled trial. EurSpine J. 2008; 17:936–943.
28. Hicks GE, Fritz JM, Delitto A, McGill SM. Preliminary development of a clinical prediction rule for determining which patients with low back pain will respond to a stabilization exercise program. Arch Phys Med Rehabil. 2005;86:1753–1762.
29. Iverson CA, Sutlive TG, Crowell MS, et al. Lumbopelvic manipulation for the treatment of patients with patellofemoral pain syndrome: Development of a clinical prediction rule. J Orthop Sports Phys Ther. 2008;38:297–309; discussion 309–212.
30. Lesher J, Sutlive T, Miller G, et al. Development of a clinical prediction rule for classifying patients with patellofemoral pain syndrome who respond to patellar taping. J Orthop Sports PhysTher. 2006;36:854–866.
31. McGinn TG, Guyatt GH, Wyer PC, et al, Evidence-Based Medicine Working Group. Users' guides to the medical literature, XXII: How to use articles about clinical decision rules. JAMA. 2000;284:79–84.
32. Stanton TR, Hancock MJ, Maher CG, Koes BW. Critical appraisal of clinical prediction rules that aim to optimize treatment selection for musculoskeletal conditions. PhysTher. 2010;90:843–854.
33. Beneciuk JM, Bishop MD, George SZ. Clinical prediction rules for physical therapy interventions: A systematic review. PhysTher. 2009;89:114–124.
34. Brunnhuber K, Nash S, Meier DE, Weissman DE, Woodcock J. *Putting Evidence into Practice: Palliative Care.* London: BMJ Publishing Group Limited; 2008.
35. Wong R, ed. *Evidence Based Healthcare Practice.* Arlington, VA: Marymount University; 2003.
36. Garg AX, Neill KJ, Adhikari NKJ, McDonald H, Rosas-Arellano MP, Devereaux PJ, Beyene J, Sam J, R. Brian Haynes RB. Effects of computerized clinical decision support systems on practitioner performance and patient outcomes: A systematic review. JAMA. 2005; 293(10):1223–1238.

37. Chaudhry B, Wang J, Wu S, Maglione M, Mojica W, Roth E, Morton SC, Shekelle PG. Systematic review: Impact of health information technology on quality, efficiency, and costs of medical care. Ann Intern Med. 2006;144:742–752.

38. Heselmans A, Van de Velde S, Doncee P, Aertgeerts B, Ramaekers D. Effectiveness of electronic guideline-based implementation systems in ambulatory care settings—A systematic review. Implementation Science. 2009; 4:82.

39. Johnston ME, Langton KB, Haynes RB, Mathieu A. Effects of computer-based clinical decision support systems on clinician performance and patient outcomes: A critical appraisal of research. Ann Intern Med. 1994;120:135–142.

40. Hunt DL, Haynes RB, Hanna SE, Smith K. Effects of computer-based clinical decision support systems on physician performance and patient outcomes: A systematic review. JAMA. 1998;280(15):1339–1346

41. Kawamoto K, Houlihan CA, Balas EA, Lobach DF. Improving clinical practice using clinical decision support systems: A systematic review of trials to identify features critical to success. BMJ. Apr 2005;330:765.

42. Halamka JD. Health information technology: Shall we wait for the evidence? Ann Intern Med. 2006;144:775–776.

43. Vreeman DJ, Taggard SL, Rhine MD, Worrell TW. Evidence for electronic health record systems in physical therapy. PhysTher. 2006;86:434–449.

44. Deutscher D, Hart DL, Dickstein R, et al. Implementing an integrated electronic outcomes and electronic health record process to create a foundation for clinical practice improvement. Phys Ther. 2008;88:270–285.

45. Committee On Quality Of Health Care In America, Institute Of Medicine. *Crossing the Quality Chasm: A New Health System for the 21st Century.* Washington, DC: National Academy Press; 2001.

Evidence-Based Practice: Does It Work in Practice?

Throughout the first three sections of this text, we have presented principles to guide us in each of the three elements of evidence-based practice. Section I focuses on our clinical judgment and decision making processes; Section II on the importance of knowing and respecting our patients' values and choices; Section III on identifying and appraising evidence from the literature. In all three sections, we have provided examples of clinical application of these principles. But a central question remains: *Can and do clinicians actually use these principles in their own clinical practices?*

In this concluding section, we explore the answers to this question. Research has shown us that human beings need time to adopt recommended changes and that there are some typical steps in that adoption process. In addition, we know that there are barriers to adoption that are also fairly consistent across all types of change in many different groups of people.[1] In Chapter 17, we present what is known about the diffusion of change in general, what we know about the adoption of evidence in health care, and the barriers to and opportunities for change in the future.

In health care we have come to rely on the patient record as *the* source of information about all aspects of patient care.[2] In Chapter 18, Kristin von Nieda discusses the importance of documentation as the basis for understanding our response to change in our practices, the importance of good outcome measures in this documentation, and the linkage of good documentation to quality measurement and improvement activities.

In Chapter 19, Christopher Bise and Anthony DeLitto delve more deeply into the connections of evidence based practice and quality improvement. They describe a successful program to assess the clinical performance of the therapists in their practice regarding a specific patient population. This example demonstrates that, indeed, we can put evidence based practice principles into practice!

References

1. Rogers EM. *Diffusion of Innovations* 4th ed. New York: The Free Press; 1995.
2. Erickson M, McKnight R, Utzman R. *Physical Therapy Documentation: From Examination to Outcome.* Slack; 2008.

chapter 17

Translating Evidence Into Practice

*Human behavior flows from three main sources:
desire, emotion and knowledge.*

—Plato

We've got to put a lot of money into changing behavior.

—Bill Gates

•

✳ Mr. Ketterman's Case

I have the sense that I'm not making use of current knowledge about Alzheimer's disease as I treat Mr. Ketterman. What's holding me back? *(See Appendix for Mr. Ketterman's health history.)*

INTRODUCTION

The previous sections have presented a foundational introduction to the three main components of evidence-based practice (EBP). Clinicians will find that most decisions required of them can benefit from the integration of sound clinical reasoning, patient-focused preferences, and critically appraised evidence. Whether you are selecting a diagnostic test or an intervention, your odds of having the best patient outcomes are enhanced when you ground your decisions in EBP. We are finding increasing evidence to support this assumption.[1,2] But knowing and doing can be miles apart when it comes to human behavior, and clinicians are susceptible to barriers that make acceptance of EBP more difficult. Understanding the slow pace of change in the health care system makes it important to identify strategies to quicken our abilities to get the right care to the right patient at the right time. Increasing the rate of change to best physical therapy practice would result in significant improvements in our patient outcomes. Evensen et al[3] refers to this as closing the evidence-practice gaps. Although most authors believe this is an appropriate goal, it will require the removal of barriers at several levels of health care, including the patient, the practitioner, and the health care organization.

Researchers and clinicians who identify problems with adherence to best practice, and who design and test interventions to decrease these barriers, are participating in what is called knowledge translation research or implementation science. The Canadian Institutes of Health Research define knowledge translation as:

> the exchange, synthesis and ethically sound application of knowledge—within a complex system of interactions among researchers and users—to accelerate the capture of the benefits of research for society through improved health, more effective services and products, and a strengthened health care system.[4]

Evensen et al[3] have described a disappointingly low amount of high-quality evidence in the past decade for guiding our understanding of how to implement the changes we hope will close the evidence-practice gap. The literature in medicine reports a preponderance of observational studies or simply papers that restate the practice guidelines or treatment recommendations.

In this chapter we will discuss three elements that can affect, in either a positive or negative manner, the process of getting evidence into practice: dissemination, practitioner acceptance, and organizational support for EBP (Fig. 17-1). We will draw from the best available evidence in physical therapy to identify barriers and recommend interventions that have been effective. For some knowledge translation, the path to the desired change is rather straightforward, whereas for other innovations the path may be more complex, as illustrated in Figure 17-2. Whether you are attempting a simple or a complex change in practice, the information in this chapter will be useful for individual clinicians as well as communities of practitioners and managers who wish to facilitate best practice in their settings.

DISSEMINATION OF INNOVATION

Perceptions of Innovation

This term, *innovation*, may sound too grand for the steady changes we hope to see. We might think it is reserved for things like the creation of the Internet, a truly innovative development in society, so that recommended changes to our practice pale by comparison.

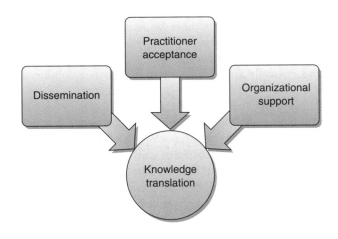

Figure 17-1 Elements of Knowledge Translation.

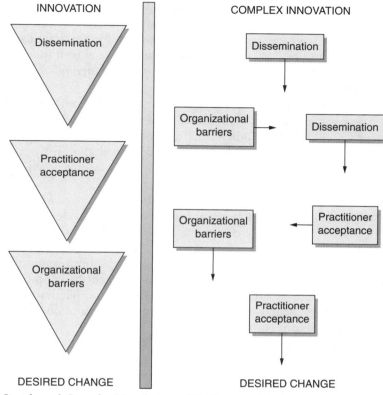

Figure 17-2 Simple and Complex Translation of Evidence to Practice.

However, any change that represents a new method or practice should be considered an innovation. Clinicians and scientists in physical therapy are innovators as they attempt to evaluate a new exercise technique or try a new position for applying joint mobilizations. Once the evidence supporting the novel approach to care of our patients has been tested and found effective, the task turns to disseminating this good news. Many say this is the point at which EBP meets a significant barrier. In a seminal paper on disseminating innovations in health, Berwick states, "In health care, invention is hard, but dissemination is even harder."[5,p1970] Jette,[6] discussing these issues in physical therapy, comments that our profession must take studies of how best to diffuse innovations just as seriously as studies that produce the innovations.

Dissemination in Physical Therapy

The Institute of Medicine has drawn our attention to the problems of dissemination of evidence in health care in its classic report entitled *Crossing the Quality Chasm*.[7] The report concludes, "Between the health care we have and the care we could have lies not just a gap, but a chasm." What do we know about the gap or chasm between the physical therapy care we have and the care we could have? Evidence supporting a diffusion of innovation problems in physical therapy is increasing. Several research studies have investigated the rate of physical therapists' adherence to professionally accepted practice guidelines.[8–14] Mikhail et al[11] documented the typical practice decisions of 100 physical therapists for patients with acute low back pain and found 68% using interventions with strong or moderate evidence of effectiveness, while 90% also used interventions for which research evidence was limited or absent. Bekkering et al[10] and Brennan et al[9] studied patient outcomes for physical therapists provided with knowledge of current practice guidelines using one of several educational strategies and found mixed results both in practitioner adherence and patient outcomes, demonstrating how complex the problem of changing practice can be.

Classic methods of dissemination of research evidence in the past century required researchers to publish their work in peer-reviewed journals and clinicians to find that work and read it. Alternatively, they could attend professional conferences, at some expense, and attend research platform or poster sessions in search of practice innovations. This approach placed a huge demand on clinicians to access published research and to improve their abilities to critically appraise the work.

In Section III we demonstrated a variety of new strategies that are now available for accessing and understanding innovations. Clinicians are calling for a broader array of methods of dissemination to enhance the speed of change in clinical practice. A consensus panel of emergency medicine physicians, working to reduce barriers to dissemination, recommends that "researchers and advocates should disseminate findings through multiple forums beyond peer-reviewed publications when an ED-based (emergency department-based) public health intervention has enough evidence to support integration into the routine practice of emergency care."[15,p1133] Professional associations are playing a role in this aspect of dissemination by using e-mail to notify practitioners of current guidelines.

What types of dissemination strategies work? Spreading carefully collected evidence throughout a profession as diverse as physical therapy is a challenge. Practitioners in our field are diversified in setting and in specialization, such that targeting the information needed by each practitioner is a challenge. New technology can be quite helpful in pushing focused knowledge to practitioners in a prescriptive manner that affords good access of just the right amount and type of information. Barriers to dissemination have included limited access as well as limitations in comprehension.

Sufficient studies of methods of dissemination in physical therapy have been conducted for a systematic review of this work. Menon et al[16] found moderate evidence from one high-quality randomized controlled trial (RCT) and two observational studies to suggest that the use of an active, multicomponent knowledge translation program to be successful in improving knowledge. They also found strong evidence to support the effectiveness of multicomponent interventions to change practice behavior, including increased self-perceived and actual adherence to practice guidelines. In this systematic review, the knowledge translation interventions used in the studies did not demonstrate significant changes in physical therapists' attitudes toward EBP.

Dissemination of Evidence to Consumers

What lies ahead in health care is an increasingly educated consumer who wishes to be an active participant in his or her health care decisions. In response, researchers have begun to study the process of creating, tailoring, and disseminating evidence to consumers. Tugwell et al state their aim this way: "to put the results of rigorous research into the hands of consumers so they can use it when making important decisions related to their health."[17,p1729] The Cochrane Consumers and Communication Review Group supports this dissemination to consumers and recommends several foci for intervention development, including interventions directed to the consumer and interventions for communication exchange between providers and consumers.[18] Some of these interventions include the development of educational materials in various formats, termed *decision aids*, to prepare people to participate in "close call" decisions that involve weighing benefits, harms, and scientific uncertainty.[19,20] It is often said that to teach someone you must master the knowledge you wish to teach, and in the teaching you enhance your knowledge further. Thus, developing decision aids is perhaps another strategy for improving the dissemination of innovation to the clinician.

PRACTITIONER ACCEPTANCE

Seminal work on diffusion of innovation comes from a broad range of theoretical frameworks developed by researchers in fields as diverse as communications, public policy, health policy, agriculture, family planning, and nutrition. Everett Rogers, a well-known diffusion scholar, published his first text on the topic in 1962. Over the past five decades, knowledge about factors that influence the rate of dissemination for a beneficial behavior have been developed from studies as diverse as new hybrid seed corn in agriculture and public health studies of water boiling in a Peruvian village.[21] Across these many studies Rogers has determined that the perception of the innovation as well as the characteristics of the individuals being encouraged to adopt an innovation can significantly affect the rate of adoption.

Practitioners' Perspectives

The perceptions of the innovations we desire in physical therapy are also likely to influence their rate of adoption. Clinicians should find the innovation to be beneficial to themselves or their patients, and the risks of adopting the innovation should not outweigh these perceived benefits. Related to the clinician's perception of benefit is the perception that the innovation is not in conflict with personal or professional values. Innovations that decrease the physical therapist's autonomy to make clinical decisions in conjunction with the patient will likely be rejected. A third perspective that can affect the rate of innovation adoption is its complexity. A complex innovation may not result in a positive cost/benefit analysis from the clinician's perspective. One solution in this situation is simplifying the innovation in some manner. Berwick states, ". . . innovations are more robust to modification than their inventors think, and local adaptation, which often involves simplification, is nearly a universal property of successful dissemination."[5,p1971]

Rogers identified two additional significant perceptions that seem very applicable in a physical therapy clinical context: trialability and observability. Trialability is described as the ease with which an adopter might test the proposed innovation in a small context to determine the outcomes before a widespread implementation. One would imagine that this is a likely first step for trying out a new patient intervention. Observability refers to the ease with which a potential adopter might observe the innovation before testing it.[21] This also may be an important and practical perception for physical therapists, who customarily discuss practice decisions with colleagues.

Practitioners' Innovation Adoption Patterns

Rogers' work identified a pattern of innovation adoption behaviors based on the proposed personal characteristics of individuals targeted for the innovation.[22] He describes five categories, based on the mean adoption time. Figure 17-3 describes these categories in relation to a statistical normal distribution. The individuals who are much above average in time to adopt an innovation are called *innovators*. These are generally individuals who have a high tolerance for risk in decision making and are very interested in novel ideas. In health care, Berwick[5] states, they might be considered as mavericks. The next group, approximately 13%, would

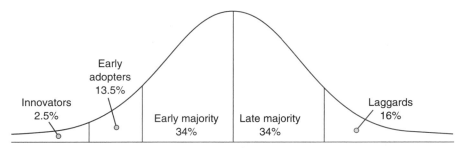

Figure 17-3 Adopter Categorization on the Basis of Innovativeness. *(Redrawn from Rogers EM.* Diffusion of Innovations, *4th ed. New York: The Free Press; 1995.)*

also adopt an innovative idea more quickly than the average person and are termed *early adopters*. This group, considered to be composed of significant opinion leaders, is willing to test innovative ideas and has little personal difficulty with changing the way things are done. They are often respected leaders, and internal and external colleagues pay attention to their opinions. The next group, the *early majority*, includes those who watch the early adopters and take their lead from them. They generally adopt an innovation at or above the mean rate of adoption. They are more risk-averse than the early adopters and value an innovative idea with strong local importance rather than testing a novel idea that does not have a direct application to their work. The last two groups will adopt innovation at a rate below the average. The *late majority* tends to watch the early majority for signs of a *"new status quo,"*[5,p1972] choosing not to change their behaviors until it is quite certain that the innovation has merit. The last group to adopt are termed *"laggards"* by Rogers or *"traditionalists"* by Berwick. These individuals are strongly connected to the status quo and tend to be reticent to adopt innovation without significant proof of concept.

What influences a physical therapist to become an early adopter or innovator? Values and beliefs might be predictors of the inclination to help spread evidence based innovations. Our professional core values include the pursuit of excellence in practice, and these are reinforced by the core values of accountability and professional duty. It is true that clinicians with similarly strong core values could fall into any of the five rate of adoption categories described by Edwards, but this provides an excellent platform for debate of a particular innovation. Clinicians whose values foster an engaged attitude toward changing practice patterns can be identified and supported in their work by an organization committed to the pursuit of best practice models, the third element of the process of diffusion.

ORGANIZATIONAL CHARACTERISTICS

Berwick[5] describes the third collection of factors that will influence the rate of dissemination as contextual or managerial influences. Health care organizations of all sizes can create nurturing environments for adoption and innovation of best practice policies. A practice or organization that wishes to allow some clinicians to pursue innovation would arrange time and resources for the creative work this entails, taking into account that productivity may be sacrificed as various new approaches are tested. Identifying a likely innovation in published and peer-reviewed literature is the first step in the process, and it is facilitated by providing resources to push these ideas out to practitioners for consideration, perhaps via automated literature searches or with the assistance of informatics professionals. Identifying and supporting a likely innovator is the second step, providing time to test the innovation on a small but particular scale in the practice.

Once the organization decides to pursue the dissemination of a particular innovation, one of several paths may be chosen: optional, recommended, or required behavior changes.[5] If the innovation will be challenging to integrate into the organization, and also of as yet unquantifiable value, an optional approach might fit best. This optional path allows the collection of additional quality improvement data to further judge the value of the innovation in the setting. Choosing to label the change in practice as either recommended or required will communicate a very different message to organization members, one that they may have difficulty distinguishing. Matching the diffusion approach to the impact of the innovation is a crucially important management decision, as the use of one predominant strategy for all innovations is unlikely to be as successful. For example, Lankshear describes a strategy with multiple options to recommend a change to encourage physicians to document the stage of disease in cancer patients, including knowledge transfer strategies such as providing advice from opinion leaders in the setting, practitioner education sessions, or audit feedback on performance.[22]

Successful research dissemination or knowledge transfer strategies are typically created to meet the needs of the clinicians who are to use the knowledge in making clinical decisions and to accommodate the environment in which they practice. MacDermit et al[22] suggest it is important to consider organizational factors that may facilitate or impede knowledge transfer. To identify some of these factors in physical and occupational therapy practice, they proposed a study of knowledge transfer in the use of standardized outcome measures in adult and pediatric patients with chronic health conditions. The knowledge transfer outcome was described as strategies to "select health status measures for clinical practice, score/interpret results, incorporate measures into clinical reasoning, and recognize and address personal and organizational barriers and facilitators of change."[22,p6] Two types of organizational interventions were planned: a 30-hour session of faculty-led tutorials combined with facilitated independent group work in a problem-based learning format and a Web-based instructional presentation over a 6-week period using a similar problem-based learning format, with the learners not in the same location. Although the results of this work are not yet available, the researchers planned to interview subjects regarding their perceptions of facilitators and barriers to knowledge transfer in their practice setting.

A variety of management strategies to enhance knowledge transfer in practice are reported in the literature. Most traditional are continuing education courses in one format or another. In the most recent Cochrane review of the effectiveness of continuing education for health professionals, the evidence is very weak regarding the effectiveness of traditional continuing education as an intervention for changing practice. Forsetlund et al report a small effect for improving patient care following continuing education interventions, similar to those found for auditing of practitioner compliance, practitioner feedback, and educational outreach.[23]

Practitioner audit and feedback are described as a process by which objective data on practitioner compliance are provided to the practitioner to enhance the quality of care given. Audits can take many forms and can be implemented electronically or in a more intense, personal counseling process. Jamveldt et al report in a Cochrane review of audit and feedback techniques for knowledge transfer that they can have a small to moderate impact on professional practice. The effects of audit and feedback were greater when the practitioner's baseline adherence to recommended practice is low and when feedback is delivered more intensively.[24] Foy et al[25] found that audit and feedback strategies are used extensively in the United Kingdom, but there is insufficient evidence regarding the best methods of applying this quality improvement technique in an organization.

Organizational strategies for quality improvement are also considered as strategies for knowledge transfer. Educational outreach visits can be targeted to a single clinical site or a community outreach to enhance the practitioner's awareness of an innovative practice. These visits often employ local opinion leaders or clinician colleagues who have been nominated or recognized as being influential in a community. The decision support systems discussed in Section III are also tools that may be structured to facilitate the adoption of a new practice guideline. For example, electronic reminders of a new initiative at a clinical site can help clinicians who wish to adhere to best practice models become compliant. Chapter 19 reports on a program instituted in one organization designed to improve the quality of care through use of clinical data and feedback to clinicians.

ADDITIONAL PERSPECTIVES ON KNOWLEDGE TRANSLATION

There may be many additional facilitators and barriers to changing practice in physical therapy than those covered in this chapter. We need additional evidence on this topic: success stories and descriptions of unique barriers in various settings or for the specific types of patients we treat. The research on knowledge translation itself must be scrutinized for criteria that indicate strength of evidence. Two journals created in the past decade are devoted to translational research: *Implementation Science* (www.implementationscience.com) and the *Journal of Translational Medicine* (www.translational-medicine.com). Majumdar[26] has reviewed three high-quality and successful knowledge-to-action studies in medicine and suggests some criteria for translational research. He recommends translational studies that provide sufficient detail for replication, indicate a clinically meaningful change score, and analyze both the process of practitioner change and the accompanying patient outcomes. He also suggests a research agenda for translational research that would investigate the persistence of practitioner change behaviors as well as the occurrence of relapse to old habits.

The barriers to implementation of physical therapy EBP are similar in many respects to those for other areas in health care. Salbach et al in a study of Canadian physiotherapists identified two organizational barriers to EBP for patients who have had a stroke: a lack of training in EBP and time in the work day to search and interpret the literature.[27] In a later study, Salbach et al reported similar organizational barriers of time and training and recommended the incorporation of technology in the form of personal digital assistants for ease of accessing evidence, as well as educational sessions led by experts with opportunities for case-based learning and skill training.[28] This combination of technology aids and face-to-face educational sessions was considered the strongest for actually changing practice.

However, in many countries physical therapists may experience a unique barrier that relates to autonomy in clinical decision making. This was a finding of a qualitative study of 43 physiotherapists in Belgium.[29] In addition to identifying obstacles to dissemination of knowledge, the physiotherapists were concerned with their limited autonomy in clinical care as compared to that of the referring physicians. This perspective is a primary barrier to knowledge translation, for a practitioner who lacks self-efficacy in clinical decision making is unlikely to risk adopting an innovation in practice. We consider autonomy in clinical decisions to be a necessary condition for knowledge translation.

In terms of access to knowledge, the clinician's dilemma is not only about having too little evidence to guide practice; it is also about the translation of the right evidence into practice in a timely manner. The practice community must depend on the research community and those who work to prepare valid and unbiased summaries of evidence for practice. Tricco et al[30] suggest that knowledge translation that depends only on individual studies runs the risk of a new practice being adopted without sufficient support and that *knowledge syntheses* should be "the basic unit of knowledge translation."[30,p.11]

Straus suggests that we are wise to avoid the knowledge translation imperative that all knowledge must be implemented.[31] Our profession will benefit from a mature and selective approach to knowledge translation so as to avoid the whiplash phenomenon associated with repeatedly contradictory health advice, such as we have experienced in human nutrition. In our profession, the now rejected "no pain, no gain" advice provides an example of the difficulty of presenting a trustworthy message to the public about exercise.

CONCLUSION

Shea,[32] reporting on a decade of knowledge translation research, points to several major success stories, including a significant reduction in heart disease attributed to a multifaceted knowledge translation project on smoking cessation. She also reminds us that in the 21st century we have many more tools available to engage a community in knowledge translation, including media and Internet social networking sites. These tools can facilitate the goal of knowledge translation to enhance the health-related decision making of all—patients, practitioners, managers, and policy makers. If we keep patients at the center of this process, as the targeted benefactors of the best evidence and clinical decision making we can provide, we can enhance physical therapy care for all.

SELF-ASSESSMENT

1. There are several studies (listed below) that support the value of exercise in people like Mr. Ketterman with or at risk of Alzheimer's disease. What barriers would you expect to find in convincing your colleagues to implement exercise programs for this patient group?
2. What strategies would you use to overcome these barriers?

References for Self-Assessment Activity

- Abbott RD, White LR, Ross GW, Masali KH, Curb JD, Petrovitch H. Walking and dementia in physically capable elderly men. JAMA. 2004;292(12):1447–1453.
- Larson EB, Wang I, Bowen JD, McCormick WC, Teri L, Crane P, Kukull WA. Exercise is associated with reduced risk for incident dementia among persons 65 years of age and older. Ann Intern Med. 2006;144:73–81.
- Scarmeas N, Luchsinger JA, Schupf N, Brickman AM, Cosentino S, Tang MX, Stern Y. Physical activity, diet, and risk of Alzheimer disease. JAMA. 2009;302(6):627–637. doi: 10.1001/jama.2009.1144.
- Teri L, Gibbons LE, McCurry SM, Logsdon LG, Buchner DM, Barlow WE, Kukull WA, LaCroix AZ, McCormick W, Larson EB. Exercise plus behavioral management in patients with Alzheimer disease. JAMA. 2003;290(15):2015–2022. doi: 10.1001/jama.290.15.2015.
- Weuve J, Kang JH, Manson JE, Breteler MMB, Ware JH, Grodstein F. Physical activity, including walking, and cognitive function in older women. JAMA. 2004;292:1454–1461.

- van Gelder BM, Tijhuis MAR, Kalmijn S, Giampaoli S, Nissinen A, Kromhout D. Physical activity in relation to cognitive decline in elderly men: The FINE Study. Neurology. 2004;63:2316–2321.

CONTINUED LEARNING

- The Agency for Healthcare Research and Quality of the U.S. Department of Health and Human Services has supported research on the concept of pay for performance (http://www.ahrq.gov/qual/pay4per.htm), which is designed to align payment incentives with appropriate care based on sound evidence. Review one of these programs and reflect on:

1. Is the evidence sound?
2. Are the incentives based on sound principles?
3. What might you do differently?

REFERENCES

1. Duncan PW, Horner RD, Reker DM, et al. Adherence to postacute rehabilitation guidelines is associated with functional recovery in stroke. Stroke. 2002;33:167–177.
2. Reker DM, Duncan PW, Horner RD, et al. Postacute stroke guideline compliance is associated with greater patient satisfaction. Arch Phys Med Rehabil. 2002;83:750–756.
3. Evensen AE, Sanson-Fisher R, D'Este C, et al. Trends in publications regarding evidence–practice gaps: A literature review. Implementation Science. 2010,5:11
4. Canadian Institutes of Health Research. CIHR knowledge translation strategy 2004–2009. http://www.cihr-irsc.gc.ca/e/26574.html#defining Accessed May 2011.
5. Berwick DM. Disseminating innovations in health care. JAMA. 2003;289:1969–1975.
6. Jette AM. Invention is hard, but dissemination is even harder. Phys Ther. 2005;85:390–391.
7. Institute of Medicine. Crossing the Quality Chasm: A New Health System for the 21st Century. Washington, DC: National Academy Press; 2001:1.
8. Poitras S, Blais R, Swaine B, et al. Management of work-related low back pain: A population-based survey of physical therapists. Phys Ther. 2005;85:1168–1181.
9. Brennan GP, Fritz JM, Hunter SJ. Impact of continuing education interventions on clinical outcomes of patients with neck pain who received physical therapy. Phys Ther. 2006;86:1251–1262.
10. Bekkering GE, van Tulder MW, Hendriks HJM, et al. Implementation of clinical guidelines on physical therapy for patients with low back pain: Randomized trial comparing patient outcomes after a standard and active implementation strategy. Phys Ther. 2005;85:544–555.
11. Mikhail C, Korner-Bitensky N, Rossingnol M, et al. Physical therapists' use of interventions with high evidence of effectiveness in the management of a hypothetical typical patient with acute low back pain. Phys Ther. 2005;85:1151–1167.
12. Harting J, Rutten GMJ, Rutten STJ, et al. A qualitative application of the diffusion of innovations theory to examine determinants of guideline adherence among physical therapists. Phys Ther. 2009;89:221–232.
13. Jette DU, Bacon K, Batty C, et al. Evidence-based practice: Beliefs, attitudes, knowledge, and behaviors of physical therapists. PhysTher. 2003;83:786–805.
14. Brown CJ, Gottschalk M, Van Ness PH, et al. Changes in physical therapy providers' use of fall prevention strategies following a multi-component behavioral change intervention. Phys Ther. 2005;85:394–403.
15. McKay MP, Vaca FE, Field C, et al. Public health in the emergency department: Overcoming barriers to implementation and dissemination. Acad Emerg Med. 2009;16:1132–1137.

16. Menon A, Korner-Bitensky N, Kastner M, et al. Strategies for rehabilitation professionals to move evidence-based knowledge into practice: A systematic review. J Rehabil Med. 2009;41:1024–1032.
17. Tugwell PS, Santesso NA, O'Connor AM, et al. Knowledge translation for effective consumers. Phys Ther. 2007;87:1728–1738.
18. Cochrane Reviews, Consumers and Communication Group. www.cochrane.org/reviews/en/subtopics/54.html Accessed February 13, 2010.
19. O'Connor AM, Bennett CL, Stacey D, et al. Decision aids for people facing health treatment or screening decisions. Cochrane Database of Syst Rev. 2009;Issue 3.
20. Lankshear S, Brierley JD, Imrie K, et al. Changing physician practice: An evaluation of knowledge transfer strategies to enhance physician documentation of cancer stage. Healthcare Quart. 2010;13(1):84–92.
21. Rogers EM: *Diffusion of Innovations*, 4th ed. New York: The Free Press; 1995.
22. MacDermid JC, Solomon, P, Law M, et al. Defining the effect and mediators of two knowledge translation strategies designed to alter knowledge, intent and clinical utilization of rehabilitation outcome measures: A study protocol. Implementation Science. 2006; 1:14.
23. Forsetlund L, Bjørndal A, Rashidian A, et al. Continuing education meetings and workshops: Effects on professional practice and health care outcomes. Cochrane Database of Syst Rev. 2009; Issue 2.
24. Jamtvedt G, Young JM, Kristoffersen DT, et al. Audit and feedback: Effects on professional practice and health care outcomes. Cochrane Database Syst Rev. 2006.
25. Foy R, Eccles MP, Jamtvedt G, et al. What do we know about how to do audit and feedback? Pitfalls in applying evidence from a systematic review. BMC Health Services Res. 2005;5:50.
26. Majumdar SR. Successful high-quality knowledge translation research: Three case studies. J ClinEpidem. 2011:64;21–24.
27. Salbach NM, Jaglal SB, Korner-Bitensky N, et al. Practitioner and organizational barriers to evidence-based practice of physical therapists for people with stroke. Phys Ther. 2007;87:1284–1303.
28. Salbach NM, Veinot P, Jaglal SB, et al. From continuing education to personal digital assistants: What do physical therapists need to support evidence-based practice in stroke management? J Eval Clin Pract. Oct. 12, 2010.
29. Hannes K, Staes F, Goedhuys J, et al. Obstacles to the implementation of evidence-based physiotherapy in practice: A focus group-based study in Belgium (Flanders). Physiother Theory and Prac. 2009;
30. Tricco AC, Tetzlaff J, Moher D. The art and science of knowledge synthesis. J Clin Epidem. 2011;64;11–20.
31. Straus SE, Tetroe JM, Graham ID. Knowledge translation is the use of knowledge in health care decision-making. J Clin Epidem. 2011:64:6–10.
32. Shea BJ. A decade of knowledge translation research—What has changed? J Clin Epidem. 2011;64:3–5.

chapter 18

Documentation as Evidence

Kristin von Nieda, PT, DPT, MEd

I write entirely to find out what I'm thinking, what I'm looking at, what I see and what it means.

— JOAN DIDION

•

✳ Mr. Ketterman's Case

Mr. Ketterman has so many issues that we are addressing. I want to be able to keep track of them all and I would like to be able to use what I learn from his care to help me with future patients. How can I manage this in my busy day? *(See Appendix for Mr. Ketterman's health history.)*

INTRODUCTION

In Section III, we discussed identifying, assessing, and applying, as appropriate, evidence from the research literature to decisions about patient care. Yet, it is apparent that the research literature does not hold all the answers to all the questions we have about patient care. In Chapter 19, Drs. Bise and Delitto discuss an approach that uses the data generated in everyday care as a source of evidence. This approach, as with many evidence based activities, relies on documentation to be successful.

The goals of this chapter are to examine the multiple purposes of documentation and how these purposes may be met in producing accurate and useful documentation about a patient's condition. Thus, improved documentation can become a source of evidence that aids in decision making.

THE HEALTH CARE RECORD

The patient/client record serves multiple purposes. According to the American Health Information Management Association (AHIMA), documentation has many purposes. For most clinicians, most of the time, the primary purpose of documentation is to *provide a basis for clinical reasoning* in planning care and assessing its success for the individual patient. Ideally, the patient/client record also serves as a *communication tool for providers* involved in the care and supports patient/client care delivery. Appropriate and meaningful documentation is important to support optimal decision making, to minimize risk, to promote continuity of care, and to determine the best plan of care for the patient/client.

Documentation is also a mandatory practice, subject to applicable jurisdictional and regulatory requirements. There are *specific legal requirements* about when and how to document patient care and charting errors. There are additional requirements for signature and other means to demonstrate the authenticity of the record. *Payment for services* is justified through documentation in the patient/client record. Different payment sources have specific mandates for documentation to justify both approval for services and to determine which, if any, services are eligible for payment.

All of these purposes matter in patient care, but the last one, *a means for data collection and retrieval*, may be the most important in terms of evidence based practice. When the clinical record contains standardized information, then these data can be retrieved and analyzed, both within and across practices. Secondary purposes are education, regulation (compliance and accreditation), research, policy making (allocating resources and business planning), and industry needs (including research and development).[1]

Standards for Quality in Documentation

AHIMA[2] has defined comprehensive guidelines the patient record should meet if it is to serve as a basis for data collection through the collection of high-quality data. The characteristics are:

- Accessibility
- Accuracy/Validity
- Comprehensiveness
- Consistency
- Currency
- Clear Definition
- Granularity (the correct level of detail)
  - Relevancy
  - Precision
- Timeliness

The purposes for which documentation is currently used extend beyond the reasons cited above and include risk assessment and management, quality assessment and improvement, peer review, and productivity measurement. When taking the manifold purposes of documentation into consideration, the task of documenting clearly, correctly, comprehensively, and meaningfully becomes even more important.

Documentation is defined in the *Guide to Physical Therapist Practice*[3] as "any entry into the client record, such as a consultation report, initial examination report, progress note, flow sheet/checklist that identifies the care/service provided, re-examination, or summation of care." The American Physical Therapy Association gives general guidelines in its *Guidelines for Physical Therapy Documentation* that expand on specific elements that may be included. (The *Guidelines* may be found at www.APTA.org and at the F.A. Davis Web site for this book.) Documentation is a complex process that has many discrete parts. The *Guidelines* provide both lists of the various types of documentation that are seen in physical therapy and guidance for the standards that should be used in creating them.[3] Standards include the need for clear authentication as to the physical therapist of record for the patient. Table 18.1 shows some of the many different kinds of documents created in the physical therapy record.

Table 18.1	**Purposes of Documentation and Elements Needing Documentation in the Physical Therapy Record**
Purpose of Documentation	Essential elements in documentation
Initial Examination and Evaluation	History Systems review Selection and administration of appropriate tests and measures Evaluation Diagnosis Prognosis Plan of care
Continuation of Care	Patient/client self-report Specific interventions Changes in patient/client status Responses to interventions Communication Re-examination Interpretation of findings Revisions to the plan of care
Summation of the Episode of Care	Criteria for discharge Current physical/functional status Degree of achievement of anticipated goals and expected outcomes Reasons for goals and outcomes not being achieved Discharge plan related to patients'/clients' continuing care

BARRIERS TO QUALITY DOCUMENTATION

If all documentation possessed the characteristics discussed above, we would be able to readily use it for developing evidence about the success of care. But there are disparities in much of the physical therapy documentation that preclude it from serving as a meaningful database. Practitioners, including physical therapists, often complain about the time needed to complete documentation as a primary reason for not producing documentation of the best quality.[4-9] Several other reasons are also apparent, as are discussed later.

Focus on Intervention

Current documentation commonly does not address all the appropriate elements listed in the APTA *Guidelines*. The examination may be limited to the identification of impairments and functional loss and may lack a meaningful, complete evaluation, diagnosis, and prognosis. Throughout the continuum of care, documentation commonly focuses on identifying impairments and listing interventions. Flow sheets and checklists are frequently used to record interventions, but there may be no additional documentation to substantiate the patient's/client's responses to the interventions and the subsequent need to revise the plan of care. Too often, the documentation lacks apparent connections between interventions, functional problems, and outcomes. Physical therapists commonly document a discharge summary but may fail to include pertinent discharge criteria about anticipated goals and expected outcomes.

Payment Incentives

Often, practitioners focus on payment for services as the primary reason for documentation of patient care. Economic factors can influence symptom reporting, as can pending litigation with potentials for monetary rewards. Payment for services may promote unfavorable behavior changes in practitioners, such as misrepresentation of information in the patient/client record to obtain reimbursement from insurance companies. Wynia and colleagues[10] surveyed 720 practicing physicians and reported that 39% used falsified patient information or exaggerated symptom severity to obtain insurance authorization. As an explanation for this deceptive documentation, the authors offered the term *covert advocacy* to describe the behavior that results from the tension between patient advocacy and cost containment,.[10]

Nadler et al (2004) reviewed documentation of a straight leg raise (SLR) test in 200 people with a diagnosis of lumbar radiculopathy or disc herniation. Documentation of a positive SLR was more likely if patients were covered under personal injury insurance programs than if they were covered under a managed care workers' compensation program. The likelihood of a positive bilateral SLR diagnosis was even more strongly associated with a personal insurance program. The authors concluded that there might be numerous explanations for these differences, including exaggeration of symptoms by participants, covert advocacy, differences in education levels of providers performing the test, and poor technique or improper interpretation.[11]

Although these studies involved physicians, not physical therapists, it is not too far a leap to imagine that deceptive documentation could occur in physical therapy practices as well. For example, many physical therapists believe that Medicare patients in the acute setting would not be admitted into a rehabilitation setting if the documentation said that they could walk more than 150 feet, so they record that the patient walks 50 feet times 3, an example of covert advocacy. Or they believe that patients would not be considered homebound if they walk more than 100 feet; therefore they may well feel the need to practice covert advocacy and record that a patient can ambulate fewer than 100 feet when this is not true.[12] Interestingly, Medicare guidelines focus on the need for skilled care but do not specify number of feet as a decision determinant.

Lack of Standardized Terminology

The lack of standardized terminology across health professions has affected the quality of documentation. Poor documentation leads to uncertainty in interpreting patient information, impairs communication among providers, and decreases the continuity of care. Müller-Staub et al (2007) evaluated the impact of an educational program to improve implementation of standardized nursing diagnoses (NANDA), interventions (NIC), and outcomes (NOC) based on the premise that standardized language would lead to improved data management and enhanced quality assessment of nursing practices in the areas of diagnosis, intervention, and outcomes. Results indicated that standardized language led to an improvement in the formulation of nursing diagnoses, identification of signs/symptoms and correct etiologies, specific nursing interventions, and documentation of nursing-sensitive patient outcomes.[13]

Oostendorp et al investigated the intrarater and interrater reliability and internal consistency of physical therapy documentation based on a set of quality indicators developed for the study. The authors also looked at the clinical utility of the set of quality indicators and evaluated the quality of physiotherapy patient documentation. They developed a set of 44 indicators, organized into six clusters, representing phases of the physical therapy examination/evaluation process. They are:

1. General (general patient information)
2. Intake
3. History taking
4. Examination
5. Treatment
6. Discharge

Three individuals, a physiotherapist/movement specialist, a physiotherapist, and a health researcher, conducted 147 chart reviews from 160 practices in the Netherlands using the set of quality indicators from the six clusters and a scoring system from 0 to 3 (0 = absent; 1 = somewhat present; 2 = mostly present; 3 = always present). After determining internal consistency, intrarater reliability, and interrater reliability, they concluded that the evaluation instrument has apparent clinical utility and that the quality of the documentation was what they termed moderate (mean score 1.6).[14]

In a pro bono clinical practice setting involving volunteer physical therapists from various facilities and student physical therapists with varying levels of clinical experience and from different academic institutions, the variety of abbreviations is noteworthy. Some examples include:

- P! (pain)
- E′ (elbow)
- S′/ (shoulder extension)
- TB ex (Theraband™ exercises)
- TAC (transverse abdominal contraction)
- DKC (Double knees to chest)
- LAD (long axis distraction)
- POE (prone on elbows)

Though it is possible to decipher the abbreviations in the context of the patient/client documentation as a whole, it is inconvenient in terms of time and inefficient in terms of communication and data collection.

IMPROVING THE UTILITY OF DOCUMENTATION AS A SOURCE OF EVIDENCE

If documentation is to become a reliable source of evidence, these barriers must be overcome. The recommendations to improve documentation, and thereby improve patient care, have two major themes in common: increasing use of electronic record keeping and improving the links between the documentation and the actual outcomes of care.

Use of Electronic Record-Keeping Systems

Electronic record keeping has been proposed as one solution for improving the quality and consistency of documentation. For example, Knaup et al developed a software system, *eardap,* that was based on an *e*xtensible *a*rchitecture for using *r*outine *d*ata for *a*dditional *p*urposes. Just as with clinical research based on a standard terminology, the impetus for the development of this software was the concept that standardized documentation would lead to effective communication through sharing of data based on standardizing terminology.[15] Medicare, along with numerous policy organizations and many insurance companies, has supported the move toward submission of electronic records for payment of services on the premise that electronic record keeping could:

- Improve the quality of documentation
- Increase the efficiency of communication, including that for payment
- Improve patient safety and therefore improve patient outcomes[16]

Despite the promise of electronic record keeping, evidence shows that computer-based systems are not yet the complete answer. A systematic review by Delpierre et al showed that while computer-based systems seem to increase practitioners and patient satisfaction, they were as likely as not to produce positive changes in practitioner behavior related to improved patient care.[17] Because of the anticipation that properly implemented computer-based documentation will have great benefits, policy groups continue to try to identify the barriers to full implementation and the means for overcoming those barriers (Box 18.1).[18–19]

A review of the available literature in physical therapy [20] summarized the benefits (improved reporting, operational efficiency, interdepartmental communication, data accuracy, and access to data for future research) and barriers (need for workflow or behavior modification, software or hardware inadequacy, inadequate staff training) found in previous research about the use of computerized record systems in physical therapy. Based on analysis of the factors that seemed to lead to better success in implementation, the authors of the review recommended

---

Box 18.1	**Principles for Success as Defined by the National Research Council in Their Report: Computational Technology for Effective Health Care: Immediate Steps and Strategic Directions**

Principles for Evolutionary Change

1. Focus on improvements in care—technology is secondary.
2. Seek incremental gain from incremental effort.
3. Record available data so that today's biomedical knowledge can be used to interpret the data to drive care, process improvement, and research.
4. Design for human and organizational factors so that social and institutional processes will not pose barriers to appropriately taking advantage of technology.
5. Support the cognitive functions of all caregivers, including health professionals, patients, and their families.

Principles for Radical Change

1. Architect information and workflow systems to accommodate disruptive change.
2. Archive data for subsequent re-interpretation, that is, in anticipation of future advances in biomedical knowledge that may change today's interpretation of data and advances in computer science that may provide new ways of extracting meaningful and useful knowledge from existing data stores.
3. Seek and develop technologies that identify and eliminate ineffective work processes.
4. Seek and develop technologies that clarify the context of data.

that the following principles be used in implementing computer-based systems for physical therapy documentation:

- Incorporate workflow analysis into the system design and implementation
- Include end users, especially clinicians, in the system development activities
- Devote significant resources to training
- Plan and test carefully to ensure adequate software and hardware system performance
- Pursue the efficient capture of coded data
- Commit to data standards

Support for more widespread adoption of computer-based systems has also been expressed in various APTA activities, including adoption of the policy Support of Electronic Health Records in Physical Therapy in 2008[21] and by support of the Physical Therapy and Society Summit (PASS) in 2009. The Summit focused on a futuristic perspective of health care, including the many opportunities for the use of computer-based systems. One of the major themes of the PASS was also the concept of "disruptive change." Similar to the recommendations from the National Research Council (see Box 18.1), this concept emphasizes the need to be able to recognize and embrace change that makes fundamental differences in current systems.[22]

Description of Actual Patient Outcomes

If documentation is to provide us with better information about patient care, one of the ways we need to improve is by using more standardized outcome measurements, when such measurement is available. By using standardized tools for measuring outcomes, the data in our documentation can be used in observational studies to describe the results of various diagnostic labels and interventions when used in actual practice, in other words, to help measure the effectiveness of our care.

There are many different kinds of outcomes in which we are interested as physical therapists. We need to measure outcomes across the disability model, starting with any changes to pathology that we might achieve, and then measure changes in function, including body structure, activity level, and participation in behaviors related to role. There are also many other areas where we would be interested in measuring outcome, including patient satisfaction, costs of care, and general, health-related quality of life. A good standardized outcome measure is based on many of the same principles discussed in Chapter 12. Standardized measures must be reliable, valid, and generalizable to the patient population for which we are documenting care. We need to know the ability of the test to measure both clinically meaningful and statistically significant change. All outcome measures should be as objective (free from measurement bias) as possible. Subjective measures are those that are much more susceptible to the bias of the observer.[23]

One of the most familiar ways to document patient care is known as the SOAP note. Laurence Weed developed the concept for the SOAP note in the 1960s as part of a documentation system. He was one of the first people to make a strong case for the relationship between clinical reasoning and the form of documentation used by practitioners. He proposed that by documenting patient data in an organized way, a person's thinking becomes apparent to others and to him- or herself, it becomes available for careful scrutiny, and thereby both the documentation and the thinking could be improved. His proposal was a fully integrated, problem-oriented patient record system, which included the patient record, regular auditing of the record, and practitioner education based on the audit. The record was to include

- An organized database for all information collected about the patient through various tests
- A list of the problems that the patient had, extending beyond pathological diagnoses (predating the concept of the disablement model)
- An initial plan for care
- Progress notes

The progress notes were to be in three forms, the narrative note, flow sheets documenting changes in data over time, and a discharge note. It is the narrative note that has come to be called the SOAP note. Each note was to include:

- **S**ubjective notes (what the patient said)
- **O**bjective notes (what the practitioner observed)
- **A**ssessment of what this meant
- **P**lan for future care

All of Weed's concerns and perspectives are still valid today, but the use of the SOAP note has become somewhat problematic. Labeling what patients report to us as "subjective" and what we observe as "objective" in the note has confused many practitioners about the true meaning of these words. Patients can report information to us that is objective (free from bias), and we can record data we collect that is quite subjective (likely to be biased). We would, perhaps, be better off thinking of the first element as symptoms—what is reported to us by the patient—and the second element as signs—what we observe. A second problem with the SOAP note is that while it has been widely adopted, all the other elements of the record system have not been, thereby significantly reducing the impact of Weed's concepts on improving patient care. But it is easy to see that Weed's ideas form the basis of the clinical decision support systems that are now beginning to be available for practitioners (see Chapter 16).[24,25]

In choosing an outcome measure, we can ask several questions:

1. **How much system specificity do we need?**
   A tool containing items that are clearly not relevant to the patient wastes time, but the more specific the measure, the more limited our ability to compare outcomes across large groups.
2. **Does the tool measure the range of outcomes in which we are interested?**
   Outcome tools have what is termed ceiling and floor effects. This means that some tools are very good at measuring outcomes in people with severe impairments and decreased function and other tools are much better at measuring outcomes in patients who started care with fewer impairments and a high level of function. Very few tools can do both.

3. **Over what time frame are we concerned about changes in performance?**

   Some tools are best at measuring change across the course of a typical episode of care, such as days or weeks. Others are best at measuring change over long periods, such as months and years, as would be appropriate for patients with long-term or chronic health problems.

4. **Are we interested in measuring changes in one person over time or in comparing the results for groups of patients?**

   This question is certainly also related to time frame but deals with another fundamental difference. Sometimes we need a tool to help us measure the individual patient's progress toward specific goals, and sometimes we are interested in comparing our overall programs, as in benchmark activities, or in creating databases for evidence based practice or clinical research.

5. **Is the tool completed by observation of patient behavior or by patient report?**

   It is not possible for a therapist to observe all behaviors, nor is it desirable. For example, we often see a patient after trauma and/or surgery and we need to rely on reports from the patient or family about prior level of function as the baseline outcome measure. Some tools, but not all, have been shown to reliably measure behavior through patient report.

6. **Was the tool really created to measure outcomes across time or did it have another purpose?**

   Many of the tools used in clinical practice have been developed for a particular purpose. For example, the Berg Balance Score was developed as a screening tool.[26] The Functional Impairment Measure (FIM) was developed as a way to compare group data across multiple rehabilitation facilities.[27] Neither of these was developed as a means to track outcomes for individual patients across time, although subsequent work has been done to assess their appropriateness as tools for this purpose.[28,29] Until the tool has been validated for our intended purpose, it is best to use it for its original, validated purpose.

7. **Can I design a tool that is specific to my practice; can I adapt an existing tool to make it more specific to my practice?**

   It is tempting, and all too common, to develop "home-grown," idiosyncratic tools for documenting outcomes in patient care. But such tools have not been studied for what is called their psychometric properties. In other words, we don't know their reliability, validity, or generalizability. Therefore, these tools may not be telling us very much at all about real changes in impairment or function based outcomes. And they certainly can't help us in developing databases for evidence based practice.

Just as with other aspects of evidence based practice, the adoption of appropriate standardized measures has been slower than would be desirable. Researchers examining the reasons for this have identified that in addition to the usual barriers, such as perceived lack of time and lack of knowledge, physical therapists also believe the standardized tools do not always provide sufficient description of the quality of movement being observed.[30–32] Stevens et al have described in a case study the adoption of more standardized outcome measures in one practice, a process very similar to that discussed in Chapter 17. They emphasized that implementation of outcome measures has to be inclusive of documentation strategies but also emphasized that the most important aspect of their plan was incorporating the use into therapists' clinical reasoning.[33] Deutcher et al described the benefits of integrating an electronic system with implementation of standardized measures. They concluded that such a system leads to the types of analysis described by Delitto and Bise in Chapter 19.[34]

New documentation systems for physical therapy have been devised that build on these principles. For example, the American Physical Therapy Association (APTA) has created, in partnership with an outcomes measurement firm, a product known as APTA CONNECT. APTA CONNECT is designed to be a point-of-care, computerized patient record system. In addition to the ability to schedule and register patients, the system contains many standardized outcome tools. The data entered into APTA CONNECT are then loaded into a national outcomes database, which is used to better understand the effect of physical therapy care. In addition, APTA is expanding this national database to allow submission of data from all physical therapists, whether or not they are using APTA CONNECT. (www.apta.org/CONNECT/)

QUALITY IMPROVEMENT SYSTEMS

A full discussion of quality measurement and improvement in health care is beyond the scope of this book. Documentation has been linked to the concept of quality for as long as health-services researchers and clinicians have been discussing quality. Avedis Donabedian is considered one of the founding theorists in this area. He contended that there are three approaches to the evaluation of quality:

• Appraisal of *structure*, including physical structures, qualifications of heath-care personnel, and administrative organization. These structural elements are seen as necessary, but *not* sufficient to assure quality care.
• Appraisal of *process,* focused primarily on what the health care practitioner does. This approach relies on being able to identify a standard for acceptable, or even best, process.
• Appraisal of *outcomes*, evaluating the end results *of care* in terms of health and satisfaction. This approach is successful only if all parties can agree on what successful outcomes actually are and is based on a belief, preferably evidence, that the outcomes are actually a result of the care provided.[35]

This model has been the basis of much of the work done about quality over the past 50 years. Evidence based practice clearly has roots in the model. Figure 18-1 shows the model as well as specific physical therapy examples in each category.

Donabedian pointed out that patient care documentation is an essential source of information for all three aspects of the model. He documented the prevailing issues of incompleteness, inaccuracy, and potential bias in the patient record, issues with which we continue to grapple today. Considerable efforts have been made at all levels of the health care enterprise (see side bar) to put in place quality assessment techniques designed for all three types of appraisal. Almost all of these techniques rely on good documentation.

Many organizations focus on the issues of quality in health care. Perhaps the two most prominent in the United States are the Agency for Healthcare Research and Quality (AHRQ), which is part of the U.S, Department of Health and Human Services (U.S. DHHS) and the Joint Commission.

As stated at the AHRQ Web site (www.ahrq.gov/), AHRQ's mission is "to improve the quality, safety, efficiency, and effectiveness of health care for all Americans." It further states that the overall focus of AHRQ is on:

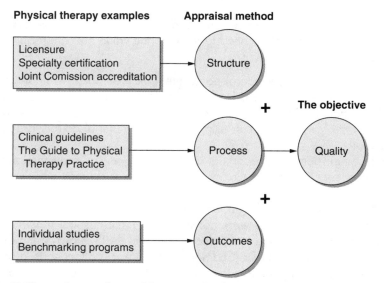

Figure 18-1 The Different Approaches to Measuring Quality.

- "Safety and quality: Reduce the risk of harm by promoting delivery of the best possible health care.
- Effectiveness: Improve health care outcomes by encouraging the use of evidence to make informed health care decisions.
- Efficiency: Transform research into practice to facilitate wider access to effective health care services and reduce unnecessary costs."

To achieve its goals AHRQ supports research in the following areas:

- **"Comparative Effectiveness ...** Comparative effectiveness research improves health care quality by providing patients and physicians with state-of-the-science information on which medical treatments work best for a given condition.
- **Patient Safety** The Patient Safety Portfolio helps identify risks and hazards that lead to medical errors and finds ways to prevent patient injury associated with delivery of health care. ...
- **Health Information Technology** Through this research Portfolio, AHRQ and its partners identify challenges to health IT adoption and use, solutions and best practices for making health IT work, and tools that will help hospitals and clinicians successfully incorporate new information technology. ...
- **Prevention/Care Management** The Prevention/Care Management Portfolio focuses on translating evidence based knowledge into current recommendations for clinical preventive services that are implemented as part of routine clinical practice to improve the health of all Americans. ...
- **Value Research** The Value Research Portfolio aims to find a way to achieve greater value in health care—reducing unnecessary costs and waste while maintaining or improving quality—by producing the measures, data, tools,

(Continued on page 314)

evidence and strategies that health care organizations, systems, insurers, purchasers, and policymakers need to improve the value and affordability of health care. ..."

In its role as an arm of the federal government, AHRQ makes its findings and those of the researchers it supports freely available through its Web site, which has material designed specifically for consumers and for practitioners. It is well worth a regular review; viewers can also request that material be forwarded to them via e-mail.

The Joint Commission, as it reports at its Web site, www.jointcommission.org/, began as a concept of Dr. Ernest Codman, an orthopedic surgeon who is widely considered to be the first major spokesman for health care quality. In 1910, he proposed that hospitals should begin tracking the end results of the care provided to patients, and when the results were not satisfactory, the hospital should endeavor to determine why and make necessary changes to improve. (Physical therapists may be familiar with Dr. Codman's name, as it is attached to a group of post-operative shoulder exercises long used in physical therapy.) Work by various physicians and hospital groups on this concept led to the formation of the Joint Commission on Accreditation of Hospitals (JCAH) in 1951, with the purpose of giving accreditation to hospitals that met certain minimum standards. Through the years, the Joint Commission's role has expanded to include many other types of health care organizations so that its current mission is stated, "All people always experience the safest, highest quality, best-value health care across all settings."

The earliest efforts of the Joint Commission focused on appraisal of structure; it subsequently has taken many initiatives related to quality assessment and improvement. This increased focus on the appraisal of process has relied on documentation to determine quality. In the 1970s, the Commission began promoting the use of the chart audit to identify if a predetermined set of activities had occurred with particular patients. Most recently it has implemented a new program stressing the use of measures for quality improvement that meet these four criteria:

- There is a strong evidence base showing that the care process leads to improved outcomes.
- The measure accurately captures whether the evidence based care process has, in fact, been provided.
- The measure addresses a process that has few intervening care processes that must occur before the improved outcome is realized.
- Implementing the measure has little or no chance of inducing unintended adverse consequences.[36]

Once again, the close interaction between evidence based practice, quality improvement activities, and documentation has been demonstrated. These two agencies, one a federal initiative and the other a voluntary initiative on the part of health care providers, lead the way in policy making in these areas.

Studies of implementing various means of improving documentation generally show some benefit. For example, Gumery et al (2000) reported the effect of chart audits done pre- and post-training on improving physical therapy documentation for patients in an adult cystic fibrosis unit in Birmingham, England. The purpose of the study was to assess adherence to professional standards of the Chartered Society of Physiotherapy (CSP) and the Association of Chartered Physiotherapists in Respiratory Care (ACPRC) by all physiotherapists working in the adult cystic fibrosis unit. The authors concluded that chart audits and training were useful tools in improving documentation and can lead to five key outcomes:

- increased knowledge and understanding of effective practice,
- increased effectiveness of service provision,
- improved practice,
- improved quality of patient care, and
- demonstration of commitment to evidence-based practice.[37]

CONCLUSION

Efforts to use documentation as a means of improving the quality of health care have been under way for at least a century, yet documentation still does not always achieve the quality required for it to be readily used as an accurate record of care, as a basis for developing evidence from practice, and as a mechanism for measuring and improving quality. What can we do to change this situation? We appear to be at the point where electronic systems can provide all of the elements needed to make documentation a successful tool for quality assessment and improvement, including ease of use, access at the point of care, and ability to document the complexity of patient care. Zhou et al[38] bring us full circle with their work showing that simply implementing electronic systems is not sufficient. Success is linked to the system's ability to help the practitioner make better decisions. Chapter 19 describes just such a program in actual physical therapy practice. Other examples will be available at the F.A. Davis Web site for this text. We can also recognize the issues discussed in Chapter 17 to help reduce barriers to successful implementation. Perhaps the growth of point-of-care decision-support systems, as discussed in Chapter 16, offer the best possibility for the future.

SELF-ASSESSMENT

1. Review the documentation provided about Mr. Ketterman in the Appendix. Although it contains more than would typically be found in a clinical chart, review those elements that would be contained in a patient chart. What suggestions can you make to improve this documentation? What can you learn from the example to improve your own documentation?
2. Review three or four clinical charts. Do they meet the standards identified in this chapter? What suggestions would you make to the clinicians who documented in the charts to improve the record?
3. Identify the documentation system used in your clinical practice or in one with which you are familiar. Is there a system that you can identify? Does the system have the right elements to support good physical therapy documentation?

CONTINUED LEARNING

- The APTA has developed Defensible Documentation as a tool to help clinicians improve their documentation skills. Downloadable documents are available to members only at www.apta.org/Documentation/DefensibleDocumentation/, and an Internet-based course is available to all at learningcenter.apta.org/. Either of these tools has a great deal of information that can be helpful in improving documentation in a wide variety of settings.
- Identify the outcome measures used in your practice. Identify what is known about the reliability, validity, and generalizability of these measures for your given patient population. The book, *Is Change Real?* by Riddle and Stratford (Philadelphia, FA Davis, 2013) can be useful in determining whether you should adopt or change outcome measures in practice.
- Review the quality-assurance activities in your practice. Determine whether they measure the quality of the structure, process, or outcome of care. Do you have ideas on how to improve these activities?

REFERENCES

1. American Health Management Information Association. Practice Brief: Definition of the Health Record for Legal Purposes. http://library.ahima.org/xpedio/groups/public/documents/ahima/bok1_009223.hcsp?dDocName=bok1_009223 Accessed February 21, 2012.
2. American Health Management Information Association. HIM Principles in Health Information Exchange: Data Quality Attributes Grid. http://library.ahima.org/xpedio/groups/public/documents/ahima/bok1_035071.pdf
3. American Physical Therapy Association. *Guidelines: Physical Therapy Documentation of Patient/Client Management.* APTA Board of Directors; 2005. www.apta.org/uploaded-Files/APTAorg/About_Us/Policies/BOD/Practice/DocumentationPatientClientMgmt.pdf#search = %22guidelines%20documentation%22
4. Oxentenko AS, West CP, Popkave C, et al. Time spent on clinical documentation: A survey of internal medicine residents and program directors. Arch Intern Med. 2010; 170(4):377–380.
5. Gottschalk A, Flocke SA. Time spent in face-to-face patient care and work outside the examination room. Ann Fam Med. 2005;3:488–493.
6. Ammenwerth E, Spötl H-P. The time needed for clinical documentation versus direct patient care: A work-sampling analysis of physicians' activities. Methods of Information in Med. 2009;1:84–91.
7. Malone DJ. The new demands of acute care: Are we ready? Editorial, PhysTher. 2010;90:1370–1373.
8. Lopopolo RB. The relationship of role-related variables to job satisfaction and commitment to the organization in a restructured hospital environment. PhysTher. 2002;82:984–999.
9. Blau R, Bolus S, Carolan T, et al. The experience of providing physical therapy in a changing health care environment. PhysTher. 2002;82:648–657.
10. Wynia MK, Cummins DS, PhVanGeest JB, et al. Physician manipulation of reimbursement rules for patients. JAMA. 2000;283(14):1858–1865.
11. Nadler SF, Malanga GA, Ciccone DS. Positive straight-leg raising in lumbar radiculopathy: Is documentation affected by insurance coverage? Arch Phys Med Rehabil. 2004;85: 1336–1338.
12. Personal communication from physical therapist students and physical therapists.
13. Müller-Staub M, Needham I, Odenbreit M, et al. Improved quality of nursing documentation: Results of a nursing diagnoses, interventions, and outcomes implementation study. Int J Nurs Terminologies and Classifications. 2007;18(1):5–17,.
14. Oostendorp RAB, Pluimers DJ, Nijhuis-van der Sanden MWG. Physiotherapy patient documentation: The Achilles heel of evidence-based practice? Nederlands Tijdschrift Voor Fysiotherapie. Juni 2006;3(116):56–61.

15. Knaupa P, Gardeb S, Merzweilerc A, et al. Towards shared patient records: An architecture for using routine data for nationwide research, Int J Med Informatics. 2006;75: 191–200.
16. The Official Web Site for the Medicare and Medicaid EHR Incentive Programs. https://www.cms.gov/EHRIncentivePrograms/ Accessed December, 2010.
17. Delpierre C, Cuzin L, Fillaux J, et al. A systematic review of computer-based patient record systems and quality of care: More randomized clinical trials or a broader approach? Int J Quality Health Care. 16(5):407–416.
18. Committee on Data Standards for Patient Safety Board on Health Care Services Institute of Medicine of the National Academy of Sciences. *Key Capabilities of an Electronic Health Record System: Letter Report.* Washington, DC: National Academies Press; 2003.
19. Stead WW, Lin HS, eds. *Computational Technology for Effective Health Care: Immediate Steps and Strategic Directions.* Washington, DC: National Academies Press; 2009.
20. Vreeman DJ, Taggard SL, Rhine MD, et al. Evidence for electronic health record systems in physical therapy. PhysTher. 2006;86:434–449.
21. American Physical Therapy Association. *Support of Electronic Health Record In Physical Therapy.* APTA; 2008.
22. Kigin CM, Rodgers MM, Wolf SL, for the PASS Committee Members. The Physical Therapy and Society Summit (PASS) meeting: observations and opportunities. PhysTher. 2010;90:1555–1567.
23. McDowell I. *Measuring Health: A Guide to Rating Scales and Questionnaires,* 3rd ed. Oxford, UK: Oxford Press; 2006.
24. Weed L. *Medical Records, Medical Education, and Patient Care.* Chicago: Year Book Medical Publishers; 1969.
25. Weed L. Quality control. In: Walker HK, Hurst JW, Woody MF, eds. *Applying the Problem-Oriented System.* New York: Medcom Press; 1973.
26. Berg K, Wood-Dauphinee S, Williams JI, et al. Measuring balance in the elderly: Preliminary development of an instrument. Physiother Can. 1989;41:304–311.
27. Hamilton BB, Granger CV, Sherwin FS, et al. A uniform national data system for medical rehabilitation. In: Fuhrer MJ, ed. Rehabilitation outcomes: Analysis and measurement. Baltimore: Paul H Brookes; 1987:137–147.
28. Blum L, Korner-Bitensky N. Usefulness of the Berg Balance Scale in stroke rehabilitation: A systematic review. PhysTher. 2008;88:559–566.
29. Chumney D, Nollinger K, Shesko K, et al. Ability of Functional Independence Measure to accurately predict functional outcome of stroke-specific population: Systematic review. J Rehab Res & Develop. 2010;47(1):17–30.
30. Copeland JM, Taylor WJ, Dean SG. Factors influencing the use of outcome measures for patients with low back pain: A survey of New Zealand physical therapists. PhysTher. 2008;88:1492–1505.
31. Jette DU, Halbert J, Iverson C, et al. Use of standardized outcome measures in physical therapist practice: Perceptions and applications. PhysTher. 2009;89:125–135.
32. McGinnis PQ, Hack LM, Nixon-Cave K, et al. Factors that influence the clinical decision making of physical therapists in choosing a balance assessment approach. PhysTher. 2009;89:233–247.
33. Stevens JGA, Beurskens AJMH. Implementation of measurement instruments in physical therapist practice: Development of a tailored strategy. PhysTher. 2010; 90:953–961.
34. Deutscher D, Hart DL, Dickstein R, et al. Implementing an integrated electronic outcomes and electronic health record process to create a foundation for clinical practice improvement. PhysTher. 2008;88:270–285.
35. Donabedian A. *A Guide to Medical Care Administration, Volume II: Medical Care Appraisal–Quality and Utilization.* New York: American Public Health Association; 1966.
36. Chassin MR, Loeb JM, Schmaltz SP, et al. Accountability measures—Using measurement to promote quality improvement. N Engl J Med. 2010;363:683–668.
37. Gumery L, Sheldon J, Bayliss H, et al. Do physiotherapy records meet professional standards? Physiother. 2000;86:655–659.
38. Zhou L, Soran CS, Jenter CA, et al. The relationship between electronic health record use and quality of care over time. J Am Med Inform Assoc. 2009;16:457–464.

chapter 19

Quality Improvement in Action

Christopher G. Bise, PT, DPT, MS
Anthony Delitto, PT, PhD, FAPTA

Things could be worse. Suppose your errors were counted and published every day, like those of a baseball player.

—UNKNOWN

•

✳ Mr. Ketterman's Case

I've worked hard to learn how to improve my care for patients like Mr. Ketterman. Is there some way I can find out if my interventions are effective over time? Should I be encouraging my colleagues to make the same changes? *(See Appendix for Mr. Ketterman's health history.)*

INTRODUCTION

In previous chapters of this book, you have had the opportunity to gain *competence* in the nuts and bolts of evidence-based practice (EBP). That is, you have used published research and other forms of evidence to increase your knowledge and skills in determining the diagnostic and prognostic value of tests and measures, evaluating clinical diagnostic strategies, making accurate prognoses, and deciding on the most efficacious treatment interventions for your patient. You are now ready for the next step in the EBP process: *implementation* of this newfound competence into your everyday practice. By implementing EBP, your increased competence and knowledge will potentially change your attitude about your approach to patients by not only considering what the latest evidence has to offer but actually realigning your behavior when appropriate, as measured by your own *clinical performance*. This EBP paradigm is illustrated in Figure 19-1.

Achieving Change in Performance

It becomes very important to distinguish between clinical competence and clinical performance in the evidence based process. We cannot assume that competence (e.g., knowledge of

319

best practice principles and skill of administering) immediately translates to evidence based clinical performance, where the latter depends on aligning clinical behavior to be consistent with best practice principles.

The evidence is very clear that the translation of evidence into clinical performance is lagging in our health care system, a fact best illustrated by the Institute of Medicine's (IOM) characterization of the "Quality Chasm."[1] The extent of disparity between best practice standards and clinical performance is an unfortunate fact that transcends all health professions, including physical therapy. For example, in 1994 the Agency for Health Care Policy and Research (now known as the Agency for Health Care Research and Quality) published evidence based practice guidelines for managing acute low back pain, some of which were highly relevant to physical therapy.[2] Among the myriad of interventions for acute low back pain, two interventional procedures were assessed that fell well within the scope of practice for physical therapy: use of physical agents (e.g., heat, cold) and manual therapy. The guideline recommended against the use of physical agents and in favor of using manipulation for acute low back pain. Several years after this guideline was published, it is clear from the literature that physical therapists' attitudes toward these interventions and subsequent clinical behaviors (e.g., choices of treatment interventions) were clearly not aligned with the recommendations. In fact, evidence related to clinical performance demonstrates that *overutilization* of physical agents and *underutilization* of manual therapy is the rule in physical therapists' management of low back pain.[2]

Although many potential barriers to translation have been proposed, some researchers point to competency shortfalls as a primary reason for clinical care not aligning optimally with best practice standards.[3] As the evidence based literature grows, clinicians are increasingly pressured to keep up-to-date and must negotiate and digest an ever increasing body of literature related to their patients and practice environments. We hope that the strategies and tools described in the preceding chapters will be helpful. In addition, we suggest strategies of lifelong learning, such as the judicious use of continuing education, can be used to stay current with contemporary knowledge and skills necessary to effectively treat patients.

An integral part of any lifelong learning plan is a candid assessment of your own performance. We are seeing competency assessment become increasingly common in graduate curriculums and ongoing assessment of advanced practice knowledge and skills in the clinic. Unfortunately, competency assessment alone does not ensure that clinical practice will be consistent with evidence-based, best practice standards.

In addition to staying up-to-date with competencies relevant to your patients and practice environments, perhaps the most important component of EBP is the implementation of newfound knowledge and skill in daily practice and *review of your performance*. Only by reviewing performance will you convince yourself that your patients are better off as a result of your efforts to implement the latest in EBP principles. The EBP paradigm (see Fig. 19-1) involves gaining new knowledge and skills from published literature through searching and evaluation that will lead to changing *attitudes* toward tests, measures, and interventions, which will eventually lead to *changing clinical behavior* (e.g., implementing tests, measures, and interventions based on evidence in lieu of those you may now be using). In order to assess performance with regard to adherence to EBP principles, you must measure it comprehensively.

The remaining portion of this chapter will focus on strategies for routinely evaluating your clinical performance with an emphasis on implementing best practice standards that are evidence based. In addition, we emphasize the importance of tracking patient outcomes.

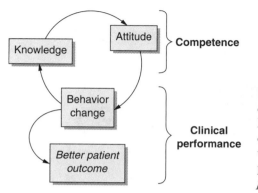

Figure 19-1 The EBP Paradigm. Knowledge obtained through the EBP process should eventually lead to attitude changes and eventually to behavior change. Knowledge, skill, and attitude can be tested through *competency assessment.* Adherence to best practice standards is best measured through *clinical performance assessment.*

Reviewing Performance: A Continuous Quality Improvement Approach

To gain *competence* in evaluating and managing patients using the best available evidence requires a framework by which you can critically appraise evidence and tools and that allows you to gather, collate, organize, and digest the ever increasing body of new evidence as it is published and disseminated. Previous chapters in this book have given you the tools with which to search, appraise, and summarize literature relevant to your practice environment. Now this information must be transformed into a measurable *process of care* for the patients that you see in everyday practice. The remaining portion of this chapter will attempt to show how quality improvement (QI) principles apply in the measurement of clinical performance.

A very simple old adage in QI literature is: you cannot manage what you do not measure. Performance assessment in any domain requires a comprehensive measurement approach. In clinical care, we attempt to measure clinical performance by routine use of chart audits, direct observation, and the use of specific clinical performance instruments. These approaches are largely unsuccessful because of unwarranted variability in the process of care and documentation of the same, both of which inhibit a comprehensive assessment of performance.

We have provided an overall framework for clinical performance appraisal and how it fits in the EBP process (see Fig. 19-1). More specific steps will allow you to collect and collate clinical data that is critical to performance appraisal. Ultimately, these steps lead to an accessible clinical database that becomes the tool used for performance appraisal.

Framework for QI-Based Performance Assessment

Figure 19-2 outlines four steps necessary for accurately evaluating clinical performance as it relates to implementing an evidence based approach to patient care in a clinical setting. The key component includes *measuring clinical performance,* with the goal of evaluating how well you are adhering to evidence based practice standards that you have set for yourself.

Step 1: Formulate the data fields for the clinical database that will be used for clinician performance assessment. This database will include patient information from the following categories:

1. Patient history (including pertinent medical history)
2. Tests and measures selected

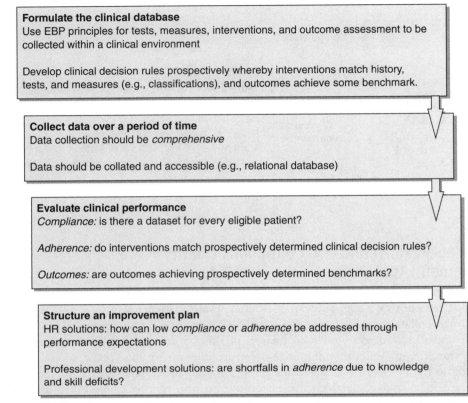

Formulate the clinical database
Use EBP principles for tests, measures, interventions, and outcome assessment to be collected within a clinical environment

Develop clinical decision rules prospectively whereby interventions match history, tests, and measures (e.g., classifications), and outcomes achieve some benchmark.

Collect data over a period of time
Data collection should be *comprehensive*

Data should be collated and accessible (e.g., relational database)

Evaluate clinical performance
Compliance: is there a dataset for every eligible patient?

Adherence: do interventions match prospectively determined clinical decision rules?

Outcomes: are outcomes achieving prospectively determined benchmarks?

Structure an improvement plan
HR solutions: how can low *compliance* or *adherence* be addressed through performance expectations

Professional development solutions: are shortfalls in *adherence* due to knowledge and skill deficits?

Figure 19-2 Four Steps to a Performance-Based Assessment of Implementing Evidence-Based Practice Within a Clinical Environment.

3. Clinical decision rules used
4. Interventions selected
5. Patient outcomes

In planning and formulating the database, it is helpful to keep in mind the end goal, which is to be able to evaluate adherence to best practice standards and clinical performance. Several factors are worth discussion:

- **Comprehensiveness versus exhaustiveness:** Whenever a clinical database is formulated, the temptation arises to collect too much information. The more data to be collected, the greater the likelihood you will not have a complete data set on all patients because of the workload involved. The collection must be precise but extensive enough to be representative of the variables being assessed. Keep in mind that in a quality improvement initiative, the tolerance for missing data must be kept at a minimum.
- **Environmental considerations:** As you prepare to collect the data, you need to consider how environmental factors can affect both the data and the collection process. Data will need to be collected and entered into a database and then monitored. Poor adherence to any one of these processes can lead to incomplete data sets, which will compromise the QI effort. Barriers to complete data sets are numerous in a fast-paced clinical environment with limited resources. To ensure completed data sets, some system of surveillance

must be incorporated. The methodology can include clerical staff or an automated information technology (IT) approach.

- **Cultural considerations:** Finally, you need to consider the culture in which you are collecting the data. As a profession, physical therapists have long relied on intuition and remain somewhat skeptical when presented with change. As you begin to collect and analyze the data, the culture around you may not embrace the process because it suggests the possibility of change.

Step 2: Collect data over time. Again, with the goal in mind, pick a defined period over which to collect the data. The duration should be of sufficient length to allow for an accurate snapshot of the behavior or practice patterns being analyzed. Keep in mind that the data collection must be comprehensive—it must include all data—and can sometimes be a tedious process. Careful attention must be given to the type of collection system used. A system that is labor-intensive might produce the most data but may begin to compete inappropriately with patients for the attention of the clinical staff. Collection that is too lean may not give the full picture of clinical performance. The optimal system will be quick and easy for clinicians to use and easy to read or input for those responsible for data input.

Once in the database, the data need to be accessible to you and your research (or QI) team and presented in a way that is easy to understand. Avoid complicated statistical computations. Try to present the facts in a format that will allow those involved with the process to evaluate the metrics being measured and then draw conclusions about performance. Businesses outside of health care have long used metrics to evaluate their performance. With the increased use of technology and the availability of real-time sales data, a "dashboard system" has become the norm in large companies. The "dashboard" presentation of the database makes the data easy to obtain, read, and analyze. You can then begin to make appropriate changes in clinical behavior based on this easily available record of performance.

Step 3: Evaluate clinical performance. After the data have been collected, collated, and presented in a useable form, you can begin to draw conclusions about clinical performance. The first component for analysis is compliance. How compliant was the individual practitioner with the data collection? Remember, data collection must be comprehensive or it doesn't reflect the true nature of performance. Second is adherence to the protocol. Our research has investigated the results of compliance with clinical decision making protocols. The data collected evaluated whether individual therapists correctly classified patients and then initiated the proper interventions regarding low back care. The final step was evaluating the outcomes achieved and their correlation with a set of predetermined benchmarks. Benchmarking is the process whereby individuals can evaluate their own personal performance against that of a group or a predetermined set of metrics. Our research specifically evaluated the downstream costs for low back care. Therapists who adhered to the protocol were compared with those who deviated from the established low back care guidelines. The established care guidelines were the benchmark. (See below for a fuller description of this research.)

Step 4: Structure an improvement plan. The final step in performance assessment is to create a plan for improvement. In the last step, compliance and adherence were evaluated. Problems in these areas could be addressed through the human resource department. Improvements in compliance allow an analysis of a comprehensive data set that more accurately reflects clinical practice.

After the first data set has been analyzed, adherence to specific treatment protocols can be ascertained. Changes in adherence can be measured over time and then compared to the baseline. The only remaining question is why clinicians do not adhere to the protocol. In our experience, most of the answers to this question can be broken down into two categories: nonadherence based on lack of knowledge and nonadherence based on lack of interest in or agreement with the QI process. The first is easily remedied: Educate the clinicians. The second, and more critical, will require an educational component but may also require the intervention of a third party. With national health care reform looming on the horizon, the third party may be the insurer or in some cases the consumer. Current research has focused on answering one question: What will it take to get clinicians to "do the right thing"?[4] (Chapter 17 discussed this issue in more detail.) In the remainder of this chapter, we will give an example of QI research and how it makes the transition from instrument of measure to instrument of change.

Continuous Quality Improvement in Action

At the University of Pittsburgh, students are involved in a clinical performance final project. The project is intended to give students a tool for evaluating their clinical performance as they become licensed therapists. Early in the evidence based practice portion of the curriculum, students begin to select interventions and outcome measures for specific pathologies based on the strength of current evidence. The intervention and its outcome are then part of the data the student collects and then uses to populate the QI database fields. Data collection occurs during the first 6 months of the final year of clinical education. After 6 months, students analyze the data for adherence to best practice standards, compliance with data collection, and patient outcomes. Each student then identifies deficiencies, makes a plan for change, and begins the data collection process again. The final step of the project is a presentation of the initial and final data sets with a critical evaluation of clinical performance and ability to evaluate and change deficiencies over the clinical year. The result is an invaluable resource for evaluating personal change. You may say at this point that this is an academic assignment, required of students, and could never be executed in a clinical situation. McGee et al showed that not only can this system of performance be implemented in clinical practice but it can actually be used to decrease the total overall cost of delivery of physical therapy care.[5]

In 2007, a research group at the University of Pittsburgh identified difficulties with therapists' adherence to a treatment protocol for low back pain (LBP). The advantages of a treatment-based classification (TBC) approach were identified as far back as 1995 and culminated in a series of articles.[6] Finally, a randomized controlled trial (RCT) published in 2006 offered undeniable evidence that a treatment-based classification system offered superior outcomes over other interventions in the treatment of LBP.[7] Despite the evidence, care for LBP by physical therapists went relatively unchanged. The 2007 University of Pittsburgh research group speculated that adherence to TBC (Fig. 19-3) would provide better outcomes while reducing total overall cost of care.

The Pittsburgh study was an excellent example of a quality improvement initiative put into practice. Let's look back at the four steps in the quality improvement process and compare it to the study. The first step is *formulation of the clinical database*. The data used in the study was gleaned from a database collected by a large health system as part of its low back initiative. This initiative began as an attempt to identify the costs associated with low back care. The data collected provided all the markers needed to identify those physical therapists who were adherent to the TBC and those that were not, as well as the patient outcomes. Step 2 involves choosing *a period of time for data collection*. The researchers chose to collect the initial data over 12 months. This allowed for an appropriate number of patients to be admitted to the data set and provided an appropriate length of time for analyzing trends that might

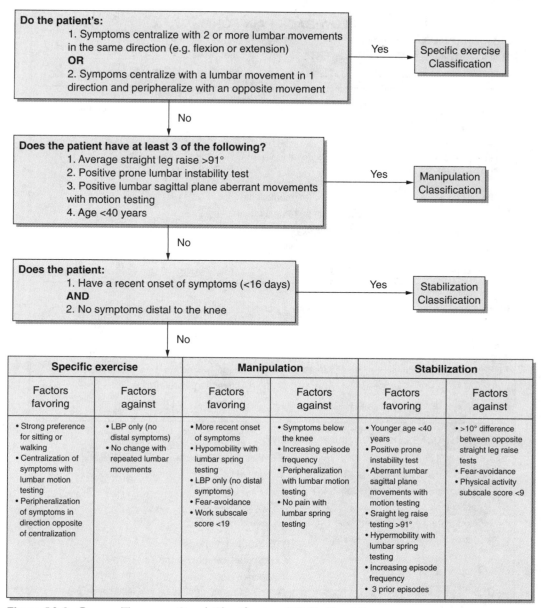

Do the patient's:
1. Symptoms centralize with 2 or more lumbar movements in the same direction (e.g. flexion or extension)
OR
2. Sympoms centralize with a lumbar movement in 1 direction and peripheralize with an opposite movement

Yes → Specific exercise Classification

No ↓

Does the patient have at least 3 of the following?
1. Average straight leg raise >91°
2. Positive prone lumbar instability test
3. Positive lumbar sagittal plane aberrant movements with motion testing
4. Age <40 years

Yes → Manipulation Classification

No ↓

Does the patient:
1. Have a recent onset of symptoms (<16 days)
AND
2. No symptoms distal to the knee

Yes → Stabilization Classification

No ↓

Specific exercise		Manipulation		Stabilization	
Factors favoring	Factors against	Factors favoring	Factors against	Factors favoring	Factors against
• Strong preference for sitting or walking • Centralization of symptoms with lumbar motion testing • Peripheralization of symptoms in direction opposite of centralization	• LBP only (no distal symptoms) • No change with repeated lumbar movements	• More recent onset of symptoms • Hypomobility with lumbar spring testing • LBP only (no distal symptoms) • Fear-avoidance • Work subscale score <19	• Symptoms below the knee • Increasing episode frequency • Peripheralization with lumbar motion testing • No pain with lumbar spring testing	• Younger age <40 years • Positive prone instability test • Aberrant lumbar sagittal plane movements with motion testing • Sraight leg raise testing >91° • Hypermobility with lumbar spring testing • Increasing episode frequency • 3 prior episodes	• >10° difference between opposite straight leg raise tests • Fear-avoidance • Physical activity subscale score <9

Figure 19-3 Current Treatment-Based Classification (TBC) Algorithm.

confound the data set. Failure of the therapist to collect or complete the minimum data set would confound further analysis.

Step 3 consists of *data analysis*. We have previously noted the importance of having complete minimum data sets (Fig. 19-4) for each patient. Early in the collection process the study coordinator noted an increase in the number of patients admitted to the study but no subsequent increase in the number of complete data sets. After the first 2 months, only 18% of the minimum data sets (MDS) had been completed. Lack of data severely compromises the

LOW BACK PAIN FORM

DEMOGRAPHICS (Initial only)

Status: ☐ Licensed PT ☐ Student PT   Date (Initial): _____

Patient ID: _____   Gender: ☐ Male   ☐ Female

HISTORY (Initial only)

Location (check one)

☐ LBP

☐ LBP and buttock/thigh symptoms (not distal to knee)

☐ LBP and leg symptoms distal to knee

Duration

☐ 15 days

☐ >15 days

Location of other symptoms (check all that apply)

☐ N/A

☐ Head/Neck

☐ Thoracic spine

☐ Upper extremity (ies)

☐ Hip(s)

☐ Knee(s)

☐ Foot/feet

FABQ

PA _____

WK _____

Post surgical

☐ Yes

☐ No

Sought medical care for this same episode in the past?

☐ Yes ☐ No

Previous episodes of LBP ☐ 0 ☐ 1–2 ☐ 3–5 ☐ >5

Frequency increasing ☐ Yes ☐ No

PHYSICAL EXAM: ☐ Initial   ☐ Follow-up   Date: _____

Avg SLR

☐ 91

☐ <91

Prone instability test

☐ Positive

☐ Negative

Mobility testing

☐ Hypo

☐ Normal

☐ Hyper

Directional preference

☐ Extension

☐ Flexion

☐ No directional preference

Aberrant movements

☐ Yes

☐ No

Pain (worst): _____   Flexion ROM: _____   Oswestry: _____

TREATMENT CLASSIFICATION (initial & weekly):

Stage I (check one)

☐ Thrust manipulation (Grade V)

☐ Non thrust manipulation (Grade I–IV)

☐ Stabilization

☐ Flexion directional preference

☐ Extension directional preference

☐ Traction

Stage II (check all that apply)

☐ Aerobic

☐ General conditioning

FABQW status (check one)

☐ Negative (<29)

☐ "At risk" (29–34)

☐ Positive (>34)

FABQPA status

☐ Positive (>14)

☐ Negative (14)

NOTE: You must check

1. One stage I category *or* one or more stage II categories ***and***

2. One FABQ status (initial only; weekly optional)

INTERVENTIONS (initial & weekly): (check all that apply)

☐ Patient education/instruction

☐ Flexion exercises

☐ Extension exercises

☐ Flexibility exercises

☐ Stabilization exercises

☐ General conditioning exercises

☐ Thrust manipulation (Grade V)

☐ Non thrust manipulation (Grade I–IV)

☐ Aerobic exercise

☐ Functional training

☐ Heat modalities

☐ Cold modalities

☐ Traction — mechanical

☐ Traction — autotraction

☐ De-weighting/unloading

☐ Behavioral exercise approach

☐ NMES (Strengthening)

☐ NMES (Pain control)

☐ Soft tissue massage

☐ Myofacial release

☐ Craniosacral therapy

☐ Other

Figure 19-4 Low Back Initiative Minimum Data Set.

ability to draw conclusions about performance. With the help of the HR department, a surveillance program was put in place to guide data collection.

This program began as a biweekly data report that identified each therapist and the number of complete vs. incomplete data sets. The facility directors were then e-mailed by the company QI officer, and the therapists who had missing data sets were asked to complete the MDS. If completion was not possible, the therapist was asked to write a short note explaining why. Through a series of accountability measures and in-service activities for clinicians, data collection slowly started to improve. Most clinicians responded to the biweekly verbal follow-up by the facility managers. As data collection improved, the frequency of verbal reminders decreased. Those clinicians who still had difficulty with collection were contacted by the directors and presented with a nonpunitive internal incentive. After 4 months of surveillance, the percentage of completed data sets rose to greater than 95%. With the increase in the number of data sets and the availability of data the study was ready to continue with the third stage of the QI process.

Analysis of the data was then completed. As Figure 19-2 shows, the three steps of evaluation of clinical performance are:

Compliance: Is there a data set for every eligible patient?
Adherence: Do interventions match prospectively determined clinical decision rules?
Outcomes: Are outcomes achieving prospectively determined benchmarks?

Compliance was addressed in the previous section. Adherence and outcomes are the final two elements that need to be addressed. The purpose of the study was to analyze the adherence to a protocol. Figure 19-5 breaks down the totals by the treatment-based classification.

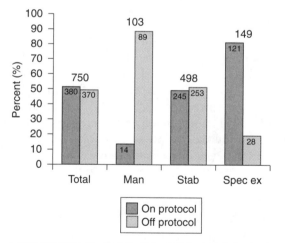

• 63.1% of 363 Stab. Neg. Prediction Rule candidates treated off-protocol
• 82.2% of 135 Stab. Prediction Rule candidates treated on-protocol

Figure 19-5 Treatment-Based Classification Cohort Compliance Breakdown. This graph outlines all patients seen during data collection. The black bars represent the patients treated on protocol, using the treatment-based classification system (TBC). The red bars represent those patients treated without regard to the TBC. Each column, excluding the "Total" column, represents a classification. Man—Manual Therapy Classification; Stab—Stabilization Classification; Spec Ex—"Specific Exercise" or Directional Preference Classification.

Of the 750 patients enrolled, just over 50% were treated with a program adhering to the guidelines outlined by the TBC, a number that certainly leaves room for improvement. However, when the numbers were broken down into their respective categories, there were opportunities for improvement in adherence to the manual therapy and the stabilization protocols: 82% of the manual therapy and just over 50% of the stabilization patients were treated in a manner that was judged nonadherent to the TBC.

The final element is outcomes. During analysis, we need to consider patient outcomes, which will then give insight into our performance. During typical analysis, the first element to be considered is, "Are our patients achieving their predetermined benchmarks?" This question can be answered using the collected data, which will allow analysis of both patient outcomes and therapist performance. To continue following the example from previous sections, we note that even though patient outcomes are evaluated, therapist compliance with the treatment-based classification (TBC) system was the variable subjected to analysis in this particular activity. Since the researchers were observing adherence to the protocol, no specific benchmarks were set with regard to patient outcomes. Rather, the benchmark being evaluated was compliance with the TBC. Again referring to Figure 19-5, areas for improvement in compliance can be easily identified. Once identified, the areas for improvement would be evaluated based on set benchmarks by comparing data previously obtained with data obtained as Steps 2 and 3 are repeated.

Step 4, the final step of the performance improvement process, is the *development of an improvement plan*. Based on the data in the example, we can speculate on a possible plan. Earlier, low compliance with data collection was addressed by implementing a system-wide surveillance program supervised by the company QI officer. The response to the program resulted in 97% compliance in completion of the MDS. The more difficult problem may be therapist adherence to a specific treatment or protocol. Why is adherence low? Data analysis reveals poor adherence when thrust procedures are indicated. This may be explained by therapists' lack of familiarity with thrust procedures; some may not be comfortable executing these treatments based on education or knowledge. Other issues identified by therapists include the opinion that benchmarks or standards infringe upon clinical autonomy.

Though these responses need to be considered, the ethical implications of nonadherence must also be considered. The TBC has been shown to provide superior outcomes and better quality of care for those with LBP.[8] If therapists are nonadherent with the classification system, are they providing the best care for patients? As the QI benchmarks are set, they will clearly address adherence to TBC. An increase in adherence is imperative for change to take place. If knowledge is the issue, further education of clinicians would augment the performance improvement process. If indifference is the issue, then a plan needs to be set in place to guide change over time. From here, we return to the clinic and start the process again.

CONCLUSION

QI may seem to be an academic debate right now, but health care is changing rapidly. The final analysis of the study described above evaluated the cost of delivery and additional downstream health care costs over the next year. During this period the authors showed a total direct health care savings in excess of $283,000 for those patients treated on protocol.[5] Remember, over 50% of the patients were treated off protocol. Imagine if adherence increased a modest 10% to 15%, increasing total overall adherence to 65%. Based on this savings we could conclude that the cost savings alone would be attractive to payers while dramatically improving quality of care for the patients involved.

The future of health care will not be built on art; rather, it will be built on evidence and performance. We can either begin to evaluate our own performance and make changes or we can let others do it for us. The QI initiative we have described continues and we are at a steady state of greater than 95% compliance with completed data sets for eligible patients. We are assessing the effectiveness of an educational program on improving adherence to TBC guidelines as well as other educational initiatives, many of which are generated by feedback to the physical therapists on their performance related to the QI initiative. Either way, quality improvement is not the wave of the future; it's the reality of now.

SELF-ASSESSMENT

1. Reflect on either a group of patients like Mr. Ketterman, a group of patients that make up a large portion of your practice, or a group you would like to treat regularly. Develop a database that contains the essential elements that would help you determine that the right care is being provided to this group of patients. As is shown in this actual case, these elements may include both the processes and the outcomes of care.
2. Using the same database, develop a minimal data set that could be used by you and your colleagues in your patient documentation to build an actual database for this group of patients.

CONTINUED LEARNING

• Examine the literature for one or two patient populations of your choice to identify therapist behaviors that you believe would result in improved care, both in process and in outcome. What benefit would you predict from implementing those behaviors?

REFERENCES

1. *Crossing the Quality Chasm: A New Health System for the 21st Century.* Washington, DC: Institute of Medicine; 2001.
2. Bigos S, Bowyer O, Braen G, et al. Acute low back problems in adults: Assessment and treatment. *Clinical Practice Guideline. Quick Reference Guide for Clinicians.* Agency for Health Care Policy and Research; 1994.
3. Kritchevsky SB, Simmons BP. Continuous quality improvement: Concepts and applications for physician care. JAMA. 1991;266(13):1817–1823.
4. Delitto A. We are what we do. Phys Ther. 2008;88(10):1219–1227.
5. McGee JC. The Cost Effectiveness of a Treatment Based Classification (TBC) Approach Compared to a Usual Care Approach in the Management of Low Back Pain in the Outpatient Physical Therapy Setting. Diss. 2009.
6. Delitto A, Erhard RE, Bowling RW. A treatment-based classification approach to low back syndrome: Identifying and staging patients for conservative treatment. Phys Ther. 1995; 75(6):470–485.
7. Brennan GP, Fritz JM, Hunter SJ, et al. Identifying subgroups of patients with acute/ subacute "nonspecific" low back pain: results of a randomized clinical trial. Spine. 2006;31(6):623–631.
8. Fritz, JM, Cleland JA, Brennan GP. Does adherence to the guideline recommendation for active treatments improve the quality of care for patients with acute low back pain delivered by physical therapists? Med Care. 2007;45(10):973–980.

Closing Words

Declare the past, diagnose the present, foretell the future; practice these acts. As to diseases, make a habit of two things—to help, or at least to do no harm. The art consists in three things—the disease, the patient, and the practitioner. The practitioner is the servant of the art, and the patient must combat the disease along with the practitioner.

—Adapted from Hippocrates, *Epidemics*, Bk. I, Sect. II

•

INTRODUCTION

We began this book with these words from Hippocrates, and they seem fitting for the book's conclusion as well. Over 2000 years ago, he identified that health care practitioners reach excellence by understanding the art of care, by recognizing the patient as a partner in care, by making accurate diagnoses and prognoses, and by knowing what helps (and harms) our patients—all the elements of evidence-based practice (EBP).

If these principles have been with us for 2000 years, one might ask why they have not been adopted fully into health care. We've discussed the barriers to individuals adopting change in Section IV, but it is also worthwhile to identify the reasons that reflective practitioners have opposed the adoption of EBP because of serious concerns about its appropriateness and the barriers that arise from the very structure of the health care system.

We will explore here the ways that EBP has been implemented by physical therapists across the country and will conclude with some thought about the possibilities for the future.

CONCERNS ABOUT ADOPTING EBP

Reasonable and reflective people have expressed some reservations about the very premises of EBP. Because these are such important issues, we will explore them here.

EBP Interferes With the Clinician's Decision Making

This concern about EBP is generally offered in one of two ways. Some complain that EBP is simply a tool of insurance companies to be used in preventing practitioners from providing the right care in order to decrease the amount spent on care.[1] While it is possible that an insurance company can misuse a particular piece of evidence to make incorrect decisions, these actions can be challenged and corrected. This possibility is far outweighed by the improvement in both quality and cost of care that can be achieved when practitioners use those tests and interventions that are shown to be more effective than others. This potential has led policy groups to recommend that the use of evidence be incorporated into health care practice. One such group is the Institute of Medicine (IOM), an independent group composed of scientists and practitioners and part of the National Academy of Sciences. They have examined the issues around EBP and have recommended that it is imperative that resources are made available to conduct systematic reviews and to develop trustworthy clinical guidelines. They state that such efforts will succeed in making health care decisions that:

- Constrain health care costs
- Reduce geographic variation in the use of health care services
- Improve quality
- Enhance consumer-directed health care[2]

Academy Health, a group designed to help move forward the principles and findings of health services research, has developed a briefing paper on how to use evidence to design health insurance benefits. They recommend developing better research to understand the effects of various coverage decisions. They also state that use of EBP to establish benefits should:

- Establish consistent expectations or standards for evaluating new treatments or technologies
- Move beyond the narrow scope of current efforts in evidence based insurance design
- Improve understanding of how different forms of incentives work
- Recognize implications of insurance coverage for health and economic equity[3]

Think tanks such as Academy Health propose a deliberative process for incorporating evidence into health insurance coverage policies, which will serve practitioners and consumers more successfully than the hit-and-miss technique followed by some individual insurers. Rapid fluctuations in covered services can have a negative effect on both quality and consumer confidence.

> "Good doctors use both individual clinical expertise and the best available external evidence, and neither alone is enough. Without clinical expertise, practice risks becoming tyrannized by evidence, for even excellent external evidence may be inapplicable to or inappropriate for an individual patient. Without current best evidence, practice risks become rapidly out of date, to the detriment of patients."[4]

A second complaint about decision making is that EBP means "cookbook" care. This complaint claims that EBP forces clinicians to use certain tests and measures, regardless of the individual patient needs, thereby depriving both the clinician and the patient of the benefits of the clinician's clinical wisdom and of personalized care.[5] We hope that this text helps to dispel at least a portion of this complaint. We have demonstrated that EBP actually means a reliance on good decision making by the practitioner. Only an astute practitioner using good decision making processes can make the decision that a particular piece of evidence actually applies to a particular patient. Another way to look at this complaint is from the perspective of unwarranted variation.[6] Variation in care can occur because of patient preference or circumstances but should not occur because practitioners have not chosen the most effective care. When the variations occur for no discernible reasons or for reasons related to poor practitioner knowledge or decision making or to financial gain, then those variations are unwarranted and the variance should be reduced. Adopting well-designed clinical guidelines is one way to reduce unwarranted variation.

What's wrong with a cookbook?

What would you do if you went home tonight and had to make dinner with a particular list of ingredients? The answer might depend on your familiarity with those ingredients and expertise as a cook. Let's suppose you are a novice in both of these areas. Your first step might be to find a recipe that contains those ingredients and then follow the recipe to prepare your meal. In other words, you would use a cookbook, because that has the best likelihood of producing an edible meal. As you become more accomplished as a cook and more familiar with the ingredients, you might start either to change some of the process, blend similar recipes, work from memory, or even develop your own, new recipe, as you learn from trial and error. Perhaps later you begin to expand to new ingredients or cooking styles, so you might well start the process of searching for an established recipe once again. As novices we typically seek out these sorts of structured guides to help us reduce the risk of failure. Should we behave differently as novice health care practitioners? Or is the question really one of making sure we pick the right recipe that matches our ingredients and our preferred outcomes?

EBP Is Unethical

This concern is a very important one to consider and address, as we owe our patients the highest possible ethical behavior. Often these concerns revolve around the injustice of applying a particular intervention to a group of patients without regard to the clinician's own judgment or the patient's own preferences. There are also concerns about adopting too rigid a definition of what acceptable evidence is, relying too heavily on the need for randomized controlled trials. There are additional concerns about the ability of even the best research to fully identify some of the more complex outcomes for care, such as reduction of pain or quality of life, and therefore lead clinicians to make decisions based on more easily measured but less relevant outcomes.[7,8]

"Evidence based medicine (EBM) is an approach to health care that promotes the collection, interpretation, and integration of valid, important and applicable patient-reported, clinician-observed, and research-derived evidence. The best available evidence, moderated by patient circumstances and preferences, is applied to improve the quality of clinical judgments."[9]

These concerns represent a view of EBP as a simple application of research results with no filter for their applicability to a particular case. A clear understanding of the need to integrate evidence with a clinician's expertise and a patient's preferences should relieve much of these concerns. They are also balanced by the perspective that ignoring what the evidence tells us may also be unethical. For example the Code of Ethics for physical therapists, promulgated by the American Physical Therapy Association, states, "Physical therapists shall demonstrate professional judgment informed by professional standards, evidence (including current literature and established best practice), practitioner experience, and patient/client values."[10]

One might argue that any practice that does not serve the patient optimally could be considered unethical practice, but such a definition excludes the motivation of the practitioner from the judgment. Clearly, a practitioner who searches diligently for the intervention that facilitates the best outcomes is practicing ethically, even if the outcomes fall short of the patient's goals. It is the practitioner's value for openness to innovations in health care that ensures ethical practice.

Evidence Is Not Always Based on Theory

Theory is focused on the reasons why a phenomenon occurs. In health care, theory attempts to explain the causes of illness and disability and the reasons why particular care meets with success. Theory is often the basis for postulating the potential of new approaches to patient care management. It is rooted in the sciences that support health care. For physical therapy, those sciences include anatomy, physiology, neuroscience, psychology, sociology, ethics, and teaching and learning.[11] In an early editorial on the issue of theory in physical therapy, the authors state, "Theory is a general, abstract body of interrelated principles, concepts, and constructs that presents a systematic, scientifically acceptable view of phenomena. Theory is conjecture that is inferred from a set of logical propositions that, in turn, are based on empirically derived evidence. Acceptable scientific theory is internally consistent, empirically testable, parsimonious, and congruous with existing knowledge. Theory also should be important scientifically."[12]

"Evidence based clinical practice is an approach to decision making in which the clinician uses the best evidence available, in consultation with the patient, to decide upon the option which suits that patient best."[13]

It is important to note that the word *theory* implies that there is an element of doubt about the accuracy of the theory. In fact, in the physical sciences, when sufficient doubt has been removed the word *theory* is often replaced with the word *law*. *Evidence*, on the other hand, is actually defined as that which tends to prove something. We have two terms that may be at odds with each other: *theory*—a not yet proved description of a phenomenon, and *evidence*—proof.

This tension between theory and evidence is well documented. There are numerous examples of interventions designed and used because they "make sense" from a theoretical perspective but are later shown to be ineffective or even harmful when tested in clinical trials.[14,15] An opposing view states,

> Good science is the best and only way to determine which treatments and products are truly safe and effective. That idea is already formalized in a movement known as evidence based medicine (EBM). EBM is a vital and positive influence on the practice of medicine, but it has limitations and problems in practice: It often overemphasizes the value of evidence from clinical trials alone, with some unintended consequences, such as taxpayer dollars spent on "more research" of questionable value. The idea of SBM (science based medicine) is not to compete with EBM, but a call to enhance it with a broader view: to answer the question "what works?" we must give more importance to our cumulative scientific knowledge from all relevant disciplines.[16-17]

One of the central concerns of these critics is the reliance of much of EBP on the randomized clinical trial (RCT). Critics believe RCTs are both too limiting for studying all the many phenomena that make up health care (see Chapters 8 and 12) and can overinflate the importance of results, particularly in studies with small numbers of subjects and small effect sizes.[16,18]

Scholars have pointed out that some of the evidence provided about interventions in physical therapy has been done in an atheoretical context, which might account for the rather small, albeit positive, effects seen in this research. For example, recent work on classification of patients with low back pain to match them to selected interventions has explicitly stated that this work is based on empirical observation, without regard for theoretical explanations of why these approaches might be successful. Researchers contend that years of seeking the mechanism of injury as a means of guiding care have not resulted in success and that this empirical approach helps patients improve. Critics of this work contend that we must do a better job of identifying the mechanisms of injury that cause the back pain if we are want to achieve the necessary level of success in identifying appropriate care.[19-21] Others have taken a more philosophical approach to their critique, noting that wholesale adoption of any single way of looking at the world leads to a loss of possibility, growth, and creativity.[22]

But rather than seeing only the tension between the two terms, they should also be seen as enlightening each other. In the best of all worlds, wouldn't a theory about how and why something works help drive the empirical research to show if it does, and wouldn't identifying that something does work help develop the theory as to why? Development of theory and production of evidence about our care should be twin goals, as together they can lead to a sound body of knowledge that matters to our patients. This really represents the inevitable link between research and practice.

Eugene Michels, one of the leaders in supporting and developing research in physical therapy, wrote about this topic often. In one letter to the editor of *Physical Therapy* he noted the deep need to develop theory in physical therapy, saying,

> . . . physical therapy research, both in its doing and in its public presentation, will continue to be eclectic and to lack direction and cohesion. . . . we will continue to admit disparate bits of research results, authoritative statements, and unfounded conclusions into our "body of knowledge," without any rules for the admission of such bits except for the apparent rule that, all other things being equal, any finding is better than none. We will have no cumulation of knowledge, if by that expression we mean enlarging or increasing our knowledge by successive additions to and corrections of existing knowledge."[23,p765,766]

In a letter to the editor a year previously, he commented, "If we are to develop our own science for understanding and doing socially useful things about human movement dysfunction, that science must first be well grounded in the definition, identification, and study of relevant, observable phenomena and variables and later explained and elaborated by appeal to more abstract and organic levels of reduction. The robust sciences work forth and back between the nonabstract and the abstract levels of reduction."[24,p1138,1139] This is all advice we would do well to heed today.

EBP, QUALITY, AND COSTS

The adoption of some specific recommendations from the evidence may actually increase the costs of care. But the hope is that widespread adoption of changes identified by trustworthy evidence will result in reduced costs of care. As we discussed in Chapter 9, the growing costs of health care in this country arouse concern about our ability to maintain those costs, about inequities in access to equivalent care across the U.S. population, and a recognition that those costs do not seem to be buying a commensurate improvement in overall quality.

"Evidence based medicine is the conscientious, explicit, and judicious use of current best evidence in making decisions about the care of individual patients. The practice of evidence based medicine means integrating individual clinical expertise with the best available external clinical evidence from systematic research. By individual clinical expertise we mean the proficiency and judgment that individual clinicians acquire through clinical experience and clinical practice. Increased expertise is reflected in many ways, but especially in more effective and efficient diagnosis and in the more thoughtful identification and compassionate use of individual patients' predicaments, rights, and preferences in making clinical decisions about their care. By best available external clinical evidence we mean clinically relevant research, often from the basic sciences of medicine, but especially from patient centered clinical research into the accuracy and precision of diagnostic tests (including the clinical examination), the power of prognostic markers, and the efficacy and safety of therapeutic, rehabilitative, and preventive regimens. External clinical evidence both invalidates previously accepted diagnostic tests and treatments and replaces them with new ones that are more powerful, more accurate, more efficacious, and safer."[25]

Gawende has identified the wide disparity in costs in specific small regions, without any positive relationship between costs and quality. He has advocated for the need to compare the effectiveness of both the specific care provided and the systems designed for the care delivery, supporting the concept that more systematic and centralized responsibility for care can help reduce costs and at least maintain, if not improve quality.[26]

The IOM has recommended that emphasis be placed on comparative effectiveness research, which can result in trustworthy clinical practice guidelines, selecting from among the array of diagnostic and prognostic tests and measures and interventions to demonstrate the best options for the entire plan of care for a patient (see Chapter 16).[2,27,28] This would meet at least part of the recommendations needed to ensure that a cost-quality balance is reached. A class of studies we have not explored, but which is important, are cost-effectiveness analyses. This line of research is designed to identify which aspects of care are able to produce the same outcomes with lower costs. Of course, the goal would be to only do cost-effectiveness studies once the actual effectiveness of various options has been identified.[2] Work has begun to more clearly identify the cost-effectiveness of physical therapy.[29] These types of studies will also contribute to achieving the cost-quality balance.

An interesting example of research designed to identify the impact of practice focused on controlling costs is a study by Milstein and Gilbertson. They identified several practices that were able, through a variety of tactics, to provide quality care at 20% or less cost than other practices, with no reduction in quality. If the 20% reduction in costs identified in this study can be extrapolated to the entire country, it would represent a saving of $640 billion, as of 2011.[30]

In Chapter 17 we discussed many of the barriers for individual clinicians and individual facilities to making changes in their practices based on the evidence. But there are also barriers that are intrinsic to the health care system in the United States that interfere with adoption of the best practices identified through the evidence. (See Chapter 9 for a discussion of the complexity of the health care system in the United States.) Why doesn't the health care system adopt these changes and realize these savings? Fuchs and Milstein[31] state that the prime reason is that the key players in the system each have their own incentives to not change. Here are some examples of the stakeholders they identify and reasons that inhibit change:

- Large insurance companies do not want to adopt standardized national benefits because that could decrease their competitive advantage in local settings, thereby decreasing profits for their shareholders.
- Large employers do not want to encourage competition among health plans so as to not alienate employees; small employers can't afford more than one plan; employers in general mistrust government solutions and recommendations that seem to restrict care. All of this means that the competition among plans based on cost reduction cannot occur.
- The general public resists change, not recognizing that health insurance benefits are actually a form of income and that carefully reducing costs could actually increase their discretionary income. In addition, the general public often has little ability to really understand the issue of risk analysis and the benefits that could arise from certain changes.
- Legislators at both the state and federal levels are influenced by the health care system lobbying effort, which can be more focused and, therefore, more successful than a diffuse effort by individuals.
- Hospital managers fear that reducing specific procedures could reduce their ability to cover the large fixed costs they have for buildings and equipment.
- Drug companies and medical equipment manufacturers believe that their best success is in developing unique products whose prices they can control and, therefore, resist attempts to standardize care.
- Health care practitioners resist change for all the reasons that we discussed in Chapter 17 and for the concerns we have discussed above.

These perspectives are primarily economic in nature and may not be the perspectives that individual health practitioners typically have, but they do describe well the difficulty in achieving system-wide changes. As health care practitioners, we are obligated to place the needs of patients first. Shouldn't we be the leaders in helping the system come together to bring about necessary and appropriate changes?[2,27]

EBP IN USE IN PHYSICAL THERAPY

While preparing this text, we asked our colleagues, through multiple listservs, for examples of the use of EBP, particularly the integration of the three elements of clinical judgment, respecting patient values, and using evidence from the literature. We received dozens of examples in a few short days.

The examples ranged from relatively small efforts, such as setting up a regular journal club using a Critically Appraised Topics (CAT) model, to developing comprehensive evidence based guidelines for use in a large facility. We will highlight just a few of these ideas here:

- Several facilities used data from their own patients to determine which particular populations were at risk for falls. They then used the literature to build better screening for fall risk, assessment of the causes of falling, and better fall prevention programs for these populations.
- Several therapists reported using specific information from the literature to explain to patients or physician colleagues the rationale for specific interventions, with increased acceptance of these changes in practice.
- The inpatient physical therapy team at one large facility holds case conferences twice a month. The first meeting is a discussion of a patient case. One week prior to that meeting, a team member provides the group with the history and tests and measures from the evaluation of one of his or her patients. The team members read this information, write their own clinical impression and plan of care, and come prepared to discuss their thoughts. In that session the group discusses differences taken by each team member. They compare evaluation statements and plans and talk about differences. At the end of the meeting (about 1 hour), they identify a clinical question that could be answered through a search of the literature. Each member of the group searches the literature, and the team leader then chooses one article in particular to use as a point of discussion at the second session. After the discussion of the article, the group asks, "Would we do something different if we saw him/her again or another, similar patient in the future?" After the second meeting, the team leader writes up a summary of the month's work and shares it electronically so all staff can access it. The team leader says, "This process has been successful and very well received by our staff. They frequently read past write-ups and those from other teams when they have a question about a patient."
- One therapist described the need to develop a specific program for care of patients with osteoporotic fractures in advance of the research evidence and base it on the known information from the study of anatomy and human movement, modifying the program as evidence became available.
- Another therapist was the first to introduce evidence based assessment tools to a group of therapists in Kenya.
- A facility developed a best practice protocol for the treatment of idiopathic toe walking. It is a treatment algorithm based on current research and clinical practice. The protocol is presented to the family with best treatment options explained based on the child's presentation. The family is then given the opportunity for input, with the goal being to educate families on current research and improved clinical outcomes as they make their decisions.
- One large inpatient facility has a practice committee. The committee has developed protocols, chronological care patterns for major patient populations seen, and standards of care documents, which include the natural history of the problem, details for the physical therapist's examination and intervention options, and copies of recommended tools and references that support the choices. What is most remarkable about this is that the committee has developed over 40 protocols and 70 standards of care. And it has made all of them publicly available at the facility's Web site, to be used by not only the therapists but patients and families and health care colleagues.
- A facility developed the position of clinical research educator (CRE), who spends 50% of his or her time on evidence-related activities. The CRE functions to identify and assess published evidence, to teach colleagues to search and appraise the literature themselves,

and to develop practice-specific evidence by collecting and analyzing data derived from their own practice.

- One facility asked the therapists to develop PICO questions based on their clinical experience and then had students participating in clinical education conduct the searches and analysis of evidence, thereby building on the strengths of each group.

- In addition to that example, several academic faculty offered examples of collaboration between the educational program and related clinical programs, where faculty offered their expertise on search and assessment and clinicians identified questions of clinical importance and their judgment in the application of the evidence to particular populations and patients.

This is a case written by a student in a course that one of us teaches in a transition Doctor of Physical Therapy Program. The assignment was to develop a marketing plan. This therapist chose to use all elements of evidence based practice to guide her plan. (It has been edited to conceal the identity of the facility and abridged for length.)

"What do you mean you have to leave that ace wrap looking like that?" Three times this past month, I found myself repeating this question to nursing staff in the vascular intensive care unit. Three times the answer was, "Because I'm under a surgeon's order that only a vascular surgeon can remove and replace this dressing." All of these patients were recipients of lower limb amputations after numerous previous revascularization procedures failed to save their limbs, young in the 40–65-year age range, and (who) wished to readily be active again. [PATIENT VALUES AND CIRCUMSTANCES] The wish to be active coupled with gaining a better quality of life, which each patient readily discussed during my initial consultation, had eluded the surgeons and to some degree the nurses. The surgeons were most concerned about limb salvage, while the nurses were most concerned about immediate bedside needs and following orders. I found myself perturbed, thinking "I need to practice best practice, and this clearly is not it."

Is a standard soft dressing like an ace wrap ultimately the most effective and efficient manner to promote faster wound healing and sooner resumption of an active lifestyle and better quality of life for the patient with an amputation? [CLINICAL QUESTION TO IDENTIFY BEST RESEARCH EVIDENCE] I turned to the literature to support my thought that these patients needed a better post-operative plan of care to allow them not only to become prosthetic candidates but also to heal and obtain a better quality of life in the most effective, efficient manner possible. Once I gathered this information, I planned to develop an education and marketing plan for the rehab management team where I work so that I would have their support as I attempted to change several aspects of the post-operative management of patients with amputations.

The online community www.360oandp.com effectively sums up what many other authors describe in more detail about the early post-operative care of the patient with an amputation, stating that it depends on the preferences of the surgeon, conditions specific to the patient, insurance coverage, and other factors. They conclude that of the numerous types of existing dressings, removable designs can benefit the patient's rehabilitation process, in addition to meeting the needs of the surgeon. With respect to other health care team members, the prosthetist can make adjustments as needed due to volumetric limb changes and effectively shape the limb, while the physical therapist can readily perform therapeutic exercise and functional progression. With more members of the team involved earlier in the process, the result is faster healing and a greater probability of successful rehabilitation.

[An ANALYSIS OF THE LITERATURE followed, showing support for the use of prefabricated removable rigid dressings (RRD).]

Given the literature's definite support for the use of a RRD and the duration it has been available, I pondered why more surgeons did not advocate this type of post-op management for their patients. The simplest yet most compelling reason that I found was, "Many of our surgeons don't want to bother with it." [CLINICAL EXPERTISE]

Would this be the case with the vascular surgeons where I work? Only discussion with them would tell, so I began to develop a marketing plan to help effectively sell the idea that the use of a prefabricated RRD system in conjunction with earlier consultation of PTs and prosthetists would ultimately promote better post-op management of these patients.

I completed a S.W.O.T. (Strengths, Weaknesses, Opportunities and Threats) Analysis to determine the potential strengths and weaknesses of implementing the use of the prefabricated RRD vs. a standard soft dressing currently used during the post-op, pre-prosthetic phase and the opportunities and threats in the environment that could help achieve the objective of changing the practice for the pre-prosthetic management of the patient with the amputation to provide best practice or improve the patient's healing time and quality of life. The analysis is a compilation of the review of several authors' works and my own experience [CLINICAL EXPERTISE]. Upon review, it does appear that pursuit of the prefabricated RRD system is an opportunity worth pursuing based on the strengths and opportunities generated. . . . The weaknesses and threats are seemingly few and can mostly be handled with effective communication among the various players on the health care team.

Next I considered a PEST (Political, Economic, Social, Technological) analysis to review the potential environmental factors. *Political*: PTs and prosthetists must receive specific MD orders. Current MD practice would need to change to include pre-op PT and prosthetist referrals to provide information to the patient and family and take initial measurements of the involved limb to begin custom RRD fabrication. The operative orders would need to include the prosthetist's application of the RRD either perioperatively or immediately post-op and PT post-op day 1, with continued follow-up by both team members until successful rehab is achieved. *Economic*: How does changing best practice encourage economic growth? Changing best practice would include earlier referral to a PT, which should theoretically generate revenue; however, our fee structure is not currently set up to recognize this gain. *Social*: ... [C]lose follow-up and education allows most patients to be fitted with an immediate post-op prosthesis (IPOP) and return to pre-amputation activities sooner, thus improving their quality of life, ... described as more efficient healing, a better chance for successful rehab, and safety, suggesting that the IPOP provides a padded environment to protect the residual limb, and with the pylon and foot attached, the patient can have a more stable bipedal gait, helping with fall prevention. *Technological*: Application of the RRD is a literal application of new technology to better manage the patients with amputations.

> Using the SWOT and PEST Analyses ... I confirmed what I wanted to achieve, which enabled me to develop goals and objectives for my marketing plan. From these, I developed this action plan:
>
> 1. To market to the rehab management team what current best practice should be in the rehab of patients with amputations;
> 2. To seek partnership with the prosthetist who currently provides service for our patients;
> 3. With the prosthetist and member(s) of the rehab management team, to meet with the vascular surgeons to discuss their perceptions of current pre- and post-op management of patients with amputations and the literature findings and to promote changing current practice; and
> 4. To implement a pathway for collaborative pre- and post-operative rehab management.
>
> ... To evaluate the effectiveness of changing our current practice in the management of patients with lower extremity amputations, recommendations include:
>
> 1. Tracking the number of new referrals received for patients in the pre- and immediate post-operative phases.
> 2. Doing a retrospective study to compare the time to ambulatory discharge, the number of post-operative falls, occurrence of skin breakdown and infections, pain ratings, gait distance, and contracture presence with a prefabricated RRD system versus a standard soft dressing. [FOLLOW-UP TO EVALUATE RESULTS OF IMPLEMENTING CHANGE]
>
> My ultimate hope is to change the way that these patients are medically managed post-operatively so that the PT staff can collaborate with the prosthetist to provide best practice. ... If I can educate and market effectively to the rehab management team and to the vascular surgeons, then I can change current practice to better reflect best practice for patients with lower extremity amputations.

As can be seen from these examples, representing all aspects of practice and all parts of the country, clinicians can find the resources to develop and utilize EBP skills.

WHAT DOES THE FUTURE HOLD?

We have emphasized the thinking processes used by clinicians in Section I. Understanding decision making is a complex science. Bell and Raiffa have identified a taxonomy used with great frequency by decision analysts, those scientists who study decision making, to clarify some of the approaches used in studying this topic. They have identified three different processes used in thinking about decision making:

- Descriptive
  1. Decisions people make
  2. How people decide
- Normative
  1. Logically consistent decision procedures
  2. How people should decide

- Prescriptive
  1. How to help people make good decisions
  2. How to train people to make better decisions.[32,p1,2]

We have discussed two sources of normative information, patient values and circumstances, in Section II, and the evidence from the literature about our tests, measures, and interventions in Section III. We have discussed descriptive information, what we learn about how clinicians actually think, in Section I. We have offered some ideas on how to improve our decision making in Section IV. But we will need to continue to test these methods, and others, as they are developed to see if they produce the changes that are desired. We hope that we will see continued growth in the study of decision making in physical therapy.

As we have discussed throughout this text, evidence based practice holds much promise to improve the care that we provide our patients. The fulfillment of this promise rests in the full integration of all three elements of EBP. Information from research is useless if thinking clinicians do not apply this information in collaboration with their patients. There continues to be growth in advocacy for the patient to be recognized as the center of our care. The federal government, as well as multiple foundations, has supported this perspective.[33–36]

At an IOM conference, placing the patient at the center was described as a Copernican shift.[37] Copernicus forced us to completely rethink our understanding of the universe. Will this focus on patients really help us change our care as completely as placing the sun in the center of the universe has done? In physical therapy, we have prided ourselves on engaging patients, because we know that our care is not passive. If the patient does not participate, then we cannot achieve reduction of impairments or improvement in function. But, have we always placed the patient really in the center? Do we collaborate in goal setting? Do we respect our patients even when they reject our advice? Have we found ways to help patients understand the evidence and judgment that (should) drive our recommendations? We hope to see continued growth in these behaviors by physical therapists and the research that demonstrates the benefits of patient-centered care.

CONCLUSION

The single best practice physical therapists can follow to improve their decision making is to reflect on decisions, individually or with colleagues or learners. This commitment to reflection in practice will never fail to provide the practitioner with more questions to pursue, strengthened values for excellence, and a stronger relationship with the patient.

Epstein, in *The Mindful Practitioner*, tells us, "Exemplary physicians seem to have a capacity for critical self-reflection that pervades all aspects of practice, including being present with the patient, solving problems, eliciting and transmitting information, making evidence based decisions, performing technical skills, and defining our own values."[38,p833] What a wonderful description of the behavior we all aspire to as clinicians who have fully embraced all aspects of evidence based practice!

REFERENCES

1. Turkelson C, Hughes, JE, Why aren't you doing evidence-based practice? AAOS Bull. June 2006;54(3).
2. Eden J, Wheatley B, McNeil B, Sox H, eds. *Knowing What Works in Health Care: A Roadmap for the Nation*. Washington, DC: National Academies Press; 2008.

3. Bernstein J. Research Insights: Using Evidence to Design Benefits. Academy Health. http://www.academyhealth.org/files/publications/RschInsightsDesignBenefit.pdf Accessed May 31, 2011.
4. Sackett, DL et al. Evidence based medicine: What it is and what it isn't. BMJ. January 13, 1996;312(7023):71–72.
5. Oostendorp RAB, Nijhuis-van der Sanden, MWG, Heerkens YF, Hendriks EJM, Huijbregts PA. Evidence-Based Rehabilitation Medicine and Physiotherapy. International Encyclopedia of Rehabilitation. http://cirrie.buffalo.edu/encyclopedia/en/article/130/ Accessed May 31, 2011.
6. Wennberg JE, Unwarranted variations in healthcare delivery: Implications for academic medical centres. BMJ. 2002;325:961–964.
7. Royeen CB. The ephemeral ethics of evidence-based practice. In: Purilo RB, Jensen GM, Royeen CB, eds. *Education for Moral Action*. Philadelphia: FA Davis; 2005.
8. Kerridge I, Lowe M, Henry D. Ethics and evidence based medicine. BMJ. 1998;316: 1151–1153.
9. McKibbon, KA et al. The medical literature as a resource for evidence based care. Working Paper from the Health Information Research Unit, McMaster University, Ontario, Canada; 1995.
10. American Physical Therapy Association. Code of Ethics for the Physical Therapist, 2010. http://www.apta.org/uploadedFiles/APTAorg/About_Us/Policies/HOD/Ethics/ CodeofEthics.pdf Accessed May 31, 2011.
11. American Physical Therapy Association. *A Normative Model of Physical Therapist Professional Education: Version 2000*. APTA; 2000.
12. Krebs DE, Harris SR. Elements of theory presentations. Phys Ther. 1988;68:690–693.
13. Muir Gray JA. *Evidence-Based Healthcare: How to Make Health Policy and Management Decisions*. London: Churchill Livingstone; 1997.
14. Facing the Evidence—Part One. http://www.abc.net.au/rn/healthreport/ stories/2006/1735075.htm Accessed May 31, 2011.
15. Facing the Evidence—Part Two. http://www.abc.net.au/rn/healthreport/ stories/2006/1740986.htm Accessed May 31, 2011.
16. Science Based Medicine. http://www.sciencebasedmedicine.org/index.php/about-science-based-medicine/ Accessed June 2, 2011.
17. Dorko B. Is Evidence Based Practice Making Us Stupid? A Thread in Barrett Dorko's Forums at Soma Simple. http://somasimple.com/forums/showthread.php?t = 5828 Accessed June 2, 2011.
18. Kristiansen IS, Mooney G. *Evidence Based Medicine: In Its Place*. London: Routledge; 2004.
19. Flynn, TW, Maher C, Riddle D. (Mod) Classification and Manipulation for Low Back Pain: Should They Be Linked? Physical Therapy Podcast. Accessed May 31, 2011.
20. Childs JD, Fritz JM, Flynn TW, et al. A clinical prediction rule to identify patients with low back pain most likely to benefit from spinal manipulation: A validation study. Ann Intern Med. 2004;141:920–928.
21. Hancock MJ, Maher CG, Latimer J, et al. Assessment of diclofenac or spinal manipulative therapy, or both, in addition to recommended first-line treatment for acute low back pain: A randomized controlled trial. Lancet. 2007;370(9599):1638–1643.
22. Holmes D, Murray SJ, Perron A, et al. Deconstructing the evidence-based discourse in health sciences: Truth, power and fascism. Int J Evid Based Healthc. 2006;4:180–186.
23. Michels E. Cumulation of Knowledge. Letter to the Editor, Phys Ther. 1995;75: 765–766.
24. Michels E. Levels of Reduction. Letter to the Editor, Phys Ther. 1994;74:1138–1139.
25. Sackett, DL et al. Evidence based medicine: What it is and what it isn't. BMJ. January 13, 1996;312(7023):71–72.
26. Gawande A. The cost conundrum. The New Yorker. June 2009;1. http://www.newyorker.com/reporting/2009/06/01/090601fa_fact_gawande Accessed on June 1, 2011.
27. Sox HC, Greenfield S. Comparative effectiveness research: A report from the Institute of Medicine. Ann Intern Med. 2009;151:203–205.

28. Freburger J, Carey TS. Comparative effectiveness research: Opportunities and challenges for physical therapy. Phys Ther. 2110;90:327.
29. Peterson LE, Goodman C, Karnes EK, et al. Assessment of the quality of cost analysis literature in physical therapy. Phys Ther. 2009;89:733–755.
30. Milstein A, Gilbertson E. American medical home runs. Health Affairs (Millwood). 2009;28:1317–1326.
31. Fuchs VR, Milstein A. The $640 billion question—Why does cost-effective care diffuse so slowly? NEJ Med. 364(21):1985–1987.
32. Bell D, Raiffa H. *Decision Making: Descriptive, Normative, and Prescriptive Interactions*. Cambridge, UK: Cambridge University Press; 1988.
33. Stanton MW. Expanding Patient-Centered Care To Empower Patients and Assist Provider. Research in Action, Issue 5. Agency for Health Care Research. http://www.ahrq.gov/qual/ptcareria.htm Accessed on June 2, 2011.
34. The Commonwealth Fund. Patient-Centered Care. http://www.commonwealthfund.org/Topics/Patient-Centered-Care.aspx Accessed June 2, 2011.
35. Olsen L, Aisner D, McGinnis JM. *The Learning Health Care System. A Workshop Summary from the IOM Roundtable on Evidence-Based Medicine*. Washington, DC: National Academies Press; 2007.
36. Taylor K. Paternalism, participation and partnership—The evolution of patient centeredness in the consultation. Pat Educ and Counsel. 2009;74:150–155.
37. Neupert PM. Information technology tools that inform and empower patients. In: McClellan, MB, McGinnis JM, Nabel EG, Olsen LM, eds. *Evidence Based Medicine and the Changing Nature of Health Care. 2007 IOM Annual Meeting Summary*. Washington, DC: National Academies Press; 2008.
38. Epstein R. Mindful practice. JAMA. 1999;282:833–839.

The Case of Sam Ketterman

Based on an actual patient, this case is described using the patient care management model; it was developed to fulfill the requirements for a course in the DPT (transition) program at MGH Institute by Dr. Hack, with thanks to the instructor in the course, Cynthia Coffin Zadai, PT, DPT, MS, CCS, FAPTA for her guidance in its development.

I Examination

1. History

General Health Status at Time of Admission

Sam Ketterman is a 90-year-old Caucasian male (DOB: 6/24/14), who was sent via ambulance for sudden onset of shortness of breath and pervasive weakness. He was subsequently admitted to the hospital through the Emergency Department with a diagnosis of congestive heart failure (CHF) and atrial fibrillation, both of new origin and unknown etiology. After an 8-day hospital stay (9/9/04–9/16/04), he was discharged from the hospital back to the assisted living facility where he previously resided. He lives in the Alzheimer's unit of that facility. Physical therapy was requested to see him to ensure safety and improve function.

Social History/Environment

Mr. Ketterman has been married for 65 years to his 92-year-old wife, who resides in the same assisted living facility in a nearby one-bedroom apartment. He is a college graduate who spent his entire career as a manager for AT&T in northern Illinois. The Kettermans retired in 1976 and moved to the western coast of Florida, where they moved to a life care community in 1990. A few years after Mr. Ketterman's diagnosis with Alzheimer's disease, Mrs. Ketterman developed severe depression and anxiety leading to paranoia. Because of this, the couple moved in 2003 to the assisted living facility in the Boston region to be closer to their family. Mr. Ketterman has bilateral hearing aids, a partial denture, and bifocals. He has a raised toilet seat and standard folding walker that were in use prior to this hospital admission. Hospital bed added post-discharge for shortness of breath. Both Mr. and Mrs. Ketterman have signed advanced directives indicating that only comfort measures should be used in the event of imminent death and have requested and received do not resuscitate orders from their physician.

Family

Mr. and Mrs. Ketterman have two sons. One lives in the Boston region with his wife. Because of their proximity to them, this son and daughter-in-law have primary responsibility for the couple's care. This son is the durable power of attorney. Their other son lives in Illinois. They have three grandchildren and a great-grandchild.

Social/Health Habits

Mr. Ketterman has never smoked and used alcohol only on social occasions. His primary activities during retirement were community service, golf, and bridge. He participated regularly in the structured exercise program at the life care community in Florida and at the assisted living facility prior to his move to the Alzheimer's unit.

Medical/Surgical History

Resolved:
Restless leg syndrome, more than 15 years, no longer treated
Colon cancer 1991, treated bowel resection and radiation
Adhesions with bowel resection, 2003
Polymyositis, 2001, cause never found, perhaps reaction to Arecept
BLE edema, 2003, due to protein deficiency, resolved
Thoracic fracture ×2, 2002, 2003, secondary to falls
Clavicle fracture, 2002, secondary to fall
Macular hole, L eye

Ongoing:
Prostatitis, more than 15 years
Hypothyroidism, more than 15 years
Continued alternating periods of diarrhea and constipation,
(possible irritable bowel syndrome, possible continued adhesions)
Basal cell carcinomas of the face and head, approx 1998, and 2004
Alzheimer's disease, since approximately 2000
Hard of hearing, corrected with bilateral hearing aids
Near-sighted, corrected by glasses, bilateral cataracts removed in the 1990s

Current Additions:
Congestive heart failure, 2004
Atrial fibrillation, 2004
Atrial stenosis, 2004
Mitral stenosis, 2004
Herpes zoster, 10/2004
Frequent skin tears, often after loss of balance

Current Condition/Chief Complaint:
Decreased independence in transfers
Decreased endurance in ambulation

Functional Status Prior to Most Recent Admission:

Independent in ambulation on levels
Close supervision for one step (no stairs)
Independent in bed, chair, toilet transfers (all raised approximately 3 inches)
Independent in eating

Moderate assistance in dressing
Maximal assistant in showering and toileting
Maximum assistance in all instrumental activities of daily living (IADLs)

Medications
Prior to Admission:
Synthroid .075 mg qd
Flomax .4 mg qd
Lasix 40 mg qd
Immodium, Allegra, and Tylenol PRN
Boost PRN

Post-admission:*
As above, plus
Lasix increased to 40 mg bid
Aspirin EC 325 mg qd
Cozaar 50 mg qd
Potassium chloride 10 mEq qd
Valtrex 500 mg bid for one week for herpes zoster
*NOTE: The family, with the physician, elected to not start Coumadin due to the adverse affects at Mr. Ketterman's age and with his comorbidities.

Other Clinical Tests (in chronological order)

TEST	DATE	RESULTS
Chest x-ray	4/03	LLL infiltrate, no CHF
Albumin	4/23/03	2.1 (low)
Albumin	8/20/03	3.4 (Within Normal Limits (WNL))
THS	6/9/04	WNL
EKG	9/9/04	Atrial fibrillation, nonspecific ST, T wave abnormality Prolonged QT
Echocardiogram	9/10/04	Aortic stenosis, mitral valve calcification, pulmonary hypertension 60 mmHg, dilated R atrium, normal systolic function left ventricle. No injection fraction noted on the exam
Abdomen series	9/9/04, 9/10/04	Evidence old surgeries, no current obstruction
Chest x-ray	9/9/04, 9/10/04	Cardiomegaly. Pulmonary congestion, B pleural effusions, consistent with CHF
US abdomen	9/10/04	Cholelithiasis, B plural effusions
CBC	9/9, 11, 12/04	RBC,HGB,PLT low, MCV,RDW high
WBC differential	9/9, 14/04	Poly high, Lymph low
Chemistry–gen'l	9/10, 11, 12/04	CL, BUN high

TEST	DATE	RESULTS
Chemistry–enzymes	9/9, 10,11,12/04	WNL
Lipid profile	9/10/04	WNL
Hepatitis markers	9/14/04	Nonreactive
TSH	9/9/04	WNL
Chest x-ray	10/1/04	B pleural effusion, cannot eval heart size
SMA-6	10/13/04	Chloride, BUN high, Protein, albumin, SGOT, SGPT low

2. Systems Review–as of 11/1/04

Neuromuscular
Gait: Ambulates with walker maximum 100' with close supervision, in stooped position, with wide base of support (BOS)

Locomotion: Transfers bed/chair/toilet to/from stand with close supervision, Needs minimal assist for shower chair transfer
Balance: Has unstable balance with loss of balance to the rear
Motor Function: No apparent alteration in tone, no apparent problems with coordination

Musculoskeletal
Appears to have significant muscle wasting throughout. All major joints appear to be limited at end range. Stands in stooped position with wide BOS, hips behind ankles, thoracic kyphosis, cervical flattening, and forward head.

Cardiovascular-Pulmonary
BP: 144/70, P: 75 (irregular), RR: 20, T: 97.8, mild edema BLE L > R

Integumentary
Skin tear posterior L upper arm, bruises across arms, herpes rash L low back, buttocks, thigh, and groin, healing excisional sites cheek and behind R ear from basal cell CA removal

Cognitive Status
Alert, oriented to person, not to place or time, reported by family to be very precise, a list maker. Needs frequent verbal cuing to carry out all activities of daily living (ADL) tasks

3. Specific Tests and Measures
Based on the data collected in the history and systems review, it was determined that specific tests and measures in the following areas are needed to fully evaluate Mr. Ketterman.

Aerobic Capacity, Endurance, & Circulation (arterial, venous, lymphatic):
BP, RR, P before activity: B/P 144/70, P: 75 (irregular), RR: 20
BP, RR, P after activity: B/P 168/84, P: 88 (irregular), RR: 28
BP, RR, P after 15 minute rest: B/P: 148/76, P: 79 (irregular), RR: 20

6 minute walk test: Not able to complete six minutes, displayed dyspnea at 4
   minutes, at a distance of 200′
Auscultation: Increased breath sounds over both lower lobes
(Oximetry not available)

Anthropometric Characteristics:
Height: approx 5′4″ (formerly approx 5′10″)
Weight: 130 lbs
Edema: 2+ pitting edema B ankles to mid tibia
BLE Girth measurements: L ankle at malleoli 11.5 inches, R ankle at malleoli
   10.75 inches

Arousal, Attention, & Cognition:
Cognitive status: Mini-mental Exam Score: 9

Assistive & Adaptive Devices:
Assessment of ADL w and w/out assistive devices in ambulation: Ambulates 2–3
   feet without walker before loss of balance posteriorly. Ambulates 200′ with
   wheeled walker with close supervision.
Assessment of ADL w and w/out bathroom equipment: Needs moderate
   assistance to rise from regular-height toilet, needs close supervision to rise
   from raised (4″) toilet. Unable to tolerate standing in shower. Able to shower
   with shower seat and moderate assistance for bathing activities

Gait, Locomotion, & Balance:
Balance/Safety: Berg Balance Score: 16
Gait: Gait Abnormality Rating Scale–Modified: 15

Integumentary Integrity:
Skin characteristics: Skin thin and dry, purpura across dorsum of hands and
   arms

Muscle Performance:
Manual muscle testing by functional groups
B shoulder flexion, extension, abduction, adduction: 3
B elbow flexion, extension: 4
B wrist flexion, extension, abduction, adduction, pronation, supination: 3+
B finger flexion, extension, abduction, adduction: 4
B hip flexion, extension, abduction, adduction: 3+
B hip internal and external rotation 3
B knee flexion, extension: 3+
B ankle dorsiflexion, plantarflexion, pronation, supination: 3+

Pain:
Pain responses: verbal report of pain in thoracic spine on contact with hard
   surfaces, verbal report of pain in groin area, sometimes associated with bowel
   movements

Posture:
Posture observation: In quiet stance,
LE: feet pronated, ankles in slight dorsiflexion, knees slightly flexed and forward
   of ankles (no varus/valgum noted), hips flexed

Spine: lumbar spine flat, thoracic spine in kyphosis, lower cervical spine flat, hyperextension of upper cervical spine
UE: shoulders elevated
All other areas WNL

Range of Motion:
Observation of range of motion showed limits at end ranges of all joints consistent with static posture described above

Self-Care & Home Management:
Functional assessment: Barthel Index score: 45

Ventilation, Respiration, & Circulation:
Observation of pulmonary pattern: Shallow intercostal breathing
Auscultation: Crackles in lower lobes consistent with recent chest x-rays

Work, Community, & Leisure Integration and Reintegration:
Observations: sits in large electric recliner chair most of day. When invited, participates in short periods (5–10 minutes) of activity one-on-one with assisted living center aide. Preferred activities include sorting and organizing. Engages in short bursts (2–3 minutes) of reminiscence. Looks at television on occasion and reads words on the screen but does not sustain attention to programming. Unable to sustain attention to participate in other activities such as cards, bingo, etc.

II Evaluation

1. Diagnosis

Based on history, systems review, and specific tests and measures, the patient has the following active diagnoses that will contribute to the design of the PT plan of care:

Pathologies:
Basal cell carcinomas of the face and head
Hypothyroidism, more than 15 years
Continued alternating periods of diarrhea and constipation,
(possible irritable bowel syndrome, possible continued adhesions)
Alzheimer's disease, since approximately 2000
Hard of hearing, corrected with bilateral hearing aids
Near-sighted, corrected by glasses, B cataracts removed in the 1990s
CHF
Atrial fibrillation
Atrial stenosis
Mitral stenosis
Frequent skin tears, often after loss of balance
Frequent falls

Impairments:
Spinal pain
Reduced range of motion all major joints
Reduced muscle strength all muscle groups

Lower extremity edema
Abnormal respiratory pattern
Decreased endurance
Increased cardiovascular and pulmonary response to workload
Increased perceived exertion with functional activities

Functional limitations:
Close supervision for all transfers
Close supervision for all ambulation
Unable to ambulate on stairs (one step only)
Maximal assistance for bathing
Moderate assistance for dressing and feeding
Maximal assistance in all IADLs

Disability:
Unable to carry out vocational or avocational roles

2. Prognosis

This 90-year-old male was in relatively good physical health prior to the acute onset of CHF, despite his worsening AD. While his CHF will not be reversed, it can be controlled. Over the course of the episode of care, Mr. Ketterman will demonstrate improved aerobic capacity, increased strength and improved balance, compared to his status at discharge from the hospital. This will result in his ability to participate more fully in his own ADLs and in physical activities in the assisted living facility.

3. Plan of Care

Interventions:
Coordination with the patient's physicians, daily caregivers, and family
Instruction to patient's caregivers and family on current condition, plan of care,
    and discharge plans, and follow-up needs
Therapeutic exercise for strength and flexibility
Functional training in self-care and ambulation
Prescription of assistive devices and equipment

Frequency and duration of the interventions:
5 weeks (2 times a week for a total of 10 visits)
In addition the patient will be seen one time every 6 weeks in the future to
    determine if further services are needed to help him and his caregivers
    manage his progressive cognitive and cardiac disease.

Anticipated goals and expected outcomes:
At the conclusion of the episode patient will have sufficient aerobic capacity to
    participate in ADLs, in community activities within the assisted living facility,
    and to ambulate distances to allow exit from the facility to visit physicians
    and family.
Because of Mr. Ketterman's age and the progressive nature of his diseases, it is
    expected that he will eventually decline. Depending on the nature of the
    decline, he may benefit from further episodes of intervention to regain
    function. Eventually he will need hospice-type care to help maintain comfort
    in the last stage of life.

Discharge plan:
Mr. Ketterman currently resides in an AD unit of an assisted living facility. It is the policy of the facility to allow aging in place and it is their intention to continue to provide services to him through the final stages of life. Therefore, he will remain in this facility. He will be discharged for this PT episode of care when the current goals are met, but because of the progressive nature of his disease, he will be placed on a schedule for regular follow-up.

III Intervention

1. Coordination, Communication, and Documentation

Confirm advanced directives
Communicate with other providers: primary care physician, cardiologist, dermatologist, and director of nursing at the assisted living facility
Communicate with family
Document instruction and supervision to day-to-day caregivers at assisted living facility
Coordinate equipment needs
Accurately document physical therapy services

2. Patient/Client-Related Instruction

Provide instruction to day-to-day caregivers
Provide instruction and information to family

3. Procedural Interventions

Therapeutic exercise for strength and flexibility
Therapeutic exercise for aerobic capacity
Functional training in self-care and ambulation

IV Reexamination

Based on initial examination and evaluation, specific tests and measures in the following areas will need to be repeated on a frequent (daily/weekly) and regular basis to monitor Mr. Ketterman's cardiovascular status, specifically to identify possible worsening of his CHF and atrial fibrillation, and to assess possible new integumentary problems, including skin tears and recurring basal cell carcinomas.

Aerobic Capacity, Endurance, & Circulation (arterial, venous, lymphatic):
To monitor blood pressure to determine if HTN remains controlled
To measure frequency and quality of pulse rate to assess worsening of atrial fibrillation

Anthropometric Characteristics:
To monitor rapid increases in weight, indicating fluid retention

Ventilation, Respiration, & Circulation:
To assess for shortness of breath, indicating worsening of CHF

Integumentary Integrity:
To determine if immediate nursing intervention is needed for skin tears
To determine if referral to dermatologist is needed for excision of more basal cell carcinomas

Based on Mr. Ketterman's ongoing pathological diagnoses, specific tests and measures in the following areas will need to be repeated on a regular basis (weekly/monthly) to determine if he needs increased social and physical support services.

Arousal, Attention, Cognition:
To determine if cognitive changes are related to the underlying progressive dementia of Alzheimer's disease or represent an acute change such as infection

Self-Care & Home Management:
To assess when further support, such as feeding, would be needed

Work, Community, & Leisure Integration and Reintegration:
To determine if activities interventions need to be modified

Based on Mr. Ketterman's ongoing diagnoses of impairments and functional limitations, specific tests and measures in the following areas will need to be repeated regularly (quarterly) to determine the need for renewed physical therapy intervention.

Gait, Locomotion, & Balance:
To assess need for an increase in assistance level

Assistive & Adaptive Devices:
To assess need for a change in assistive device or supportive equipment

Muscle Performance:
To make changes in exercise program

Pain:
To assess need for change in seating to accommodate spinal deformity or other palliative pain relief

Posture:
To assess for possible changes that can decrease postural control, resulting in need for increased assistance in locomotion

Range of Motion:
To assess for changes that put patient at increased risk for falls and for skin breakdown

V Outcomes

Outcomes will be measured by repeated use of the test and measures identified above. While it is expected that Mr. Ketterman will show some improvement in the short run following an episode of care, since his diseases are progressive, he will eventually continue to deteriorate. The essential outcome is to maintain the highest possible quality of pain-free and functional life for as long as possible and then to provide appropriate palliative care.

Specifically I will use the following tests of

Impairments:
Vital signs
Six-minute walk test
MMT

Functional limitations:
Berg Balance Scale
Gait Abnormality Rating Scale
Barthel Index

Measures of quality of life are best used to measure responses in groups of patients rather than in individuals and need appropriate cognitive status for response. Therefore no measures of quality of life were used for Mr. Ketterman. Similar issues apply to measures of patient satisfaction.

VI Termination of Services

Because Mr. Ketterman's diseases are progressive, it is anticipated that he will need periodic episodes of physical therapy care throughout the expected remainder of his life (less than 12 months) to provide appropriate care to maintain his function as much as possible, to instruct caregivers in his management, and to provide palliative care during the final stage of life.

INDEX